Clostridioides difficile Infection

Clostridioides difficile Infection

Editor

Guido Granata

MDPI • Basel • Beijing • Wuhan • Barcelona • Belgrade • Manchester • Tokyo • Cluj • Tianjin

Editor
Guido Granata
Clinical and Research
Department
National Institute for Infectious
Diseases "L. Spallanzani"
Rome
Italy

Editorial Office
MDPI
St. Alban-Anlage 66
4052 Basel, Switzerland

This is a reprint of articles from the Special Issue published online in the open access journal *Antibiotics* (ISSN 2079-6382) (available at: www.mdpi.com/journal/antibiotics/special_issues/clostri_difficile).

For citation purposes, cite each article independently as indicated on the article page online and as indicated below:

LastName, A.A.; LastName, B.B.; LastName, C.C. Article Title. *Journal Name* **Year**, *Volume Number*, Page Range.

ISBN 978-3-0365-3878-5 (Hbk)
ISBN 978-3-0365-3877-8 (PDF)

Contents

About the Editor vii

Preface to "*Clostridioides difficile* Infection" ix

Guido Granata and Davide Roberto Donno
Introduction to the Special Issue on *Clostridioides difficile*
Reprinted from: *Antibiotics* **2021**, *10*, 1233, doi:10.3390/antibiotics10101233 1

Supapit Wongkuna, Tavan Janvilisri, Matthew Phanchana, Phurt Harnvoravongchai, Amornrat Aroonnual and Sathid Aimjongjun et al.
Temporal Variations in Patterns of *Clostridioides difficile* Strain Diversity and Antibiotic Resistance in Thailand
Reprinted from: *Antibiotics* **2021**, *10*, 714, doi:10.3390/antibiotics10060714 5

Elena Novakova, Zuzana Stofkova, Vladimira Sadlonova and Lukas Hleba
Diagnostic Methods of *Clostridioides difficile* Infection and *Clostridioides difficile* Ribotypes in Studied Sample
Reprinted from: *Antibiotics* **2021**, *10*, 1035, doi:10.3390/antibiotics10091035 21

Guido Granata, Davide Mariotti, Paolo Ascenzi, Nicola Petrosillo and Alessandra di Masi
High Serum Levels of Toxin A Correlate with Disease Severity in Patients with *Clostridioides difficile* Infection
Reprinted from: *Antibiotics* **2021**, *10*, 1093, doi:10.3390/antibiotics10091093 31

Jacek Czepiel, Marcela Krutova, Assaf Mizrahi, Nagham Khanafer, David A. Enoch and Márta Patyi et al.
Mortality Following *Clostridioides difficile* Infection in Europe: A Retrospective Multicenter Case-Control Study
Reprinted from: *Antibiotics* **2021**, *10*, 299, doi:10.3390/antibiotics10030299 43

Mirela Nicoleta Voicu, Florica Popescu, Dan Nicolae Florescu, Ion Rogoveanu, Adina Turcu-Stiolica and Dan Ionut Gheonea et al.
Clostridioides difficile Infection among Cirrhotic Patients with Variceal Bleeding
Reprinted from: *Antibiotics* **2021**, *10*, 731, doi:10.3390/antibiotics10060731 55

Lara Šamadan, Mia Jeličić, Adriana Vince and Neven Papić
Nonalcoholic Fatty Liver Disease—A Novel Risk Factor for Recurrent *Clostridioides difficile* Infection
Reprinted from: *Antibiotics* **2021**, *10*, 780, doi:10.3390/antibiotics10070780 69

Suvash Chandra Ojha, Matthew Phanchana, Phurt Harnvoravongchai, Surang Chankhamhaengdecha, Sombat Singhakaew and Puey Ounjai et al.
Teicoplanin Suppresses Vegetative *Clostridioides difficile* and Spore Outgrowth
Reprinted from: *Antibiotics* **2021**, *10*, 984, doi:10.3390/antibiotics10080984 83

Hans-Jürgen Heidebrecht, Ilias Lagkouvardos, Sandra Reitmeier, Claudia Hengst, Ulrich Kulozik and Michael W. Pfaffl
Alteration of Intestinal Microbiome of *Clostridioides difficile*-Infected Hamsters during the Treatment with Specific Cow Antibodies
Reprinted from: *Antibiotics* **2021**, *10*, 724, doi:10.3390/antibiotics10060724 95

Abraham Joseph Pellissery, Poonam Gopika Vinayamohan, Deepa Ashwarya Kuttappan, Neha Mishra, Breno de Oliveira Fragomeni and Kendra Maas et al.
Protective Effect of Baicalin against *Clostridioides difficile* Infection in Mice
Reprinted from: *Antibiotics* **2021**, *10*, 926, doi:10.3390/antibiotics10080926 . . . . **109**

Muni Kumar Mahadari, Sreenu Jennepalli, Andrew J. Tague, Papanin Putsathit, Melanie L. Hutton and Katherine A. Hammer et al.
Cationic Peptidomimetic Amphiphiles Having a *N*-Aryl- or *N*-Naphthyl-1,2,3-Triazole Core Structure Targeting *Clostridioides* (*Clostridium*) *difficile*: Synthesis, Antibacterial Evaluation, and an In Vivo *C. difficile* Infection Model
Reprinted from: *Antibiotics* **2021**, *10*, 913, doi:10.3390/antibiotics10080913 . . . . **131**

Pei-Wen Wang, Wei-Ting Lee, Ya-Na Wu and Dar-Bin Shieh
Opportunities for Nanomedicine in *Clostridioides difficile* Infection
Reprinted from: *Antibiotics* **2021**, *10*, 948, doi:10.3390/antibiotics10080948 . . . . **149**

About the Editor

Guido Granata

Guido Granata, M.D., Ph.D., Infectious Disease Specialist. Allergology and Clinical Immunology Specialist. Consultant in Infectious Diseases.

In 2010, Medical Degree, "Sapienza" University in Rome, Italy.

In 2016, Board Certification in Allergology and Clinical Immunology, "Sapienza" University in Rome, Italy.

In 2016, Visiting Research Fellow at the Rheumatology Research Group, Institute of Infection,Inflammation and Ageing, University of Birmingham, UK.

In 2017, Research Fellow at the Italian National Institute for Infectious Diseases "L. Spallanzani", Rome, Italy.

In 2017, Collaborator, "CCM 2016" Project: "Clostridium difficile: good practices for the diagnosis, surveillance, communication and the infection control" funded by the Italian Ministry of Health.

In 2018, Consultant in Infectious Diseases, Severe and Immunocompromised Host Infections Unit, National Institute for Infectious Diseases "L. Spallanzani", Rome, Italy.

In 2019, Principal Investigator in the project "ReCloDi–Real Incidence of Clostridioides difficile infection in Italy", winner of the Italian Society of Anti-Infective Therapy 2019 Young Investigator Grant.

In 2020, Doctor of Philosophy degree "Monocytes surface expression of FFA4, a G Protein coupled, free fatty acid sensing receptor in HIV infected subjects", Department of Clinical Medicine, "Sapienza" University of Rome.

In 2021, Principal investigator of the study: "A prospective study on incidence, risk factors and outcome of recurrent Clostridioides difficile infection: the ReCloDi study", Winner of the 31s European Society of Clinical Microbiology and Infectious Diseases ECCMID 2021 Travel Grant.

Research activity on infection control, *Clostridioides difficile* infection, antimicrobial treatment and antimicrobial resistance. Clinical and Research Department, National Institute for Infectious Diseases "L. Spallanzani" IRCCS, Rome, Italy.

Preface to "*Clostridioides difficile* Infection"

This book collects multidisciplinary research articles focused on *Clostridioides difficile* infection. The contributions collected here shed some light on grey areas of our knowledge of *Clostridioides difficile*, including regional *Clostridioides difficile* phenotypic and genotypic patterns, the *Clostridioides difficile* infection clinical course and the mortality rate in different settings and patient case-mix, the levels of *Clostridioides difficile* toxins in patients' sera, and novel, promising therapeutic approaches. This collection serves as a valuable reservoir of knowledge for scientists and researchers in the field of infectious diseases.

I would like to thank the scientific community who showed interest in and submitted manuscripts to this collection. I am grateful to the Editor-in-Chief of *Antibiotics*, Professor Nicholas Dixon, and to the Managing Editor, Ms. Monica He, for her unvaluable support. Special thanks go to my mentor, Professor Nicola Petrosillo, who introduced and always supported me in my career and research interests, and to my beloved family, Patricia and Meletta-Flaminia.

Guido Granata
Editor

antibiotics

MDPI

Editorial

Introduction to the Special Issue on *Clostridioides difficile*

Guido Granata * **and Davide Roberto Donno**

Clinical and Research Department for Infectious Diseases, National Institute for Infectious Diseases L. Spallanzani, IRCCS, 00149 Rome, Italy; davideroberto.donno@inmi.it

* Correspondence: guido.granata@inmi.it

Citation: Granata, G.; Donno, D.R. Introduction to the Special Issue on *Clostridioides difficile*. *Antibiotics* **2021**, *10*, 1233. https://doi.org/10.3390/antibiotics10101233

Received: 26 September 2021
Accepted: 5 October 2021
Published: 11 October 2021

The Gram-positive, anaerobic bacterium *Clostridioides difficile* (CD) represents the most common cause of nosocomial diarrhea worldwide and is responsible for increased morbidity and mortality, and prolonged hospital stays [1,2]. Indeed, despite the large number of scientific publications exploring the epidemiology and the clinical management of *Clostridioides difficile* infection (CDI), there is still a huge need for studies that could clarify some important aspects of this complex disease.

First, the clinical spectrum of CDI varies in severity from asymptomatic carriage and self-limited, mild diarrhea to severe colitis, toxic megacolon, and death [3]. Mortality rates in CDI vary widely between studies, from less than 2% up to 17% [4–6]. Besides the well-known risk factors for CDI, there is a need for tools to early identify CDI patients, particularly patients at high risk for severe CDI, and recurrence of CDI [4,7].

Another issue is hospital spreading of CD. Understanding the routes of in-hospital and community CD transmission is crucial to develop specific interventions to reduce the spread of CDI. The definition and validation of antimicrobial stewardship programs on CD prevention may reduce CDI incidence, even during the COVID-19 pandemic [8].

A further uncertainty is placed on the molecular pathogenesis of CDI, including a more exhaustive description of the interplay between CD, the gut microbiota, and host immunity, as well as the exact role of CD toxins, i.e., toxin A, toxin B, and binary toxin.

Finally, no less important is the high recurrence rate observed with the currently available CDI therapy. Recurrences currently represent one of the major challenges in the management of CDI, resulting in higher hospitalization costs and in increased morbidity and mortality rates [3,4,9]. The currently recommended first-line antimicrobial therapy is represented by oral vancomycin or fidaxomicin for the first episode. Recently, new innovative approaches, based on non-antimicrobial compounds, i.e., monoclonal anti-toxin antibodies, fecal microbiota transplantation, live bacterial vaccines, and CD vaccines, have been developed. However, further studies are needed to confirm the efficacy and safety of these approaches.

This Special Issue includes ten full research articles and one review article. These contributions shed rays of light on several gray areas of our knowledge of CDI, including regional CD phenotypic and genotypic patterns, the CDI clinical course and the mortality rate in different settings and patient case-mix, the levels of CD toxin A and toxin B in the serum of CDI patients, and several novel therapeutic approaches.

The report by Wongkuna et al. showed data addressing ribotypes, toxigenicity, and antimicrobial susceptibility profiles of two series of CD isolates in Thailand [10]. The authors compared two series of CD isolates, including 50 isolates collected from 2006 to 2009 and 26 isolates collected from 2010 to 2012. Interestingly, as ribotype 017 was the most common in both groups, 18 ribotyping patterns previously unknown were identified in the region. This work provides evidence of temporal changes in CD strains in Thailand [10].

The contribution by Novakova et al. reported the local phenotypic (toxigenicity, antimicrobial susceptibility) and genotypic (PCR ribotypes, genes for binary toxins) patterns of CD isolates from CDI patients hospitalized in the region of northern Slovakia, reporting a high prevalence of CD ribotype 176 and ribotype 001 [11].

Regarding CDI pathogenesis, the work by Di Masi et al. presented a novel semi-quantitative diagnostic method to measure the serum levels of CD toxins, i.e., toxin A and toxin B [12]. By the use of this new assay, the authors report the detection of toxemia in 33 out of the 35 CDI cases included in the study. The relationship between toxin A serum levels and CDI severity was also assessed, reporting that, at the time of CDI diagnosis, the proportion of severe CDI cases with a toxin A serum level >60 pg/μL was higher than in mild CDI cases (29.4% versus 66.6%, $p = 0.04$) [12]. Of interest, this study showed that toxemia is much more frequent than expected in CDI patients, and that high serum levels of toxin A correlate with CDI severity [12].

Among the contributions included in this Special Issue, a large multicenter study was performed by members of the European Society of Clinical Microbiology and Infectious Diseases (ESCMID) Study Group for CD [13]. This retrospective, case–control study aimed to describe the risk factors, clinical presentation, and management of patients with CDI as well as reporting factors associated with mortality in the 90-day period after diagnosis. In this study, 415 CDI patients hospitalized between January 2011 and December 2019 who died within 90 days following a CDI diagnosis formed the case group that was compared in a 2:1 ratio to 209 control CDI patients hospitalized in the same wards over the same time period who survived. The study found that older age, inadequate CDI therapy, cachexia, malignancy, Charlson index, long-term facility care, elevated white blood cells, elevated C-reactive protein, bacteremia, and cognitive impairment were independent risk factors for mortality at day 90 [13]. Notably, the authors concluded that CDI prevention should be primarily focused on hospitalized elderly people receiving antibiotics. For these patients, the available preventive measures should be used all the time, instead of only after CDI diagnosis.

Regarding the risk for the development of CDI, patients with liver dysfunction, including nonalcoholic fatty liver disease patients and cirrhotic patients, deserve attention. Cirrhotic patients are vulnerable to developing CDI due to their frequent admission and infections, as well as dysbiosis and a low immune system. Considering this, variceal bleeding secondary to cirrhosis requires antibiotics to prevent bacterial translocation, and thus patients become susceptible to CDI. The study by Voicu et al. aimed to investigate the risk factors for CDI in cirrhotic patients with variceal bleeding and the mortality risk in this patient population [14]. This retrospective cohort study included 367 cirrhotic patients with variceal bleeding, from which 25 patients were confirmed to have CDI. The authors reported that a higher age, longer hospital stay, higher level of urea, higher Charlson index, and the use of proton pump inhibitors were risk factors for CDI in cirrhotic patients [14]. Moreover, the authors confirmed that the MELD score was a predictor for mortality in cirrhotic patients with CDI. Moreover, the authors proposed a model of four predictors (age, days of admission, Charlson index, Child–Pugh score) to assess the risk of CDI in cirrhotic patients. Of note, in this study, cirrhotic patients with CDI had significantly higher costs compared with those without CDI [14].

The study by Šamadan et al. evaluated patients with nonalcoholic fatty liver disease and CDI, with the aim to determine whether nonalcoholic fatty liver disease is an independent risk factor associated with CDI recurrence [15]. This retrospective cohort study included 329 hospitalized CDI patients. Of the 329 patients included, 107 patients (32.5%) experienced recurrence of CDI. The statistical analysis identified that Charlson age–comorbidity index >6, age >75 years, nonalcoholic fatty liver disease, chronic kidney disease, and immobility were risk factors associated with recurrence of CDI [15]. Therefore, the authors identified nonalcoholic fatty liver disease as a possible new host-related risk factor associated with recurrence of CDI and suggested that changes in the intestinal microbiota linked to the development and progression of nonalcoholic fatty liver disease are a possible explanation of the increased risk of CDI in these patients.

Regarding the therapeutic approaches to CDI, a contribution by Ojha et al. highlighted that teicoplanin, an antimicrobial agent approved for the treatment of other bacterial infections, prevents the outgrowth of CD vegetative cells [16].

Intriguingly, the manuscript by Heidebrecht et al. proposed, again, the idea to use specific polyclonal antibodies isolated from the milk of immunized cows to treat CDI, in contrast to the standard administration of antibiotics [17]. In this study, the authors focused on the role of the microbiome, collecting stool samples of hamsters with CDI treated with either bovine antibodies or vancomycin. The regeneration of the microbiome instantly begins with the start of the antibody treatment, in contrast to the vancomycin-treated mice, where the diversity decreased significantly during the treatment duration. Of importance, the authors underlined that the regeneration of the microbiome was not an antibody-induced regeneration, but a natural regeneration that occurred because no microbiota-inactivating substances were administered [17].

This Special Issue also includes the trial by Pellissery et al. to investigate the prophylactic and therapeutic efficacies of baicalin, a plant-derived flavone glycoside, in reducing the severity of CDI [18]. In the prophylactic trial, mice were provided with baicalin from 12 days before CD challenge through the end of the experiment, whereas baicalin administration started on day 1 post-challenge in the therapeutic trial. The authors reported that both prophylactic and therapeutic supplementation of baicalin significantly reduced the severity of colonic lesions and improved CDI clinical progression and outcome compared with the control. Moreover, the authors highlighted that baicalin supplementation favorably altered the mice microbiome composition [18].

Another innovative anti-CDI compound was described in the contribution by Mahadari et al. [19]. This research group synthesized a compound with acceptable water solubility and a CD-selective antibacterial activity. Promisingly, this novel compound exhibited mild efficacy in an in vivo murine model of CDI, reducing the severity and slowing the onset of disease [19].

Finally, in a review article, Shieh and coworkers described the current state of our knowledge about the molecular pathogenesis of CDI and the perspectives of the application of nanotechnologies for the management of CDI, including advantages and limitations. This review highlighted the great potential of nanomedicine as a novel strategy in the future management of CDI [20].

This Special Issue collects multidisciplinary research focused on CDI. The contributions here collected constitute a valuable knowledge reservoir for scientists working in this field. The Guest Editor thanks the scientific community who showed interest in and submitted manuscripts to this collection.

Funding: This research received no external funding.

Conflicts of Interest: The authors declare no conflict of interest.

References

1. Magill, S.S.; O'Leary, E.; Janelle, S.J.; Thompson, D.L.; Dumyati, G.; Nadle, J.; Wilson, L.E.; Kainer, M.A.; Lynfield, R.; Greissman, S.; et al. Changes in prevalence of health care-associated infections in U.S. Hospitals. *N. Engl. J. Med.* **2018**, *379*, 1732–1744. [CrossRef] [PubMed]
2. Suetens, C.; Latour, K.; Kärki, T.; Ricchizzi, E.; Kinross, P.; Moro, M.L.; Jans, B.; Hopkins, S.; Hansen, S.; Lyytikäinen, O.; et al. Prevalence of healthcare-associated infections, estimated incidence and composite antimicrobial resistance index in acute care hospitals and long-term care facilities: Results from two European point prevalence surveys, 2016 to 2017. *Eurosurveillance* **2018**, *23*, 1800516. [CrossRef] [PubMed]
3. McDonald, L.C.; Gerding, D.N.; Johnson, S.; Bakken, J.S.; Carroll, K.C.; Coffin, S.E.; Dubberke, E.R.; Garey, K.W.; Gould, C.V.; Kelly, C.; et al. Clinical practice guidelines for Clostridium difficile infection in adults and children: 2017 update by the Infectious Diseases Society of America (IDSA) and Society for Healthcare Epidemiology of America (SHEA). *Clin. Infect. Dis.* **2018**, *66*, e1–e48. [CrossRef] [PubMed]
4. Granata, G.; Petrosillo, N.; Adamoli, L.; Bartoletti, M.; Bartoloni, A.; Basile, G.; Bassetti, M.; Bonfanti, P.; Borromeo, R.; Ceccarelli, G.; et al. Prospective Study on Incidence, Risk Factors and Outcome of Recurrent Clostridioides difficile Infections. *J. Clin. Med.* **2021**, *10*, 1127. [CrossRef] [PubMed]
5. Kwon, J.H.; Olsen, M.A.; Dubberke, E.R. The morbidity, mortality, and costs associated with Clostridium difficile infection. *Infect. Dis. Clin. N. Am.* **2015**, *29*, 123–134. [CrossRef] [PubMed]
6. Cataldo, M.A.; Granata, G.; Petrosillo, N. Clostridium difficile infection: New approaches to prevention, non-antimicrobial treatment, and stewardship. *Expert Rev. Anti Infect. Ther.* **2017**, *15*, 1027–1040. [CrossRef] [PubMed]

7. Cataldo, M.A.; Granata, G.; D'Arezzo, S.; Tonziello, G.; Vulcano, A.; De Giuli, C.; Meledandri, M.; Di Caro, A.; Petrosillo, N. Hospitalized patients with diarrhea: Rate of Clostridioides difficile infection underdiagnosis and drivers of clinical suspicion. *Anaerobe* **2021**, *70*, 102380. [CrossRef] [PubMed]
8. Granata, G.; Bartoloni, A.; Codeluppi, M.; Contadini, I.; Cristini, F.; Fantoni, M.; Ferraresi, A.; Fornabaio, C.; Grasselli, S.; Lagi, F.; et al. The Burden of Clostridioides Difficile Infection during the COVID-19 Pandemic: A Retrospective Case-Control Study in Italian Hospitals (CloVid). *J. Clin. Med.* **2020**, *9*, 3855. [CrossRef] [PubMed]
9. Petrosillo, N.; Granata, G.; Cataldo, M.A. Novel Antimicrobials for the Treatment of Clostridium difficile Infection. *Front. Med.* **2018**, *5*, 96. [CrossRef] [PubMed]
10. Wongkuna, S.; Janvilisri, T.; Phanchana, M.; Harnvoravongchai, P.; Aroonnual, A.; Aimjongjun, S.; Malaisri, N.; Chankhamhaengdecha, S. Temporal Variations in Patterns of Clostridioides difficile Strain Diversity and Antibiotic Resistance in Thailand. *Antibiotics* **2021**, *10*, 714. [CrossRef] [PubMed]
11. Novakova, E.; Stofkova, Z.; Sadlonova, V.; Hleba, L. Diagnostic Methods of Clostridioides difficile Infection and Clostridioides difficile Ribotypes in Studied Sample. *Antibiotics* **2021**, *10*, 1035. [CrossRef]
12. Granata, G.; Mariotti, D.; Ascenzi, P.; Petrosillo, N.; di Masi, A. High Serum Levels of Toxin A Correlate with Disease Severity in Patients with Clostridioides difficile Infection. *Antibiotics* **2021**, *10*, 1093. [CrossRef]
13. Czepiel, J.; Krutova, M.; Mizrahi, A.; Khanafer, N.; Enoch, D.A.; Patyi, M.; Deptuła, A.; Agodi, A.; Nuvials, X.; Pituch, H.; et al. Mortality Following Clostridioides difficile Infection in Europe: A Retrospective Multicenter Case-Control Study. *Antibiotics* **2021**, *10*, 299. [CrossRef]
14. Voicu, M.N.; Popescu, F.; Florescu, D.N.; Rogoveanu, I.; Turcu-Stiolica, A.; Gheonea, D.I.; Iovanescu, V.F.; Iordache, S.; Cazacu, S.M.; Ungureanu, B.S. Clostridioides difficile Infection among Cirrhotic Patients with Variceal Bleeding. *Antibiotics* **2021**, *10*, 731. [CrossRef]
15. Šamadan, L.; Jeličić, M.; Vince, A.; Papić, N. Nonalcoholic Fatty Liver Disease—A Novel Risk Factor for Recurrent Clostridioides difficile Infection. *Antibiotics* **2021**, *10*, 780. [CrossRef] [PubMed]
16. Ojha, S.C.; Phanchana, M.; Harnvoravongchai, P.; Chankhamhaengdecha, S.; Singhakaew, S.; Ounjai, P.; Janvilisri, T. Teicoplanin Suppresses Vegetative Clostridioides difficile and Spore Outgrowth. *Antibiotics* **2021**, *10*, 984. [CrossRef] [PubMed]
17. Heidebrecht, H.-J.; Lagkouvardos, I.; Reitmeier, S.; Hengst, C.; Kulozik, U.; Pfaffl, M.W. Alteration of Intestinal Microbiome of Clostridioides difficile-Infected Hamsters during the Treatment with Specific Cow Antibodies. *Antibiotics* **2021**, *10*, 724. [CrossRef] [PubMed]
18. Pellissery, A.J.; Vinayamohan, P.G.; Kuttappan, D.A.; Mishra, N.; Fragomeni, B.d.O.; Maas, K.; Mooyottu, S.; Venkitanarayanan, K. Protective Effect of Baicalin against Clostridioides difficile Infection in Mice. *Antibiotics* **2021**, *10*, 926. [CrossRef] [PubMed]
19. Mahadari, M.K.; Jennepalli, S.; Tague, A.J.; Putsathit, P.; Hutton, M.L.; Hammer, K.A.; Knight, D.R.; Riley, T.V.; Lyras, D.; Keller, P.A.; et al. Cationic Peptidomimetic Amphiphiles Having a N-Aryl- or N-Naphthyl-1,2,3-Triazole Core Structure Targeting Clostridioides (Clostridium) difficile: Synthesis, Antibacterial Evaluation, and an In Vivo C. difficile Infection Model. *Antibiotics* **2021**, *10*, 913. [CrossRef] [PubMed]
20. Wang, P.-W.; Lee, W.-T.; Wu, Y.-N.; Shieh, D.-B. Opportunities for Nanomedicine in Clostridioides difficile Infection. *Antibiotics* **2021**, *10*, 948. [CrossRef] [PubMed]

antibiotics

MDPI

Article

Temporal Variations in Patterns of *Clostridioides difficile* Strain Diversity and Antibiotic Resistance in Thailand

Supapit Wongkuna [1], Tavan Janvilisri [1], Matthew Phanchana [2], Phurt Harnvoravongchai [3], Amornrat Aroonnual [4], Sathid Aimjongjun [5], Natamon Malaisri [3] and Surang Chankhamhaengdecha [3,*]

1 Department of Biochemistry, Faculty of Science, Mahidol University, Bangkok 10400, Thailand; supapit.won@gmail.com (S.W.); tavan.jan@mahidol.ac.th (T.J.)
2 Department of Molecular Tropical Medicine and Genetics, Faculty of Tropical Medicine, Mahidol University, Bangkok 10400, Thailand; matthew.pha@mahidol.edu
3 Department of Biology, Faculty of Science, Mahidol University, Bangkok 10400, Thailand; phurt.har@mahidol.edu (P.H.); nattamon.nut.ma@gmail.com (N.M.)
4 Department of Tropical Nutrition and Food Science, Faculty of Tropical Medicine, Mahidol University, Bangkok 10400, Thailand; amornrat.aro@mahidol.edu
5 Graduate Program in Molecular Medicine, Faculty of Science, Mahidol University, Bangkok 10400, Thailand; sathid.ex@gmail.com
* Correspondence: surang.cha@mahidol.ac.th

Citation: Wongkuna, S.; Janvilisri, T.; Phanchana, M.; Harnvoravongchai, P.; Aroonnual, A.; Aimjongjun, S.; Malaisri, N.; Chankhamhaengdecha, S. Temporal Variations in Patterns of *Clostridioides difficile* Strain Diversity and Antibiotic Resistance in Thailand. *Antibiotics* **2021**, *10*, 714. https://doi.org/10.3390/antibiotics10060714

Academic Editor: Guido Granata

Received: 13 May 2021
Accepted: 8 June 2021
Published: 13 June 2021

Abstract: *Clostridioides difficile* has been recognized as a life-threatening pathogen that causes enteric diseases, including antibiotic-associated diarrhea and pseudomembranous colitis. The severity of *C. difficile* infection (CDI) correlates with toxin production and antibiotic resistance of *C. difficile*. In Thailand, the data addressing ribotypes, toxigenic, and antimicrobial susceptibility profiles of this pathogen are scarce and some of these data sets are limited. In this study, two groups of *C. difficile* isolates in Thailand, including 50 isolates collected from 2006 to 2009 (THA group) and 26 isolates collected from 2010 to 2012 (THB group), were compared for toxin genes and ribotyping profiles. The production of toxins A and B were determined on the basis of toxin gene profiles. In addition, minimum inhibitory concentration of eight antibiotics were examined for all 76 *C. difficile* isolates. The isolates of the THA group were categorized into 27 $A^-B^+CDT^-$ (54%) and 23 $A^-B^-CDT^-$ (46%), while the THB isolates were classified into five toxigenic profiles, including six $A^+B^+CDT^+$ (23%), two $A^+B^+CDT^-$ (8%), five $A^-B^+CDT^+$ (19%), seven $A^-B^+CDT^-$ (27%), and six $A^-B^-CDT^-$ (23%). By visually comparing them to the references, only five ribotypes were identified among THA isolates, while 15 ribotypes were identified within THB isolates. Ribotype 017 was the most common in both groups. Interestingly, 18 unknown ribotyping patterns were identified. Among eight *tcdA*-positive isolates, three isolates showed significantly greater levels of toxin A than the reference strain. The levels of toxin B in 3 of 47 *tcdB*-positive isolates were significantly higher than that of the reference strain. Based on the antimicrobial susceptibility test, metronidazole showed potent efficiency against most isolates in both groups. However, high MIC values of cefoxitin (MICs 256 µg/mL) and chloramphenicol (MICs $\geq$ 64 µg/mL) were observed with most of the isolates. The other five antibiotics exhibited diverse MIC values among two groups of isolates. This work provides evidence of temporal changes in both *C. difficile* strains and patterns of antimicrobial resistance in Thailand.

Keywords: *C. difficile* infection; molecular analysis; toxin production; antibiotic resistance

1. Introduction

Clostridioides difficile (formerly *Clostridium difficile*), belonging to the family *Clostridiaceae* and genus *Clostridioides*, is an obligate anaerobic, Gram-positive, spore-forming, toxin-producing bacillus [1,2]. This organism is well known to cause infectious diarrhea in humans, ranging from mild diarrhea to severe pseudomembranous colitis [3]. *C. difficile* infection (CDI) has been primarily a healthcare-associated illness, which can occur during antibiotic treatment. Furthermore, the ability of *C. difficile* to form spores leads to the problem of recurring infection. The persistence of spores in the physical environment facilitates its transmission [4]. The pathogenesis of CDI is attributed to the production of two major toxins: toxins A and B. Toxin A is an enterotoxin encoded by *tcdA*, and toxin B is a cytotoxin encoded by *tcdB*. Both toxins belong to the family of large clostridial toxins (LCTs) and are located within a 19.6 kb pathogenicity locus (PaLoc) [5]. In addition to toxins A and B, some strains of *C. difficile* also produce a binary toxin (CDT) encoded by two genes, *cdtA* and *cdtB*, on CdtLoc, a separate pathogenicity island [6]. Although CDTs are not directly required for diseases, they have been known to promote the virulence of *C. difficile* by impairing host immunity and acting in synergy with toxins A and B, exacerbating toxicity [7].

Over the recent decades, the epidemiology of CDI has dramatically changed. The epidemiology in North America and Europe and some parts of Asia is well-documented. While ribotype 027 causes major outbreaks in North America and Europe, ribotype 017 is the most dominant ribotype in Asia [8,9]. In Thailand, tcdA-negative, tcdB-positive ribotype 017 is the most prevalent *C. difficile* strain [10–12]. However, the occurrence of *C. difficile* has not been studied in all regions of Thailand. Recently, the diversity and prevalence of *C. difficile* have increased and influenced the incidence of CDI in many areas. Several ribotypes have emerged and lead to epidemic infections across the world; for example, ribotype 014/20 in Australia [13,14], ribotype 369 in Japan [15], and ribotype 078 in China [16].

Antibiotic use plays a major role in the development of CDI and recurrent diseases by disrupting the normal flora in the gut and allowing the invasion of *C. difficile* [17,18]. The first-line treatment for CDI is the use of antibiotics, including vancomycin, fidaxomicin, and metronidazole [19,20]. However, drug resistance has become one contributing factor that drives the global prevalence of CDI [21–24]. Although information on *C. difficile* has been globally expanded, little knowledge of antibiotic susceptibility of *C. difficile* in Thailand is available. Previous studies showed that *C. difficile* isolates in Thailand were susceptible to vancomycin and metronidazole. However, a high resistance level against multiple antibiotics, such as clindamycin, erythromycin, and moxifloxacin has been reported [25,26]. This study was conducted to compare two groups of *C. difficile* clinical isolates collected in different time periods from a University-affiliated tertiary hospital and the National Institute of Health of Thailand. To describe the diversity of *C. difficile* clinical isolates during 2006–2009 and 2010–2012, the presence of toxin genes and ribotype, including toxin levels and antimicrobial susceptibility patterns, were characterized using molecular techniques.

2. Results

2.1. Toxin Gene Profiles of *C. difficile* Isolates

The multiplex PCR was employed to identify the toxin gene profiles of *C. difficile* isolates. Seventy-six *C. difficile* isolates were classified into five profiles based on the presence of toxin genes. Only two toxigenic types were observed in the THA group. Twenty-seven THA isolates (54%) were characterized as $A^-B^+CDT^-$ (toxigenic), and 23 THA isolates (46%) were $A^-B^-CDT^-$ (non-toxigenic) (Figure 1A). All 27 isolates in the THA group that were previously positive for *tcdA* carried the *tcdA* 3′-end deletion (Supplementary Table S1). Later, they were grouped as *tcdA*-negative isolates instead. Thus, none of the toxigenic isolates in the THA group were *tcdA*-positive. In the THB group, six isolates (23%) were classified as $A^+B^+CDT^+$, five isolates (19%) as $A^-B^+CDT^+$, two isolates (8%) as $A^+B^+CDT^-$, seven isolates (27%) as $A^-B^+CDT^-$, and six isolates (23%) as $A^-B^-CDT^-$ (Figure 1B). Among *tcdA*-negative isolates in the THB group, in 12 isolates (63%) were found the deletion regions within the 3′-end (Table S1). Based on the molecular analysis, around 54% of the THA isolates and 77% of the THB isolates were toxigenic (Figure 1). The most dominant toxigenic type was A^-B^+, which was about 54% of THA isolates and 46% of THB isolates.

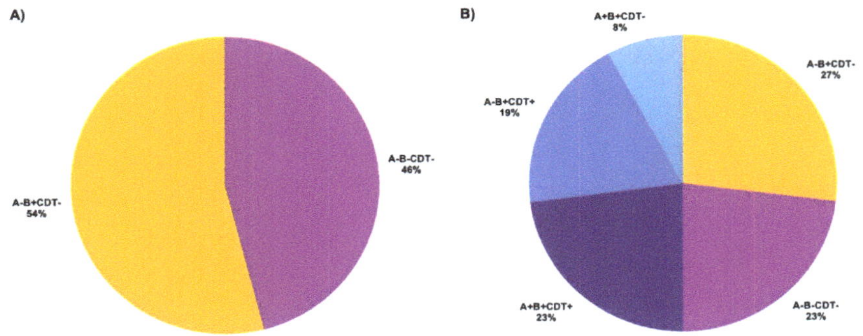

Figure 1. Toxin gene analysis of *C. difficile* isolates. The distribution of toxin profiles in *C. difficile* isolates from (**A**) THA group, which contained *C. difficile* isolates collected from 2006 to 2009 (n = 50) and (**B**) THB group, which contained *C. difficile* isolates collected from 2010 to 2012 (n = 26). Toxin profiles were characterized based on the presence of toxin genes and the deletion of *tcdA* 3′-end. A, B, and CDT represent *tcdA*, *tcdB*, and *cdtAB*.

2.2. Ribotypes of *C. difficile* Isolates

The band patterns of 16S and 23S rRNA PCR products were compared to the reference *C. difficile* ribotypes (Figure S1). Based on PCR ribotyping, THA isolates were separated into five ribotypes (Figure 2A). Ribotype 017 was the only standard ribotype found in the THA group, whereas the other four ribotypes showed different patterns from the standards (NN or NT). The dominant ribotype was NN05, followed by ribotype 017 and NN07. Even though the number of isolates in the THB group was lower compared to the THA group, THB isolates were classified into 15 ribotypes (Figure 2B). Ribotype 017 had the highest prevalence in the THB group with seven isolates (27%). Only one isolate (4%) was classified as ribotype 020. Alternatively, the other 14 isolates in the THB group showing distinct ribotyping patterns compared to the references were classified into 13 unknown ribotypes. The distribution of toxin gene profiles and ribotyping profiles is elaborated in Table 1. Diverse ribotypes were observed with each toxin gene profile; for instance, the $A^{+}B^{+}CDT^{+}$ group was composed of five ribotyping patterns, RT020, NT01, NT03, NT05, and NT06 (Table 1). These results suggest a high diversity of *C. difficile* isolates in Thailand.

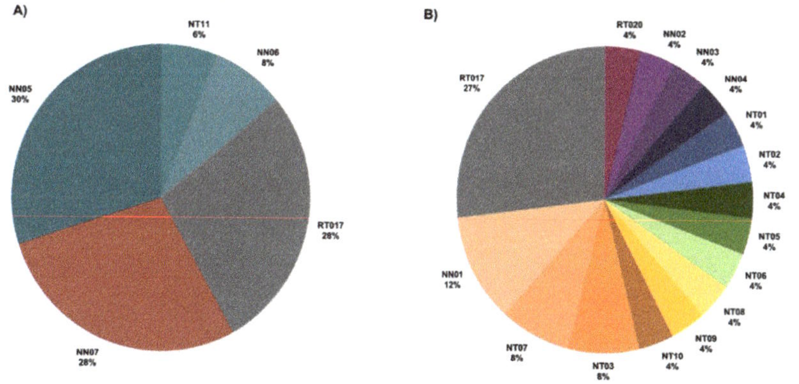

Figure 2. Ribotypes of *C. difficile* isolates using PCR ribotyping method. (**A**) The distribution of ribotypes among *C. difficile* isolates in the THA group (n = 50). (**B**) The distribution of ribotypes among *C. difficile* isolates in the THB group (n = 26). PCR ribotyping was performed on 16S and 23S rRNA genes. Ribotypes were assigned based on the band patterns of gel electrophoresis. RT017 and RT020 represent the standard *C. difficile* ribotypes. NT and NN represent new ribotype patterns of *C. difficile* toxigenic and non-toxigenic isolates, respectively.

Table 1. Summary of toxin gene profiles and ribotyping profiles of 76 *C. difficile* isolates in Thailand.

Toxigenic Profile	No. of Isolates		No. of Isolates of																			
	THA (n = 50)	THB (n = 26)	RT017	RT020	NN01	NN02	NN03	NN04	NN05	NN06	NN07	NT01	NT02	NT03	NT04	NT05	NT06	NT07	NT08	NT09	NT10	NT11
$A^+B^+CDT^+$		6		1								1		2		1	1					
$A^+B^+CDT^-$		2																2				
$A^-B^+CDT^+$		5	1										1		1				1		1	
$A^-B^+CDT^-$	27	7	20						9	1										1		3
$A^-B^-CDT^-$	23	6			3	1	1	1	6	3	14											

2.3. Toxin Production of *C. difficile* Isolates

Toxin production of *C. difficile* is a significant factor causing CDI [27]. In this study, toxin production of toxigenic *C. difficile* isolates, including A^+B^+, A^+B^-, and A^-B^+, was accessed using indirect ELISA. The toxin levels of individual isolates were compared to the toxin production of *C. difficile* R20291 ($A^+B^+CDT^+$), a recent emergence of a highly virulent bacterium. The unique ability of hypervirulent strain R20291 is associated with an increase in toxin production [28]. The amounts of toxins A and B were similar among toxigenic isolates in the THA and THB groups. Notably, four toxin-positive isolates, THB1, THB38, THB156, and THB376, significantly increased toxin A levels (2–9 folds) compared to R020291 (Figure 3A). Toxigenic THA isolates were found to produce similar levels of toxin B to the reference strain. Three isolates, THB2, THB136, and THB156, significantly produced greater levels of toxin B (3–6 folds) compared to the reference strain (Figure 3B). Interestingly, THB156 was the only toxigenic isolate that produced a significantly high level of toxin A and B. On the basis of these results, many THB isolates represented high toxin producers, suggesting increased toxin production of toxigenic *C. difficile* isolates in Thailand.

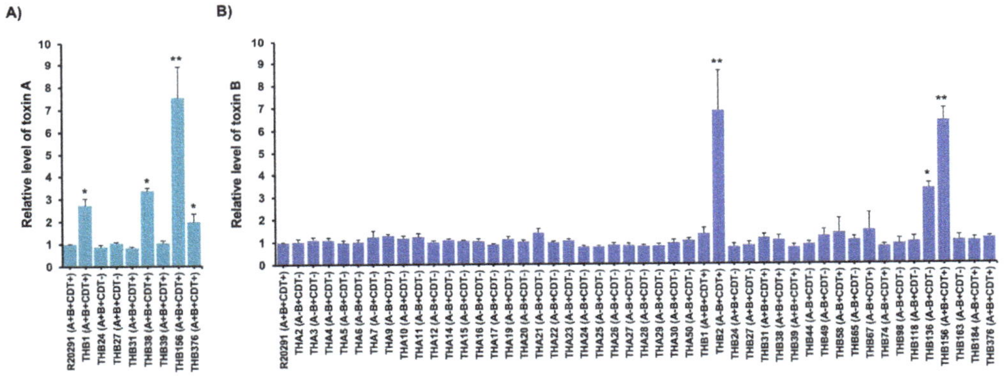

Figure 3. The relative level of toxin A and B production of *C. difficile* isolates. Toxigenic *C. difficile* isolates in the THA group; B^+ (n = 27) and the THB group; A^+ (n = 8) and B^+ (n = 20) were subjected to indirect ELISA. (**A**) The light blue bars represent toxin A, and (**B**) the dark blue bars represent toxin B. The graph shows average values of 3 independent samples in the experiments. Error bars refer to mean ± SEM, $p < 0.05$, *, and $p < 0.01$, **.

2.4. Antimicrobial Resistance Profiles of *C. difficile* Isolates

Antibiotic resistance has become one of the major challenges of CDI treatment. In this study, the antimicrobial susceptibility of the 76 *C. difficile* isolates was determined using the minimum inhibitory concentration (MIC) method. A variety of MIC values of eight antibiotics were observed across *C. difficile* isolates (Figure 4). Antibiotic susceptibility patterns of two groups of isolates are summarized in Table 2. In the THA group, 48 isolates (96%) were susceptible to amoxicillin with an MIC_{90} of 2 μg/mL, while 46 isolates (92%) were susceptible to ampicillin with an MIC_{90} of 4 μg/mL. All THA isolates were resistant to chloramphenicol with an MIC_{90} of $\geq$ 64 μg/mL. In addition, all THA isolates were resistant to cefoxitin, except one isolate with an MIC_{90} of 256 μg/mL. Conversely, all isolates in the THA group were susceptible to metronidazole with an MIC_{90} of 4 μg/mL. Amoxicillin and ampicillin showed potent activity against all THB isolates with an MIC_{90} of 2 and 4 μg/mL, respectively. Additionally, most THB isolates were resistant to chloramphenicol with an MIC_{90} of $\geq$ 64 μg/mL (96.15%), followed by cefoxitin with an MIC_{90} of 256 μg/mL (92.31%). None of the isolates in the THB group were resistant to metronidazole and only three THB isolates (11.54%) were resistance to vancomycin. In addition, three (11.54%) and two (7.69%) of THB isolates were resistant to levofloxacin and rifampicin, respectively. Minor differences in the MIC range between THA and THB isolates were observed (Table 3). For instance, chloramphenicol showed an MIC range of 32- ≥ 64 μg/mL in THA isolates, and 16- ≥ 64 μg/mL in THB isolates. A slightly greater ratio of resistant isolates was shown in THA isolates compared to THB isolates. Overall, two groups of isolates showed similar patterns of MIC values. Most THA and THB isolates were susceptible to all antibiotics, except cefoxitin and chloramphenicol, which showed the highest MIC ranges and resistance rates (Table 2). In total, 49 (98%) of the THA isolates and 23 (88.46%) of the THB isolates were resistant to more than one antibiotic. Most of them were resistant to chloramphenicol, cefoxitin, and levofloxacin, which belong to different antibiotic classes. These findings demonstrated multidrug-resistant (MDR) strains among Thai *C. difficile* isolates (Table S2).

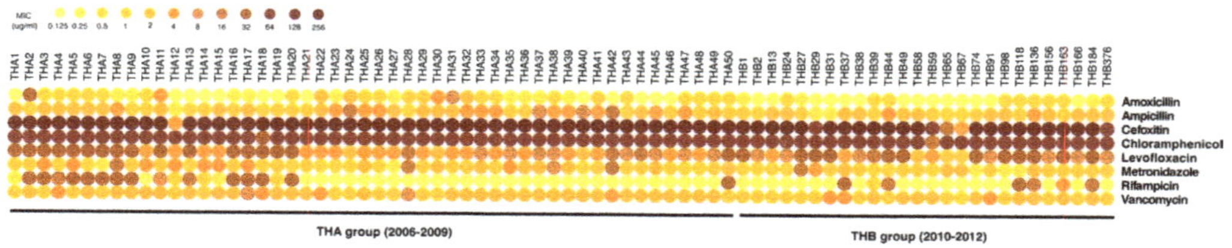

Figure 4. The MIC values of *C. difficile* isolates in Thailand. Eight antibiotics were used to investigate MIC values of *C. difficile* isolates in THA group (n = 50) and THB group (n = 26) using broth dilution method. The colors represent different MIC values.

Table 2. Antibiotic susceptibility patterns of *C. difficile* isolates in Thailand.

Antibiotics	MIC Range (μg/mL)		MIC_{50} (μg/mL)		MIC_{90} (μg/mL)		Breakpoints (μg/mL)	Susceptible (%)		Intermediate (%)		Resistant (%)	
	THA (n = 50)	THB (n = 26)	THA	THB	THA	THB	S/I/R	THA	THB	THA	THB	THA	THB
Amoxicillin	≤0.125-32	≤0.125-0.5	0.5	≤0.125	2	0.5	≤4/8/≥ 16 ≤2/4/≥ 8	96	100	2	0	2	0
Ampicillin	0.25-16	0.25-4	2	2	4	2	≤0.5/1/≥ 2	92	100	4	0	4	0
Cefoxitin	4-256	4-256	256	256	256	256	≤16/32/≥ 64	2	7.69	0	0	98	92.31
Chloramphenicol	32- ≥ 64	16- ≥ 64	≥64	≥64	≥64	≥64	≤8/16/≥ 32	0	0	0	3.85	100	96.15
Levofloxacin	2- ≥ 32	1- ≥ 32	8	8	≥32	≥32	-/-/≥8 [a]	-	-	-	-	56	11.54
Metronidazole	0.25-16	0.25- ≥ 16	1	1	4	2	≤8/16/≥ 32	96	96.15	4	3.85	0	0
Rifampicin	≤0.125- ≥ 32	≤0.125- ≥ 32	≤0.125	≤0.125	≥32	≥32	≤0.06/0.012-16/≥ 32 [b]	0	0	74	92.31	26	7.69
Vancomycin	1-8	0.5-4	2	1	4	4	≤2/-/> 2 [c]	88	88.46	-	-	12	11.54

* Clinical breakpoints determining the susceptibility categories: S; susceptible, I; intermediate, and R; resistance. All breakpoints were recommended by CLSI, except [a] breakpoint for levofloxacin by published data [29], [b] breakpoint for rifampicin by published data [30], and [c] breakpoint for vancomycin by EUCAST.

Table 3. Sequences of primers for amplifying toxin genes of *C. difficile* and amplicon size.

Analysis	Target Gene	Primer Name	Sequence (5′-3′)	Amplicon Size (bp)
Multiplex PCR	*tcdA*	tcdA-F	GTATGGATAGGTGGAGAAGTCAGTG	632
		tcdA-R	CGGTCTAGTCCAATAGAGCTAGGTC	
	tcdB	tcdB-F	GAAGATTTAGGAAATGAAGAAGGTGA	441
		tcdB-R	AACCACTATATTCAACTGCTTGTCC	
	cdtA	cdtA-F	ATGCACAAGACTTACAAAGCTATAGTG	260
		cdtA-R	CGAGAATTTGCTTCTATTTGATAATC	
	cdtB	cdtB-F	ATTGGCAATAATCTATCTCCTGGA	179
		cdtB-R	CTTGTTCTGGTACCAAATAATCCG	
	16S rRNA	UFU-L	GCCTAACACATGCAAGTCGA	800
		802-R	TACCAGGGTATCTAATCC	
tcdA 3′-end deletion	*tcdA*	NK9	CCACCAGCTGCAGCCATA	2535
		NKV011	TTTTGATCCTATAGAATYTAACTTAGTAAC	

3. Discussion

C. difficile infection (CDI) has occurred worldwide over recent decades. The prevalence and epidemiology of *C. difficile* in many regions are well documented [31,32]. However, information on *C. difficile* occurrences in Thailand remains limited. This work was conducted to continuously update information on *C. difficile* clinical isolates in Thailand by comparing two groups of clinical isolates that were collected in different time periods. *C. difficile* isolates were classified based on molecular features, including toxin genes and the 16S–23S rRNA intergenic spacer regions [33,34]. Normally, three major toxigenic types (A^+B^+, A^+B^-, A^-B^+) cause clinical incidences of CDI. The toxigenic type A^+B^+ is the most common among toxigenic types [35,36]. However, the presence of *tcdA* 3′-end deletion has been detected in many clinical isolates, resulting in toxin A-negative *C. difficile* isolates [37,38]. About half of *C. difficile* isolates collected during 2006–2009 (THA group) were toxigenic with the highest occurrence of A^-B^+ isolates (Figure 1A). Although isolates used in this study were obtained from the patients with CDI, consistent with previous studies, non-toxigenic strains were highly detected from clinical samples due to the mix of both the non-toxigenic and toxigenic populations and isolation method [10,39,40]. The population sizes of non-toxigenic and toxigenic *C. difficile* isolates in Thailand during 2006–2018 were comparable. The most dominant toxigenic isolates were tcdA-negative and tcdB-positive (A^-B^+) [10]. In contrast, the majority of *C. difficile* isolates collected during 2010–2012 (THB group) were toxigenic, and toxin gene profiles increased to five types, $A^-B^-CDT^-$, $A^-B^+CDT^-$, $A^+B^+CDT^-$, $A^-B^+CDT^+$, and $A^+B^+CDT^+$ (Figure 1B). However, no $A^-B^-CDT^+$ was detected in this study, corresponding to the previous study showing low prevalence of binary toxin-positive but toxin A- and B-negative *C. difficile* strains in France [41]. Some *C. difficile* isolates have the binary toxin gene (*CDT*), an actin-specific ADP-ribosyl transferase encoded by two genes, *cdtA* and *cdtB* on the CDT locus (CdtLoc) [6,42]. The binary toxins are widely observed in hypervirulent *C. difficile*, such as the ribotypes 027 and 078, which cause higher severity of CDI [43,44]. Therefore, the binary toxin may serve as an additional virulent factor by enhancing the production of toxins A and B. Our findings indicate a higher prevalence of toxigenic isolates in Thailand from 2010 to 2012.

Currently, PCR ribotyping is a general technique for epidemiological distinction of *C. difficile* isolates. This method amplifies polymorphic sequences between 16S and 23S intergenic spacer regions, which vary among strains [33,45,46]. It is the most common method employed for molecular analysis of *C. difficile* strains and is considered the gold standard method for *C. difficile* typing [10,11,33,47]. A similar incidence shown in the analysis of toxin genes was also observed with the ribotyping profiles. The number of ribotypes found during 2010–2012 was up to 16 ribotypes, from five ribotypes identified during 2006–2009 (Figure 2). *C. difficile* ribotype 017 has been recognized as a major cause of CDI outbreaks in Asia, and ribotype 020 is also a common strain [12,48]. Ribotype 017 was also the most frequently found in Thailand [11]. Consistent with this study, the most common ribotype in both groups was ribotypes 017. Besides, there were unknown ribotypes which showed different amplified patterns compared to the references between the two groups. However, we could not compare the PCR ribotyping patterns of the unknown ribotypes to other unknown ribotypes discovered in the previous studies in Thailand due to the limitation of this method. Other techniques, including pulse-field gel electrophoresis (PFGE), restriction endonuclease analysis (REA), and multilocus variable-number tandem-repeat analysis (MLVA), can be applied to improve typing of *C. difficile* strains [49,50]. Based on PCR ribotyping, molecular epidemiology of *C. difficile* isolated in Thailand significantly differs from other regions where ribotypes 027, 014/20, 002, 106, and 001 have dominated in North America and ribotypes 027, 014, 001, and 078 have frequently been isolated in Europe [51,52]. On the basis of toxin genes and ribotype identification, the diversity of *C. difficile* isolates in Thailand has increased over time.

Toxins A and B are the primary virulence factors contributing to the pathogenesis of CDI. They are considered to cause severe diseases [53]. Several studies have revealed that A^-B^+ strains can cause the same range of disease as isolates producing both, but a few pathogenic isolates have been found as A^+B^- [54–56]. In the current study, none of the toxigenic isolates were classified as A^+B^-, supporting the finding that toxin B is important for the pathogenesis of *C. difficile* without the presence of toxin A. This implied that pathogenic *C. difficile* isolates in Thailand were mainly influenced by the production of toxin B. Based on the relative quantification of toxins in this study, three of eight *tcdA*-positive (A^+) isolates showed significantly greater production of toxin A compared to a recent hypervirulent *C. difficile* strain. Most *tcdB*-positive (B^+) isolates produced toxin B at the same level as the reference strain, of which only three *tcdB*-positive isolates in the THB group significantly increased the level of toxin B (Figure 3). Remarkably, most isolates that produced high levels of toxins A and B were binary toxin-positive (CDT^+) isolates. A high toxin production is one of the features of hypervirulent strains associated with severity of disease [57–59]. Markedly, an increase in toxin production is influenced by binary toxins [6,60]. Therefore, the higher amount of toxins produced by isolates in this study might be associated with the presence of binary toxin genes.

Antibiotic resistance has become one of the most important virulence factors associated with the development of CDI. The expansion of strain diversity advocates antibiotic resistance in *C. difficile* [24,61,62]. To determine the direction of the antibiotic susceptibility of Thai *C. difficile* isolates, two groups of isolates were tested against several classes of antibiotics, which are recommended in infectious diarrhea [63,64]. None of the isolates fully resisted metronidazole, but three isolates showed intermediate resistance. However, 9 of 76 isolates had full resistance to vancomycin. This incidence was also observed in several studies with reduced susceptibility to vancomycin [22,65]. Our observations suggest a high efficiency of metronidazole for treating CDI, that also relates to the previous studies in Thailand [25,26]. Beta-lactam groups of antibiotics are most frequently correlated with CDI [66]. Several studies reported a low level of resistance to this antibiotic group [61,62]. In this study, amoxicillin and ampicillin also showed potent action against *C. difficile* isolates in Thailand. This supported the fact that antibiotics in the same class provide equal efficacy. Nevertheless, fluoroquinolones (ciprofloxacin, levofloxacin, moxifloxacin, norfloxacin) and cephalosporins (cefazolin, cefepime, ceftazidime, ceftriaxone, cefuroxime, cefotetan, cefoxitin) are common antibiotic groups used for treating bacterial infection in the clinical setting, and they continue to promote CDI [67,68]. The same incidence was detected in this study, in which the majority of *C. difficile* isolates were resistant to levofloxacin and cefoxitin. Resistance to chloramphenicol is rare in *C. difficile*. Only a small number of isolates have been reported to be chloramphenicol resistant [24,69]. Contrary to our observations, all isolates fully resisted chloramphenicol, except for one that showed intermediate resistance. In addition, the reduced susceptibility to rifampicin in *C. difficile* clinical strains has been reported in Asia, Europe, and North America [69–71]. Correspondingly, rifampicin-resistant isolates were detected in the current study. On the basis of antibiotic resistance analysis, most *C. difficile* isolates in this study were resistant to multiple antibiotics, increasing the chance of treatment failure. Although *C. difficile* isolates between two periods showed distinct diversity, the difference in the patterns of antibiotic resistance was not observed in this study.

In summary, *C. difficile* isolates from patients diagnosed with diarrhea during 2006–2009 and 2010–2012 were characterized for toxigenic types, ribotypes, toxin production, and antibiotic resistance. The toxigenic profiles found in Thailand rose to five types, including $A^-B^+CDT^-$, $A^+B^+CDT^+$, $A^+B^+CDT^-$, $A^-B^+CDT^+$, and $A^-B^-CDT^-$. In particular, ribotype 017 was predominant among clinical isolates in Thailand. Additionally, 18 unknown ribotypes were discovered in Thai isolates. Some *C. difficile* isolates in Thailand were able to produce similar levels of toxins A and B to the toxins of the hypervirulent *C. difficile* strain, R20291. There was no difference in susceptibility to vancomycin and metronidazole between two periods, supporting the fact that they are primary antibiotics for CDI therapy. In addition, amoxicillin, ampicillin, and rifampicin also had an effective impact on treating isolates in Thailand. Based on these findings, this study presents temporal changes in C.

difficile strain diversity and patterns of antimicrobial resistance in Thailand, which will be useful for surveillance.

4. Materials and Methods

4.1. Sample Collection and Bacterial Culture

In total, 76 *C. difficile* clinical isolates were obtained from a University-affiliated tertiary hospital and the National Institute of Health of Thailand. The isolation of *C. difficile* from stool samples of diarrheal patients was performed in previous studies [39,40]. These isolates were separated into 2 groups based on collection periods. The THA group was composed of 50 isolates collected from 2006 to 2009, and the THB group contained 26 isolates collected from 2010 to 2012. Each isolate was cultured on cycloserine–cefoxitin fructose agar (CCFA) for 24 h at 37 °C under anaerobic conditions (Coy Laboratory Products, Glass Lake, MI, USA) supplemented with 0.1% taurocholate to recover and enrich *C. difficile* cells. A single colony was cultured in fresh brain heart infusion (BHI) broth and incubated in an anaerobic chamber at 37 °C for 24–48 h. The culture was preserved with 10% (v/v) glycerol at −80 °C for further use.

4.2. Toxin Genotyping

Genomic DNA of *C. difficile* isolates was extracted from BHI culture using an E.Z.N.A.® Stool DNA kit (Omega Bio-tek, Norcross, GA, USA), according to the manufacturer's instructions. DNA purity and concentration were assessed by NanoDrop™ spectrophotometer (Thermo Fisher Scientific, Waltham, MA, USA). Toxigenic profiles of all *C. difficile* isolates were analyzed by multiplex PCR with 5 specific primer pairs, *tcdA, tcdB, cdtA, cdtB*, and 16S rDNA (Table 3). The PCR reaction was conducted in a total volume of 20 µL containing 25–200 ng of genomic DNA, 0.8 mM dNTPs, 5 mM $MgCl_2$, 1× PCR buffer, (500 mM KCl, 100 mM tris-HCl, pH 9.1), 1U *Taq* DNA polymerase (Vivantis, kuala Lumpur, Malaysia), and 0.2 µM primers. Amplification was performed under a thermal cycler with cycling conditions including a predenaturation at 92 °C for 5 min, 30 cycles of denaturation at 92 °C for 20s, an annealing at 58 °C for 65s, and an extension at 68 °C for 90s, and a final extension at 60 °C for 5 min.

In addition, the deletion in repeating regions at the 3′ end of the *tcdA* gene was investigated using the NK9 and NKV011 primers (Table 3) by Kato et al. 1999 [72]. PCR reaction was performed under the same conditions of the multiplex PCR. The thermocycler conditions included a predenaturation at 94 °C for 6 min, followed by 37 cycles of denaturation at 94 °C for 20 s, an annealing at 55 °C for 30 s, and an extension at 60 °C for 120 s, and a final extension at 60 °C for 10 min. The PCR products were visualized using electrophoresis with 1.2% agarose gel and strained with ethidium bromide.

4.3. PCR Ribotyping

PCR ribotyping was performed based on the 16S–23S rRNA intergenic spacer regions described by Bidet et al. 1999 [73]. The primer sequences were 5′-GTGCGGCTGGATCACCT CCT-3′ (16S primer) and 5′-CCCTGCACCCTTATTACCTTGACC-3′ (23S primer). The PCR reaction was conducted in a total volume of 20 µL composed of 25–200 ng genomic DNA, 0.2 mM dNTPs, 0.2 µM primers, 1.5 mM $MgCl_2$, 10× PCR buffer (500 mM KCl, 100 mM Tris-HCl, pH 9.1), 1U *Tag* DNA polymerase, and deionized water. The thermocycler profile consisted of an initial denaturation at 95 °C for 5 min, followed by 35 cycles at 95 °C for 1 min, 57 °C for 1 min, and 72 °C for 1 min, and a final extension at 72 °C for 10 min. Amplification products were separated by electrophoresis in 3% agarose gel for 6 h with 85 V in 1× Tris-borate EDAT (TBE) buffer. The electrophoresis patterns were visualized under UV light after staining with ethidium bromide. The high-resolution image was captured and analyzed with a gel documentation system. The resulting band patterns were visually compared to PCR ribotypes of the reference strains, *C. difficile* PCR ribotypes 001, 012, 017, 020, 023, 027, 046, 056, 077, 081, 095, 106, and 117.

4.4. Quantification of Toxins A and B

Toxigenic *C. difficile* isolates (n = 47) and the reference strain, *C. difficile* R20291, were inoculated on CCFA agar plates. A single colony was cultured in fresh BHI media. A total of 1% of bacterial culture was sub-cultured into fresh BHI media for 48 h at 37 °C. The supernatant was collected from the culture using centrifugation at 5000× *g* for 10 min and sterilized by passing through a 0.22 µm membrane. Total protein was measured using Bradford's assay (Clive G et al., 1989). Indirect enzyme-link immunosorbent assay (ELISA) was performed to quantify the level of toxins A and B. Initially, 96-well polystyrene microtiter plates were coated with 100 µL of 5 mg/mL supernatant in 0.5 M carbonate buffer (pH 9.4) and incubated overnight at 4 °C. The plates were washed three times with 200 µL of 1× PBS. Then, 200 µL of blocking solution (1% BSA) was added to wells. The plates were incubated for 1 h at room temperature and washed with PBS-T (0.05% Tween-20, pH 7.4). The 100 µL final 1:500 dilution of mouse anti-toxin A (Abcam, Cambridge, UK) or 1:250 dilution of mouse anti-toxin B (Bio-Rad, Hercules, CA, USA) was added to wells. The plates were incubated for 1 h at 37 °C and washed three times with 100 µL of PBS-T at room temperature. Finally, 50 µL of 1:4 dilution of Equilibrate SignalStain® Boost IHC Detection Reagent (HRP, anti-mouse) (Cell Signaling, Beverly, MA, USA) was added to wells. The plates were then incubated for 1 h at 37 °C and washed three times with 1× PBS. Finally, 100 µL TMB (3,3′,5,5′-tetramethylbenzidine) substrate (Seracare, Milford, MA, USA) was added to wells. After 10 min of incubation at 37 °C, the reaction was stopped by addition of 100 µL of 2 N hydrochloric acid. The absorbance at 450 nm was measured by microplate reader (Tecan, Switzerland). The relative levels of toxin production were compared to the reference strain, *C. difficile* R20291.

4.5. Minimal Inhibitory Concentration (MIC) Testing

The minimal inhibitory concentration (MIC) testing was performed using 96-well broth dilution in triplicate. Nine antibiotics, including metronidazole (0.0625–16 µg/mL), vancomycin (0.0625–16 µg/mL), amoxicillin (0.125–32 µg/mL), ampicillin (0.125–32 µg/mL), cefoxitin (2–256 µg/mL), chloramphenicol (0.25–32 µg/mL), levofloxacin (0.125–32 µg/mL), and rifampicin (0.125–32 µg/mL) were subjected to MIC testing. A single colony of *C. difficile* on CCFA was inoculated into fresh BHI medium. After overnight incubation, *C. difficile* culture was transferred to freshly prepared Wilkins-Chalgren broth until the OD_{600} reached 0.6 (~10^8 CFU/mL). Two-fold serial dilutions of antibiotics (0.125–512 µg/mL) were prepared in a 96-well plate at a total volume of 200 µL. A total of 10 µL of bacterial suspension (~10^6 CFU/mL) was then inoculated into antibiotic plates. The 96-well microplates were incubated at 37 °C under anaerobic conditions for 48 h. The OD_{600} at the end point was measured using a spectrophotometer. The MIC values were defined as the lowest concentration of antibiotic where no growth of bacteria was observed. The MIC results were categorized according to the guidelines of the Clinical and Laboratory Standards Institute (CLSI), http://www.clsi.org/ accessed on 1 June 2021; the European Committee on Antimicrobial Susceptibility Testing (EUCAST), http://www.eucast.org/ accessed on 1 June 2021; and published data [29,30].

Supplementary Materials: The following are available online at https://www.mdpi.com/article/10.3390/antibiotics10060714/s1, Figure S1: PCR ribotyping of (A) standard *C. difficile* strains and (B) *C. difficile* isolates in this study, Table S1: Toxigenic profiles and ribotype of 76 *C. difficile* clinical isolates from Thailand, Table S2: Antimicrobial susceptibility of 76 *C. difficile* clinical isolates from Thailand against 8 antibiotics.

Author Contributions: Conceptualization, S.C.; data curation, S.W.; formal analysis, S.W. and N.M.; methodology, S.W, N.M., M.P., A.A., P.H., and S.A.; investigation, S.C; validation, T.J.; writing—original draft preparation, S.W.; writing—review and editing, T.J. and S.C.; project administration, S.C. and T.J. All authors have read and agreed to the published version of the manuscript.

Funding: This project is funded by the National Research Council of Thailand (NRCT) and Mahidol University (NRCT5-RSA63015) to S.C., and Research Cluster: Multi-Generation Researchers Grant from Mahidol University to S.C., T.J., and P.H.

Data Availability Statement: Data are contained within the article.

Acknowledgments: The authors thank Piyada Wangroongsarb, Department of Medical Sciences, National Institute of Health, Ministry of Public Health, for *C. difficile* THA isolates and Nigel Minton, University of Nottingham, for *C. difficile* reference ribotype strains.

Conflicts of Interest: The authors declare no conflict of interest.

References

1. Kelly, C.P.; Pothoulakis, C.; LaMont, J.T. Clostridium difficile colitis. *N. Engl. J. Med.* **1994**, *330*, 257–262. [CrossRef]
2. Oren, A.; Rupnik, M. Clostridium difficile and Clostridioides difficile: Two validly published and correct names. *Anaerobe* **2018**, *52*, 125–126. [CrossRef] [PubMed]
3. Jawa, R.S.; Mercer, D.W. Clostridium difficile-associated infection: A disease of varying severity. *Am. J. Surg.* **2012**, *204*, 836–842. [CrossRef] [PubMed]
4. Zhu, D.; Sorg, J.A.; Sun, X. Clostridioides difficile Biology: Sporulation, Germination, and Corresponding Therapies for C. difficile Infection. *Front. Cell. Infect. Microbiol.* **2018**, *8*, 29. [CrossRef] [PubMed]
5. Burnham, C.A.; Carroll, K.C. Diagnosis of Clostridium difficile infection: An ongoing conundrum for clinicians and for clinical laboratories. *Clin. Microbiol. Rev.* **2013**, *26*, 604–630. [CrossRef] [PubMed]
6. Gerding, D.N.; Johnson, S.; Rupnik, M.; Aktories, K. Clostridium difficile binary toxin CDT: Mechanism, epidemiology, and potential clinical importance. *Gut Microbes* **2014**, *5*, 15–27. [CrossRef]
7. Cowardin, C.A.; Buonomo, E.L.; Saleh, M.M.; Wilson, M.G.; Burgess, S.L.; Kuehne, S.A.; Schwan, C.; Eichhoff, A.M.; Koch-Nolte, F.; Lyras, D.; et al. The binary toxin CDT enhances Clostridium difficile virulence by suppressing protective colonic eosinophilia. *Nat. Microbiol.* **2016**, *1*, 16108. [CrossRef]
8. He, M.; Miyajima, F.; Roberts, P.; Ellison, L.; Pickard, D.J.; Martin, M.J.; Connor, T.R.; Harris, S.R.; Fairley, D.; Bamford, K.B.; et al. Emergence and global spread of epidemic healthcare-associated Clostridium difficile. *Nat. Genet.* **2013**, *45*, 109–113. [CrossRef]
9. Borren, N.Z.; Ghadermarzi, S.; Hutfless, S.; Ananthakrishnan, A.N. The emergence of Clostridium difficile infection in Asia: A systematic review and meta-analysis of incidence and impact. *PLoS ONE* **2017**, *12*, e0176797. [CrossRef]
10. Imwattana, K.; Wangroongsarb, P.; Riley, T.V. High prevalence and diversity of tcdA-negative and tcdB-positive, and non-toxigenic, Clostridium difficile in Thailand. *Anaerobe* **2019**, *57*, 4–10. [CrossRef]
11. Putsathit, P.; Maneerattanaporn, M.; Piewngam, P.; Kiratisin, P.; Riley, T.V. Prevalence and molecular epidemiology of Clostridium difficile infection in Thailand. *New Microbes New Infect.* **2017**, *15*, 27–32. [CrossRef] [PubMed]
12. Imwattana, K.; Knight, D.R.; Kullin, B.; Collins, D.A.; Putsathit, P.; Kiratisin, P.; Riley, T.V. Clostridium difficile ribotype 017-characterization, evolution and epidemiology of the dominant strain in Asia. *Emerg. Microbes Infect.* **2019**, *8*, 796–807. [CrossRef] [PubMed]
13. Umeki, S.; Niki, Y.; Soejima, R. Angiotensin-converting enzyme activity and steroid therapy in sarcoidosis. *Arch. Intern. Med.* **1987**, *147*, 2056. [CrossRef]
14. Collins, D.A.; Putsathit, P.; Elliott, B.; Riley, T.V. Laboratory-based surveillance of Clostridium difficile strains circulating in the Australian healthcare setting in 2012. *Pathology* **2017**, *49*, 309–313. [CrossRef]
15. Senoh, M.; Kato, H.; Fukuda, T.; Niikawa, A.; Hori, Y.; Hagiya, H.; Ito, Y.; Miki, H.; Abe, Y.; Furuta, K.; et al. Predominance of PCR-ribotypes, 018 (smz) and 369 (trf) of Clostridium difficile in Japan: A potential relationship with other global circulating strains? *J. Med. Microbiol.* **2015**, *64*, 1226–1236. [CrossRef]
16. Jin, H.; Ni, K.; Wei, L.; Shen, L.; Xu, H.; Kong, Q.; Ni, X. Identification of Clostridium difficile RT078 From Patients and Environmental Surfaces in Zhejiang Province, China. *Infect. Control. Hosp. Epidemiol.* **2016**, *37*, 745–746. [CrossRef]
17. Rupnik, M.; Wilcox, M.H.; Gerding, D.N. Clostridium difficile infection: New developments in epidemiology and pathogenesis. *Nat. Rev. Microbiol.* **2009**, *7*, 526–536. [CrossRef] [PubMed]
18. Loo, V.G.; Bourgault, A.M.; Poirier, L.; Lamothe, F.; Michaud, S.; Turgeon, N.; Toye, B.; Beaudoin, A.; Frost, E.H.; Gilca, R.; et al. Host and pathogen factors for Clostridium difficile infection and colonization. *N. Engl. J. Med.* **2011**, *365*, 1693–1703. [CrossRef]
19. Bagdasarian, N.; Rao, K.; Malani, P.N. Diagnosis and treatment of Clostridium difficile in adults: A systematic review. *JAMA* **2015**, *313*, 398–408. [CrossRef]
20. Ofosu, A. Clostridium difficile infection: A review of current and emerging therapies. *Ann. Gastroenterol.* **2016**, *29*, 147–154. [CrossRef]
21. Goudarzi, M.; Goudarzi, H.; Alebouyeh, M.; Azimi Rad, M.; Shayegan Mehr, F.S.; Zali, M.R.; Aslani, M.M. Antimicrobial susceptibility of clostridium difficile clinical isolates in iran. *Iran. Red Crescent Med. J.* **2013**, *15*, 704–711. [CrossRef]

22. Adler, A.; Miller-Roll, T.; Bradenstein, R.; Block, C.; Mendelson, B.; Parizade, M.; Paitan, Y.; Schwartz, D.; Peled, N.; Carmeli, Y.; et al. A national survey of the molecular epidemiology of Clostridium difficile in Israel: The dissemination of the ribotype 027 strain with reduced susceptibility to vancomycin and metronidazole. *Diagn. Microbiol. Infect. Dis.* **2015**, *83*, 21–24. [CrossRef] [PubMed]
23. Jin, D.; Luo, Y.; Huang, C.; Cai, J.; Ye, J.; Zheng, Y.; Wang, L.; Zhao, P.; Liu, A.; Fang, W.; et al. Molecular Epidemiology of Clostridium difficile Infection in Hospitalized Patients in Eastern China. *J. Clin. Microbiol.* **2017**, *55*, 801–810. [CrossRef]
24. Peng, Z.; Addisu, A.; Alrabaa, S.; Sun, X. Antibiotic Resistance and Toxin Production of Clostridium difficile Isolates from the Hospitalized Patients in a Large Hospital in Florida. *Front. Microbiol.* **2017**, *8*, 2584. [CrossRef] [PubMed]
25. Putsathit, P.; Maneerattanaporn, M.; Piewngam, P.; Knight, D.R.; Kiratisin, P.; Riley, T.V. Antimicrobial susceptibility of Clostridium difficile isolated in Thailand. *Antimicrob. Resist. Infect. Control.* **2017**, *6*, 58. [CrossRef]
26. Imwattana, K.; Putsathit, P.; Leepattarakit, T.; Kiratisin, P.; Riley, T.V. Mild or Malign: Clinical Characteristics and Outcomes of Clostridium difficile Infection in Thailand. *J. Clin. Microbiol.* **2020**, *58*. [CrossRef] [PubMed]
27. Shen, A. Clostridium difficile toxins: Mediators of inflammation. *J. Innate Immun.* **2012**, *4*, 149–158. [CrossRef]
28. Åkerlund, T.; Persson, I.; Unemo, M.; Norén, T.; Svenungsson, B.; Wullt, M.; Burman, L.G. Increased Sporulation Rate of Epidemic *Clostridium difficile* Type 027/NAP1. *J. Clin. Microbiol.* **2008**, *46*, 1530. [CrossRef] [PubMed]
29. Chow, V.C.Y.; Kwong, T.N.Y.; So, E.W.M.; Ho, Y.I.I.; Wong, S.H.; Lai, R.W.M.; Chan, R.C.Y. Surveillance of antibiotic resistance among common Clostridium difficile ribotypes in Hong Kong. *Sci. Rep.* **2017**, *7*, 17218. [CrossRef]
30. O'Connor, J.R.; Galang, M.A.; Sambol, S.P.; Hecht, D.W.; Vedantam, G.; Gerding, D.N.; Johnson, S. Rifampin and rifaximin resistance in clinical isolates of Clostridium difficile. *Antimicrob. Agents Chemother.* **2008**, *52*, 2813–2817. [CrossRef]
31. Robinson, C.D.; Auchtung, J.M.; Collins, J.; Britton, R.A. Epidemic Clostridium difficile strains demonstrate increased competitive fitness compared to nonepidemic isolates. *Infect. Immun.* **2014**, *82*, 2815–2825. [CrossRef] [PubMed]
32. Freeman, J.; Bauer, M.P.; Baines, S.D.; Corver, J.; Fawley, W.N.; Goorhuis, B.; Kuijper, E.J.; Wilcox, M.H. The changing epidemiology of Clostridium difficile infections. *Clin. Microbiol. Rev.* **2010**, *23*, 529–549. [CrossRef] [PubMed]
33. Martinez-Melendez, A.; Morfin-Otero, R.; Villarreal-Trevino, L.; Baines, S.D.; Camacho-Ortiz, A.; Garza-Gonzalez, E. Molecular epidemiology of predominant and emerging Clostridioides difficile ribotypes. *J. Microbiol. Methods* **2020**, *175*, 105974. [CrossRef] [PubMed]
34. Schumann, P.; Pukall, R. The discriminatory power of ribotyping as automatable technique for differentiation of bacteria. *Syst. Appl. Microbiol.* **2013**, *36*, 369–375. [CrossRef]
35. Wultanska, D.; Pituch, H.; Obuch-Woszczatynski, P.; Meisel-Mikolajczyk, F.; Luczak, M. Profile of toxigenicity of Clostridium difficile strains isolated from paediatric patients with clinical diagnosis of antibiotic associated diarrhea (AAD). *Med. Dosw. Mikrobiol.* **2005**, *57*, 377–382. [PubMed]
36. Deniz, U.; Ulger, N.; Aksu, B.; Karavus, M.; Soyletir, G. Investigation of toxin genes of Clostridium difficile strains isolated from hospitalized patients with diarrhoea at Marmara University Hospital. *Mikrobiyol. Bul.* **2011**, *45*, 1–10.
37. Aliramezani, A.; Talebi, M.; Baghani, A.; Hajabdolbaghi, M.; Salehi, M.; Abdollahi, A.; Afhami, S.; Marjani, M.; Golbabaei, F.; Boroumand, M.A.; et al. Pathogenicity locus determinants and toxinotyping of Clostridioides difficile isolates recovered from Iranian patients. *New Microbes New Infect.* **2018**, *25*, 52–57. [CrossRef] [PubMed]
38. Persson, S.; Torpdahl, M.; Olsen, K.E. New multiplex PCR method for the detection of Clostridium difficile toxin A (tcdA) and toxin B (tcdB) and the binary toxin (cdtA/cdtB) genes applied to a Danish strain collection. *Clin. Microbiol. Infect.* **2008**, *14*, 1057–1064. [CrossRef]
39. Chankhamhaengdecha, S.; Hadpanus, P.; Aroonnual, A.; Ngamwongsatit, P.; Chotiprasitsakul, D.; Chongtrakool, P.; Janvilisri, T. Evaluation of multiplex PCR with enhanced spore germination for detection of Clostridium difficile from stool samples of the hospitalized patients. *BioMed Res. Int.* **2013**, *2013*, 875437. [CrossRef]
40. Chotiprasitsakul, D.; Janvilisri, T.; Kiertiburanakul, S.; Watcharananun, S.; Chankhamhaengdecha, S.; Hadpanus, P.; Malathum, K. A superior test for diagnosis of Clostridium difficile-associated diarrhea in resource-limited settings. *Jpn. J. Infect. Dis.* **2012**, *65*, 326–329. [CrossRef]
41. Eckert, C.; Emirian, A.; Le Monnier, A.; Cathala, L.; De Montclos, H.; Goret, J.; Berger, P.; Petit, A.; De Chevigny, A.; Jean-Pierre, H.; et al. Prevalence and pathogenicity of binary toxin-positive Clostridium difficile strains that do not produce toxins A and B. *New Microbes New Infect.* **2015**, *3*, 12–17. [CrossRef]
42. McGovern, A.M.; Androga, G.O.; Knight, D.R.; Watson, M.W.; Elliott, B.; Foster, N.F.; Chang, B.J.; Riley, T.V. Prevalence of binary toxin positive Clostridium difficile in diarrhoeal humans in the absence of epidemic ribotype 027. *PLoS ONE* **2017**, *12*, e0187658. [CrossRef] [PubMed]
43. Xu, X.; Godoy-Ruiz, R.; Adipietro, K.A.; Peralta, C.; Ben-Hail, D.; Varney, K.M.; Cook, M.E.; Roth, B.M.; Wilder, P.T.; Cleveland, T.; et al. Structure of the cell-binding component of the Clostridium difficile binary toxin reveals a di-heptamer macromolecular assembly. *Proc. Natl. Acad. Sci. USA* **2020**, *117*, 1049–1058. [CrossRef] [PubMed]
44. Aktories, K.; Papatheodorou, P.; Schwan, C. Binary Clostridium difficile toxin (CDT)–A virulence factor disturbing the cytoskeleton. *Anaerobe* **2018**, *53*, 21–29. [CrossRef]
45. Stubbs, S.L.; Brazier, J.S.; O'Neill, G.L.; Duerden, B.I. PCR targeted to the 16S-23S rRNA gene intergenic spacer region of Clostridium difficile and construction of a library consisting of 116 different PCR ribotypes. *J. Clin. Microbiol.* **1999**, *37*, 461–463. [CrossRef]

46. Gurtler, V. Typing of Clostridium difficile strains by PCR-amplification of variable length 16S-23S rDNA spacer regions. *J. Gen. Microbiol.* **1993**, *139*, 3089–3097. [CrossRef]
47. Indra, A.; Schmid, D.; Huhulescu, S.; Hell, M.; Gattringer, R.; Hasenberger, P.; Fiedler, A.; Wewalka, G.; Allerberger, F. Characterization of clinical Clostridium difficile isolates by PCR ribotyping and detection of toxin genes in Austria, 2006-2007. *J. Med. Microbiol.* **2008**, *57*, 702–708. [CrossRef]
48. Hung, Y.P.; Huang, I.H.; Lin, H.J.; Tsai, B.Y.; Liu, H.C.; Liu, H.C.; Lee, J.C.; Wu, Y.H.; Tsai, P.J.; Ko, W.C. Predominance of Clostridium difficile Ribotypes 017 and 078 among Toxigenic Clinical Isolates in Southern Taiwan. *PLoS ONE* **2016**, *11*, e0166159. [CrossRef]
49. Killgore, G.; Thompson, A.; Johnson, S.; Brazier, J.; Kuijper, E.; Pepin, J.; Frost, E.H.; Savelkoul, P.; Nicholson, B.; van den Berg, R.J.; et al. Comparison of seven techniques for typing international epidemic strains of Clostridium difficile: Restriction endonuclease analysis, pulsed-field gel electrophoresis, PCR-ribotyping, multilocus sequence typing, multilocus variable-number tandem-repeat analysis, amplified fragment length polymorphism, and surface layer protein A gene sequence typing. *J. Clin. Microbiol.* **2008**, *46*, 431–437. [CrossRef]
50. Tanner, H.E.; Hardy, K.J.; Hawkey, P.M. Coexistence of multiple multilocus variable-number tandem-repeat analysis subtypes of Clostridium difficile PCR ribotype 027 strains within fecal specimens. *J. Clin. Microbiol.* **2010**, *48*, 985–987. [CrossRef] [PubMed]
51. Gonzales-Luna, A.J.; Carlson, T.J.; Dotson, K.M.; Poblete, K.; Costa, G.; Miranda, J.; Lancaster, C.; Walk, S.T.; Tupy, S.; Begum, K.; et al. PCR ribotypes of Clostridioides difficile across Texas from 2011 to 2018 including emergence of ribotype 255. *Emerg. Microbes Infect.* **2020**, *9*, 341–347. [CrossRef]
52. Tenover, F.C.; Akerlund, T.; Gerding, D.N.; Goering, R.V.; Bostrom, T.; Jonsson, A.M.; Wong, E.; Wortman, A.T.; Persing, D.H. Comparison of strain typing results for Clostridium difficile isolates from North America. *J. Clin. Microbiol.* **2011**, *49*, 1831–1837. [CrossRef]
53. Elliott, B.; Androga, G.O.; Knight, D.R.; Riley, T.V. Clostridium difficile infection: Evolution, phylogeny and molecular epidemiology. *Infect. Genet. Evol.* **2017**, *49*, 1–11. [CrossRef] [PubMed]
54. Drudy, D.; Fanning, S.; Kyne, L. Toxin A-negative, toxin B-positive Clostridium difficile. *Int. J. Infect. Dis.* **2007**, *11*, 5–10. [CrossRef] [PubMed]
55. Shin, B.M.; Kuak, E.Y.; Yoo, S.J.; Shin, W.C.; Yoo, H.M. Emerging toxin A-B+ variant strain of Clostridium difficile responsible for pseudomembranous colitis at a tertiary care hospital in Korea. *Diagn. Microbiol. Infect. Dis.* **2008**, *60*, 333–337. [CrossRef] [PubMed]
56. Ling, Z.; Liu, X.; Jia, X.; Cheng, Y.; Luo, Y.; Yuan, L.; Wang, Y.; Zhao, C.; Guo, S.; Li, L.; et al. Impacts of infection with different toxigenic Clostridium difficile strains on faecal microbiota in children. *Sci. Rep.* **2014**, *4*, 7485. [CrossRef]
57. Fatima, R.; Aziz, M. The Hypervirulent Strain of Clostridium Difficile: NAP1/B1/027–A Brief Overview. *Cureus* **2019**, *11*, e3977. [CrossRef]
58. Merrigan, M.; Venugopal, A.; Mallozzi, M.; Roxas, B.; Viswanathan, V.K.; Johnson, S.; Gerding, D.N.; Vedantam, G. Human hypervirulent Clostridium difficile strains exhibit increased sporulation as well as robust toxin production. *J. Bacteriol.* **2010**, *192*, 4904–4911. [CrossRef]
59. Warny, M.; Pepin, J.; Fang, A.; Killgore, G.; Thompson, A.; Brazier, J.; Frost, E.; McDonald, L.C. Toxin production by an emerging strain of Clostridium difficile associated with outbreaks of severe disease in North America and Europe. *Lancet* **2005**, *366*, 1079–1084. [CrossRef]
60. Lyon, S.A.; Hutton, M.L.; Rood, J.I.; Cheung, J.K.; Lyras, D. CdtR Regulates TcdA and TcdB Production in Clostridium difficile. *PLoS Pathog.* **2016**, *12*, e1005758. [CrossRef]
61. Buchler, A.C.; Rampini, S.K.; Stelling, S.; Ledergerber, B.; Peter, S.; Schweiger, A.; Ruef, C.; Zbinden, R.; Speck, R.F. Antibiotic susceptibility of Clostridium difficile is similar worldwide over two decades despite widespread use of broad-spectrum antibiotics: An analysis done at the University Hospital of Zurich. *BMC Infect. Dis.* **2014**, *14*, 607. [CrossRef] [PubMed]
62. Knight, D.R.; Giglio, S.; Huntington, P.G.; Korman, T.M.; Kotsanas, D.; Moore, C.V.; Paterson, D.L.; Prendergast, L.; Huber, C.A.; Robson, J.; et al. Surveillance for antimicrobial resistance in Australian isolates of Clostridium difficile, 2013–2014. *J. Antimicrob. Chemother.* **2015**, *70*, 2992–2999. [CrossRef]
63. Kim, Y.J.; Park, K.H.; Park, D.A.; Park, J.; Bang, B.W.; Lee, S.S.; Lee, E.J.; Lee, H.J.; Hong, S.K.; Kim, Y.R. Guideline for the Antibiotic Use in Acute Gastroenteritis. *Infect. Chemother.* **2019**, *51*, 217–243. [CrossRef] [PubMed]
64. Riddle, M.S.; DuPont, H.L.; Connor, B.A. ACG Clinical Guideline: Diagnosis, Treatment, and Prevention of Acute Diarrheal Infections in Adults. *Am. J. Gastroenterol.* **2016**, *111*, 602–622. [CrossRef]
65. Spigaglia, P. Recent advances in the understanding of antibiotic resistance in Clostridium difficile infection. *Ther. Adv. Infect. Dis.* **2016**, *3*, 23–42. [CrossRef] [PubMed]
66. Leffler, D.A.; Lamont, J.T. Clostridium difficile infection. *N. Engl. J. Med.* **2015**, *372*, 1539–1548. [CrossRef]
67. Slimings, C.; Riley, T.V. Antibiotics and hospital-acquired Clostridium difficile infection: Update of systematic review and meta-analysis. *J. Antimicrob. Chemother.* **2014**, *69*, 881–891. [CrossRef] [PubMed]
68. Johanesen, P.A.; Mackin, K.E.; Hutton, M.L.; Awad, M.M.; Larcombe, S.; Amy, J.M.; Lyras, D. Disruption of the Gut Microbiome: Clostridium difficile Infection and the Threat of Antibiotic Resistance. *Genes* **2015**, *6*, 1347–1360. [CrossRef]

69. Freeman, J.; Vernon, J.; Morris, K.; Nicholson, S.; Todhunter, S.; Longshaw, C.; Wilcox, M.H.; Pan-European Longitudinal Surveillance of Antibiotic Resistance among Prevalent Clostridium difficile Ribotypes' Study, G. Pan-European longitudinal surveillance of antibiotic resistance among prevalent Clostridium difficile ribotypes. *Clin. Microbiol. Infect.* **2015**, *21*, 248.e9–248.e16. [CrossRef]
70. Kim, J.; Kang, J.O.; Pai, H.; Choi, T.Y. Association between PCR ribotypes and antimicrobial susceptibility among Clostridium difficile isolates from healthcare-associated infections in South Korea. *Int. J. Antimicrob. Agents* **2012**, *40*, 24–29. [CrossRef]
71. Obuch-Woszczatynski, P.; Dubiel, G.; Harmanus, C.; Kuijper, E.; Duda, U.; Wultanska, D.; van Belkum, A.; Pituch, H. Emergence of Clostridium difficile infection in tuberculosis patients due to a highly rifampicin-resistant PCR ribotype 046 clone in Poland. *Eur. J. Clin. Microbiol. Infect. Dis.* **2013**, *32*, 1027–1030. [CrossRef] [PubMed]
72. Kato, H.; Kato, N.; Katow, S.; Maegawa, T.; Nakamura, S.; Lyerly, D.M. Deletions in the repeating sequences of the toxin A gene of toxin A-negative, toxin B-positive Clostridium difficile strains. *FEMS Microbiol. Lett.* **1999**, *175*, 197–203. [CrossRef] [PubMed]
73. Bidet, P.; Barbut, F.; Lalande, V.; Burghoffer, B.; Petit, J.C. Development of a new PCR-ribotyping method for Clostridium difficile based on ribosomal RNA gene sequencing. *FEMS Microbiol. Lett.* **1999**, *175*, 261–266. [CrossRef] [PubMed]

antibiotics MDPI

Article

Diagnostic Methods of *Clostridioides difficile* Infection and *Clostridioides difficile* Ribotypes in Studied Sample

Elena Novakova [1], Zuzana Stofkova [1,*], Vladimira Sadlonova [1] and Lukas Hleba [2]

[1] Jessenius Faculty of Medicine in Martin, Comenius University in Bratislava, Mala Hora 4A, 03601 Martin, Slovakia; elena.novakova@uniba.sk (E.N.); vladimira.sadlonova@uniba.sk (V.S.)
[2] Faculty of Biotechnology and Food Sciences, Slovak University of Agriculture in Nitra, A. Hlinku 610/4, 94901 Nitra, Slovakia; lukas.hleba@gmail.com
* Correspondence: zuzana.stofkova@gmail.com

Abstract: Background: *Clostridioides* (*Clostridium*) *difficile* is the most common nosocomial pathogen and antibiotic-related diarrhea in health-care facilities. Over the last few years, there was an increase in the incidence rate of *C. difficile* infection cases in Slovakia. In this study, the phenotypic (toxigenicity, antimicrobial susceptibility) and genotypic (PCR ribotypes, genes for binary toxins) patterns of *C. difficile* isolates from patients with CDI were analyzed, from July to August 2016, taken from hospitals in the Horne Povazie region of northern Slovakia. The aim of the study was also to identify hypervirulent strains (e.g., the presence of RT027 or RT176). Methods: The retrospective analysis of biological samples suspected of CDI were analyzed by GDH, anaerobic culture, enzyme immunoassay on toxins A/B, multiplex "real-time" PCR and PCR capillary-based electrophoresis ribotyping, and by MALDI TOF MS. Results: *C. difficile* isolates (n = 44) were identified by PCR ribotyping, which revealed five different ribotypes (RT001, 011, 017, 081, 176). The presence of hypervirulent RT027 was not identified. The *C. difficile* isolates (RT001, 011, 081, 176) were susceptible to metronidazole and vancomycin. One isolate RT017 had reduced susceptibility to vancomycin. A statistically significant difference between the most prevalent PCR ribotypes, RT001 and RT176, regarding variables such as albumin, CRP, creatinine, the length of hospitalization (p = 0.175), and glomerular filtration (p = 0.05) was not found. Conclusion: The results of PCR capillary-based electrophoresis ribotyping in the studied samples showed a high prevalence of RT176 and 001.

Keywords: *Clostridioides difficile* infection; multi-step algorithm; multiplex "real-time" PCR; PCR capillary-based electrophoresis ribotyping

Citation: Novakova, E.; Stofkova, Z.; Sadlonova, V.; Hleba, L. Diagnostic Methods of *Clostridioides difficile* Infection and *Clostridioides difficile* Ribotypes in Studied Sample. *Antibiotics* **2021**, *10*, 1035. https://doi.org/10.3390/antibiotics10091035

Academic Editor: Marc Maresca

Received: 21 May 2021
Accepted: 19 August 2021
Published: 25 August 2021

1. Introduction

Clostridioides (*Clostridium*) *difficile* is the most common nosocomial pathogen and antibiotic-related diarrhea. It causes and poses a significant medical and economic burden in healthcare facilities [1]. According to the European Centre for Disease Control and Prevention's (ECDC) point prevalence survey of healthcare-associated infections (HAI), C. difficile was the eighth most frequently found microorganism [2]. In Europe, over the last two decades, there has been an increase in the incidence of *Clostridioides difficile* infection (CDI) cases and severity of CDI infections, and new highly virulent *C. difficile* strains (e.g., RT027) and other hypervirulent strains have emerged. [1] The ECDC started coordinating the surveillance of CDI in EU countries in 2016 [3]. The overall mean CDI density was 2.8 (95% CI 1.8–3.9) cases per 10,000 patients/days and community-associated CDI (CA-CDI) with an incidence density of 0.4 (95% CI 0.2–0.6) cases per 10,000 patients/days [4]. From 2010 to 2017, the incidence of CDI in Slovakia increased from 0.9 to 20.6/10,000 hospitalized patients [5]. The diagnosis of CDI is based on clinical symptoms accompanied by microbiological evidence of toxins produced by *C. difficile* or toxigenic strains of *C. difficile* [6]. The disease is multifactorial and environmental factors seem to set the conditions for *C. difficile* development [7].

The accurate and fast diagnosis of CDI is essential for optimal patient care and preventing the spread of infection [8]. Diagnostic methods for the identification of different targets determine the presence of free toxins or toxigenic strains in the diarrheal feces. The methods that detect the presence of *C. difficile* include evidence of glutamate dehydrogenase enzyme (GDH) and anaerobic culture, and methods that detect the presence of a toxigenic *C. difficile* [6]. The importance of the real-time PCR (polymerase chain reaction) method implementation lies in the high sensitivity and specificity of the testing method. The assay has high negative predictive value (NPV) and, therefore, can be used to accelerate the exclusion of *C. difficile* infection. The PCR can help early diagnostics and the early recognition of patients with *C. difficile* before complications occur [9]. The European Society of Clinical Microbiology and Infectious Diseases (ESCMID) recommends a multi-step algorithm for the CDI diagnosis [10]. ESCMID's recommendations about multistep algorithm testing describe how a positive first test should be confirmed with one or two confirmatory tests—glutamate dehydrogenase enzyme (GDH), toxins A and B, or a polymerase chain reaction (PCR test) [11]. The controversy remains about the need to treat patients with evidence of *C. difficile* and negative toxin A/B enzyme immunoassay (EIA), as they might have undetectable toxin levels or asymptomatic colonization with *C. difficile* [12]. Hypervirulent RT027, which is also characterized by the high production of toxins A and B, is a more severe disease course with more frequent recurrences, and higher morbidity and mortality have been reported in relation with this strain. Further analyses have shown that there are more ribotypes with similar properties [13] as the RT176.

The strain BI/NAP1/027 contains a nucleotide mutation at position 117 on the *tcdC* gene that encodes the protein C, which causes the suppression of genes for A/B toxins. In addition, RT027 produces so-called binary toxins [14].

The purpose of the paper was also to identify the presence of hypervirulent strains, such as RT176 and RT027. The RT027 strain is referred to as *C. difficile* BI/NAP1/027 in the studied sample and the circulation of ribotypes among departments of in- and out-patients was monitored [15]. In a recent extensive study [16], it was shown that the effect of individual ribotypes on overall disease progression, mortality and biomarkers varied. In addition to *C. difficile* PCR ribotype 027, there are other strains that are associated with epidemics and a severe course of *C. difficile* infection. Despite the increased virulence of certain ribotypes, the PCR ribotype value as a predictor of disease severity is limited because the ribotype involved in the infection is not known until it is diagnosed. However, in epidemics, the ribotype could be considered when deciding on the choice of empirical treatment [10]. According to the data reported to the Epidemiological Intelligence Information System (EPIS) in the Horne Povazie region of northern Slovakia, the incidence of reported CDI cases had increased. In 2015, there were four patients/10,000 population reported. In 2017, the incidences doubled and, in 2018, the incidences increased up to 10 per 10,000 inhabitants. In 2019, this number remained approximately on the same level with 10.2 CDI patients per 10,000 inhabitants. About 84% of CDI patients were hospital-associated infections (HAI-CDI), and 16% of CDI patients were community associated (CA-CDI). In 2019, HAI-CDI cases from internal medicine, long-term care, intensive care unit, surgery, infectious diseases, and other wards were reported in Slovakia in 2019 (in a population of 100,000)—Figure 1. This increased incidence rate lies also in the higher testing rate and conscientious reporting to the Epidemiological Information System (EPIS) since 2016.

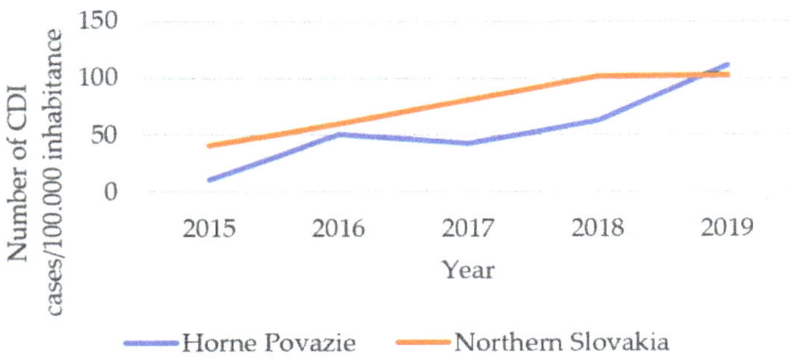

Figure 1. Number of CDI cases/100,000 inhabitants. Source: own processing according EPIS, 2020.

2. Results

Sixty *C. difficile* isolates included in the studied samples were tested for the presence of toxin genes by multiplex real-time PCR assay. [17] Twenty-eight isolates were from males and thirty-two isolates were from females. The median age was 77 years. The *C. difficile* isolates were taken from patients from the internal medicine (29 samples), long-term care (26), and surgery (1) wards, and from non-hospitalized patients (4). The average length of patient hospitalization was 40 days.

Eighteen isolates (18) had positive results for the B toxin gene (*tcdB*), and genes for binary toxins (*cdtA* and *cdtB*) and the presence of nucleotide deletion 117 on the *tcdC* regulatory gene were negative. Forty-one (41) isolates carried both the B toxin gene and the binary toxin genes (*cdtA* and *cdtB*), as well as the presence of nucleotide deletion 117 on the *tcdC* regulatory gene for B toxin. Another investigated sample was negative for all investigated toxin genes—Figure 2.

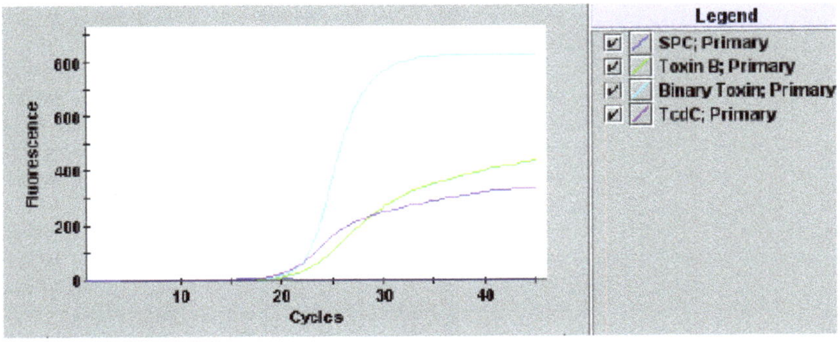

Figure 2. Positive result for toxigenic *C. difficile*, presumptive of 027/NAP1/BI [17].

Due to the severe course of the disease, the *C. difficile* isolates were further analyzed by PCR capillary-based electrophoresis ribotyping. In the studied samples, five (5) different ribotypes of *C. difficile* isolates were revealed (RT001, 011, 017, 081, 176), which were identified by PCR ribotyping. The proportion of *C. difficile* in 44 isolates was: RT176 (n = 27; 69.5%), RT001 (n = 13; 23.7%), RT011 (n = 1; 1.7%), RT081 (n = 1; 1.7%), RT017 (n = 2; 3.39%)—Figure 3.

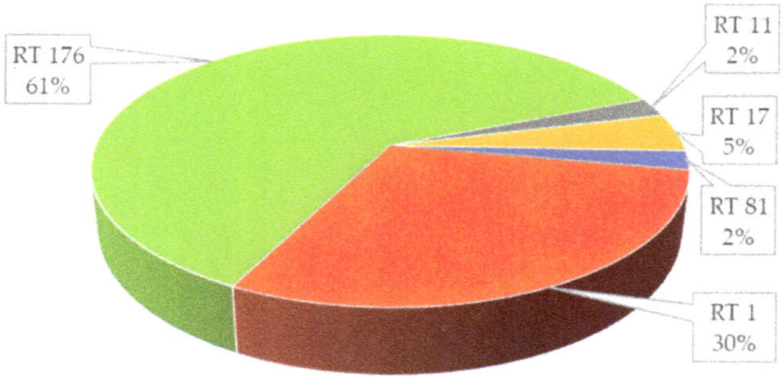

Figure 3. The proportion of ribotypes in *Clostridioides difficile* isolates (n = 44).

The PCR capillary-based electrophoresis ribotypes of *C. difficile* isolates on the strain level in patients (n = 44) were from internal medicine RT001 (6), RT176 (15), RT011 (1), RT081 (1); long-term care RT 001 (6), RT176 (12), RT017 (2); and surgery RT001 (1).

The most frequently occurring PCR ribotypes in the studied samples were RT176 and RT001. These ribotypes were present in patients' samples from in-patient departments (internal medicine, long-term care ward) but also in outpatients that had a history of prior hospitalization.

The presence of RT027 was not confirmed in any tested *C. difficile* isolate. The presence of RT176 (genetically very close to RT027) was confirmed in 27 samples—Figure 4. The importance of anaerobic cultivation resides in the determination of *C. difficile* susceptibility on antimicrobial agents. The *C. difficile* isolates (RT001, 011, 081, 176) were susceptible to metronidazole and vancomycin. One isolate RT017 had reduced susceptibility to vancomycin (Table 1).

The patients were typically hospitalized several times with chronic diseases, such as cardiovascular (29%), gastro-intestinal (24%), pulmonary (11%), renal (5%) and oncological diseases (1%), and other chronic diseases.

In the selected samples of patients, *C. difficile* isolates (n = 44) were analyzed following laboratory parameters, such as values of serum creatinine, total proteins, albumin, CRP, glomerular filtration and other parameters, such as the length of hospitalization. These parameters were compared between patients with ribotype RT001 and RT176. The dependent variable was the PCR ribotype and independent variables were the laboratory and other parameters such as the length of hospitalization.

The group infected with RT176 did not have a significantly different total protein level or level of albumin versus the group infected with RT001 (p = 0.300 and p = 0.682). Patients with RT001 had a lower level of glomerular filtration than those with RT176 (p = 0.054). There was no significant difference in the proportion of patients with an increase in serum creatinine concentration between RT001 and RT176.

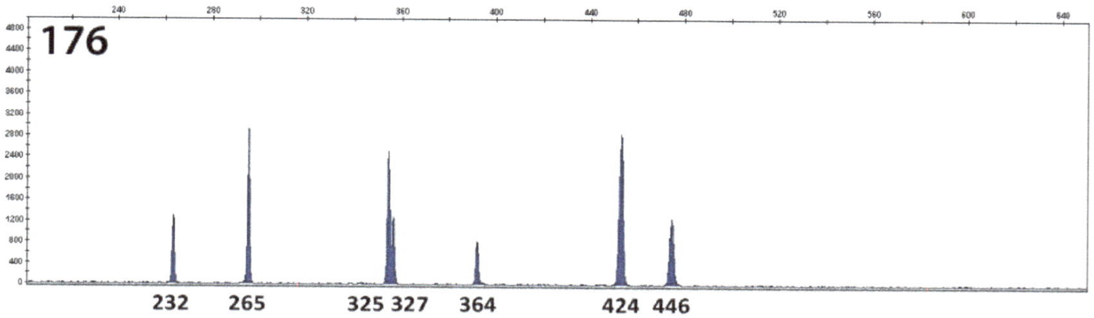

Figure 4. PCR capillary-based electrophoresis ribotyping on the strain level-RT176.

Table 1. Genotypic and phenotypic characteristics of *Clostridioides difficile* in the studied sample.

Number of *C. difficile* Isolates	Fenotype Characteristics of *C. difficile* isolates				Genotype Characteristics of *C. difficile* isolates			
	GDH/ Culture	Toxins A/B (Rapid Test, ELISA)	MIC_{90} µg/mL MTZ	MIC_{90} µg/mL VAN	Gene for B Toxin (*tcdB*)	Genes *cdtA*, *cdtB* for Binary Toxins	Deletion of nt 117 in *tcdC* Gene (Susp. RT 027)	RT Ribotypes
13	positive	positive	0.047	1.5	positive	Negative	Negative	001
27	positive	positive	0.5	1.0	positive	Positive	Positive	176
1	positive	positive	0.125	0.5	positive	Negative	Negative	011
2	positive	positive	0.125	2.0	positive	Negative	Negative	017
1	positive	positive	0.125	0.5	positive	Negative	Negative	081

Serum creatinine concentration data were also analyzed by gender. The different reference ranges were taken into account for the analyte in males and females. There was no significant difference in the level of CRP concentration between patients with RT176 isolates and RT001 isolates ($p = 0.295$).

There was a difference in the length of hospitalization ($p = 0.175$) between patients with RT001 and RT176. The mean duration of hospitalization for RT001 and RT176 patients was 44 and 35 days, respectively. Statistically significant dependence on identified ribotypes RT001 and RT176 were not found among the independent variables, serum creatinine ($p = 0.524$), total proteins ($p = 0.300$), albumin ($p = 0.682$), and CRP ($p = 0.295$) Table 2.

Table 2. *Clostridioides difficile* isolates RT001 and RT176 and selected laboratory parameters in the studied samples.

Laboratory and Other Variables	Ribotypes	Mean (Median) Years	95% Confidence Interval for Mean	Pearson $p < 0.001$
Total proteins g/L	001 176	61.10 (60.0) 57.27 (59.0)	(56.1–66.1) (51.2–63.0)	0.300
Albumin g/L	001 176	29.39 (28.95) 28.65 (28.95)	(27.56–31.21) (24.94–32.36)	0.682
CRP mg/L	001 176	78.07 (82.0) 56.75 (26)	(54.80–101.32) (18.36–95.14)	0.295
Glomerular filtration mL/s	001 176	0.861 (0.73) 1.156 (1.32)	(0.687–1.034) (0.875–1.436)	0.054
Length of hospitalization days	001 176	43.78 (44.0) 35.10 (30.5)	(36.04–51.52) (23.72–46.47)	0.175
Creatinine µmol/L	001 176	122.21 (112.0) 106.85 (76.0)	(90.6–153.7) (66.9–146.8)	0.524

All laboratory variables were analyzed by gender as well. There were no differences between male and female patients in four studied variables. The all-cause mortality was 11/14 (79%) in patients with RT001 and 18/41 (67%) in patients with RT176, respectively.

3. Discussion

Multi-step diagnostic algorithms combining GDH and toxin EIA with PCR are recommended for CDI's diagnosis [18].

The PCR tests are very sensitive to *C. difficile* but do not distinguish between symptomatic CDI and asymptomatic colonization, as they determine the genes for the production of toxins [9]. Genetic evidence of the toxigenic strain does not automatically mean that toxins are produced [19,20].

According to ESCMID, the use of one standalone CDI test is not recommended due to the low positive predictive value at low CDI prevalence [8].

The PCR ribotyping is essential for monitoring the spread of CDI and the course of the disease, as well as the detection of resistance to antimicrobial agents. This method is performed to identify individual strains, and to carry out surveillance of CDI spreading. According to the largest pan-European study of *C. difficile*, closER (2011–2015), 264 distinct ribotypes were revealed. The diversity between ribotypes varied markedly between countries and the years of the study. Epidemic and highly prevalent ribotypes included:RT027—prevalence 11.04%, RT014—9.1%, RT001—8.0%, RT078—6.5%, RT017—1.7%, RT176—1.3%, RT 011—1.1%, RT081—1.1%, and other ribotypes. The predominance of RT001 was reported in 2011 in Slovakia. The higher RT diversity was identified in 2012 (RT001, 014, 017, 081 and other ribotypes). This indicated lower antimicrobial resistance levels in countries with a greater *C. difficile* RT diversity [21]. In previous CDI studies, RT001 was also identified as predominant in Slovakia [22,23]. The new epidemic strains are less sensitive to antibiotics, e.g., resistant to fluoroquinolones. For many *C. difficile* strains, VAN susceptibility decreases gradually, which can be demonstrated by the increasing MIC. Reduced MTZ susceptibility was mainly observed in RT027 and RT198, and VAN resistance was observed in RT018 [21]. The occurrence of this ribotype 027/NAP1/BI *C. difficile* was also identified in countries in Central Europe [24]. The epidemic ribotypes exhibited a high level of antimicrobial resistance (RT017, 018 a 356) [25]. According to a study carried out in Slovakia, 2016, the occurrence of RT001 (59%), RT176 (23%), and RT027 (in 1 isolate) was found in 78 isolates [4]. The incidence of RT176 was also found in the Czech Republic [26]. The reduced susceptibility to moxifloxacin was identified in RT001, 017, 027, 176, in studies carried out by Krutova et al. and Freemann et al. [21,27].

Due to the epidemic situation during the period of our studied sample collection, there was a higher proportion of RT176 than RT001 identified. There was no RT027 identified in the studied sample. RT176 is close to ribotype RT027 and can be misidentified by commercial assays aimed at the deletion of one base pair at nucleotide 117 in the *C. difficile tcdC* gene that causes the suppression of genes for A and B toxins. The RT176 is also associated with a more severe course of the disease. RT176 is suggested to be related to RT027, since they belong to the same multilocus sequence [28].

Antimicrobial susceptibility testing investigated susceptibility to metronidazole in all *C. difficile* isolates. There was no confirmed reduced susceptibility or resistance to vancomycin in *C. difficile* isolates. Only one *C. difficile* isolate (RT017) had reduced susceptibility to vancomycin.

The link between clinical courses and specific ribotypes is still being investigated [29]. A hypervirulent RT027 is known worldwide. Some studies point to a more severe course of CDI disease when this ribotype occurs. The hypervirulent strain is referred to as *C. difficile* BI/NAP1/027 [15].

Some study results have supported that there may be other attributes of the *C. difficile* genome. These can significantly affect virulence (not only binary toxins and *tcdC* deletion), and hence the clinical course of the disease, which should be taken into account in the treatment strategy management [30]. In our studied sample, the RT027 was identified.

4. Materials and Methods

4.1. Sampling

The *C. difficile* strains isolated from 60 patients were analyzed in the laboratory in Klinicka Biochemia, Inc., Zilina, Slovakia which received fecal samples of patients suspected of CDI from 2 hospitals in northern Slovakia (with 1250 patient beds) and outpatients from a region which is inhabited by 251,202 citizens. The study investigated the prevalence of genotypic features (PCR ribotypes, genes for toxins A and B, and binary toxins), and phenotypic (toxigenicity, antimicrobial susceptibility) patterns of *C. difficile* isolates from a region of northern Slovakia were analyzed retrospectively from July to August 2016, by following multiple laboratory methods. There was no post-discharge follow up regarding readmission of the patients.

4.2. Enzymatic and Immunoenzymatic Assays and Cultivation

The samples were tested by direct diagnostic methods for *C. difficile* using the detection of GDH by the immunochromatographic method for toxins A or B (CERTEST *C. difficile* Toxin A/B), enzyme immunoassay methods ELISA (ProSpectT *C. difficile* Toxin A/B Microplate assay) to determine toxins A and B. The samples were mixed with an equal volume of 100% ethyl alcohol for 60 min at room temperature. One hundred microliters of the mixture was inoculated into *C. difficile* selective media (cycloserine-cefoxitin-fructose agar) (Brazier, Oxoid, Hampshire, UK). The plates were incubated at 37 °C for 72 h under anaerobic conditions [31].

4.3. MALDI-TOF MS Identification

The colonies of *C. difficile* were identified at the species level by Matrix Assisted Laser Desorption/Ionization Time-of-Flight Mass Spectrometry (MALDI-TOF MS), with the use of MALDI Biotyper v 3.0 system (Brucker Daltonics, Billerica, MA, USA). Intact proteins were isolated by the standard procedure with ethanol/formic acid/acetonitril extraction. *C. difficile* samples were overlaid with 1 µL of a matrix solution (HCCA = α-cyano-4-hydroxy-cinnamic acid saturated in solution containing 50% acetonitrile, 47.5% ultra-pure distillated water, and 2.5% trifluoracetic acid). Samples were dried at room temperature.

4.4. Antibiotic Susceptibility Testing

The clinical *C. difficile* isolates were also analyzed by E-tests (Oxoid) with a defined Minimal Inhibitory Concentration (MIC) for vancomycin (VAN) and metronidazole (MTZ). The Minimal Inhibitory Concentration breakpoints for MTZ (2 mg/L), VAN (2 mg/L) were applied and evaluated according to the European Committee on Antimicrobial Susceptibility Testing (EUCAST) [25,32].

4.5. Polymerase Chain Reaction PCR Ribotyping

The isolated *C. difficile* strains were analyzed also by the multiplex "real-time" PCR - GeneXpert *C. difficile*/Epi PCR assay (Cepheid, Sunnyvale, CA, USA) for the detection of the B toxin gene (*tcdB*), the binary toxin genes (*cdtA* and *cdt B*), and the deletion of the *tcdC* gene on nucleotide 117(Δ117), which allowed the presumptive identification of 027/NAP1/BI with reported sensitivities and specificities of 96.6% to 99.7% and 93.0% to 98.6%, respectively [17]. The strains were only isolated from diarrheal stool samples from patients with a severe course of the disease and were analyzed by PCR capillary-based electrophoresis ribotyping.

The PCR capillary-based electrophoresis ribotyping was performed according to the protocol [32]. In the studied isolates, multi-locus sequence typing using seven house-keeping genes (MLST) was also carried out [26]. The molecular typing of *C. difficile* was carried out in a specialized reference laboratory. The PCR capillary-based electrophoresis ribotyping patterns of investigated ribotypes and fragment analysis were performed by a DNA analyzer and by Gene Mapper v5.0 which were kindly provided by the Department of Microbiology of 2nd Faculty of Medicine of Charles University, and Motol University Hospital in Prague. This method is performed in CDI epidemics to identify individual strains, and to perform surveillance for the spread of CDI [33,34].

The samples were collected from patients in internal wards and wards for long-term care (wards from the higher occurrence of CDI). The stool samples were sent to the laboratory according to the criteria for testing (Bristol scale 5–7). The selected patient samples were analyzed for *C. difficile* isolates (n = 44) following laboratory parameters, such as values of serum creatinine, albumin, CRP, and the length of hospitalization. Laboratory parameters were compared between patients´ samples with ribotype RT001 and RT176.

4.6. Statistical Analysis

Group statistics were used to describe the basic features of the data. Independent sample tests, including the Leven´s test for Equality of Variances and the *t*-test for Equality of means, were used. The Pearson correlation method was used to determine the dependency between two variables and statistical significance was set as $p < 0.001$. Descriptive statistical tools, as well as frequency of infection by frequency histograms, statistical programs were utilized.

5. Conclusions

Accurate and fast diagnostics of CDI are essential for optimal patient care and preventing the spread of infection. Laboratory diagnosis involving a high-sensitivity screening assay, followed by a high specificity assay, is important for the treatment and diagnosis of the disease. This study investigates the prevalence, genotypic features (PCR ribotypes, genes for toxins A and B, and binary toxins) and phenotypic (toxigenicity, antimicrobial susceptibility) patterns of *C. difficile* isolated from patients with confirmed CDI. We identified the presumptive identification of 027/NAP1/BI in stool specimens, which contained toxigenic *C. difficile* but not 027/NAP1/BI. *C. difficile* isolates were investigated by PCR ribotyping, which identified five different ribotypes in forty-four isolates (RT176, 001, 011, 017, 081). The presence of the RT176 was confirmed in 27 isolates. In our studied samples, there was a higher proportion of RT176 identified than RT001 due to the epidemic situation in this period. The *C. difficile* isolates (ribotypes 001, 011, 081, 176) were susceptible to MTZ and VAN. One isolate RT017 had reduced susceptibility to VAN. Despite the limitation of the study, it highlights the prevalence of *C. difficile* RT176 in the epidemic situation during the studied period. A further study is needed to help clarify the interaction between ribotypes and other predictors and laboratory parameters.

Author Contributions: Conceptualization, E.N., Z.S., V.S. and L.H.; methodology, E.N. and L.H.; software, Z.S. and V.S.; validation, E.N. and Z.S.; formal analysis, E.N., Z.S., V.S. and L.H.; investigation, E.N., V.S. and Z.S.; resources, E.N., L.H. and Z.S.; data curation, E.N., Z.S. and V.S.; writing—original draft preparation, E.N., V.S. and L.H.; writing—review and editing, Z.S. and E.N. All authors have read and agreed to the published version of the manuscript.

Funding: This research received no external funding.

Institutional Review Board Statement: Not applicable.

Informed Consent Statement: Not applicable.

Data Availability Statement: Data are available from the corresponding author upon reasonable request.

Conflicts of Interest: The authors declare no conflict of interest.

References

1. Davies, K.A.; Longshaw, C.; Davis, G.L.; Bouza, E.; Barbut, F.; Barna, Z.; Delmée, M.; Fitzpatrick, F.; Ivanova, K.; Kuijper, E.; et al. Underdiagnosis of Clostridium difficile across Europe: The European, multicentre, prospective, biannual, point-prevalence study of Clostridium difficile infection in hospitalised patients with diarrhoea (EUCLID). *Lancet Infect. Dis.* **2014**, *14*, 1208–1219. [CrossRef]
2. European Centre for Disease Prevention and Control. *European Surveillance of Clostridium Difficile Infections*; Surveillance Protocol Version 2.3.; ECDC: Stockholm, Sweden, 2017.
3. Krůtová, M.; Wilcox, M.; Kuijper, E. The pitfalls of laboratory diagnostics of Clostridium difficile infection. *Clin. Microbiol. Infect.* **2018**, *24*, 682–683. [CrossRef]
4. Novakova, E.; Stefkovicova, M.; Kopilec, M.G.; Novak, M.; Kotlebová, N.; Kuijper, E.; Krutova, M.; Garabasova, M.K. The emergence of Clostridium difficile ribotypes 027 and 176 with a predominance of the Clostridium difficile ribotype 001 recognized in Slovakia following the European standardized Clostridium difficile infection surveillance of 2016. *Int. J. Infect. Dis.* **2020**, *90*, 111–115. [CrossRef]
5. Mazakova, I.; Sadlonova, V.; Cervenova, T.; Hudeckova, H. Appearance of Clostridium difficile infections in health care institutions in Slovakia and in the district of martin. *Acta Med. Martiniana* **2018**, *18*, 5–12. [CrossRef]
6. Crobach, M.; Planche, T.; Eckert, C.; Barbut, F.; Terveer, E.; Dekkers, O.; Wilcox, M.; Kuijper, E. European Society of Clinical Microbiology and Infectious Diseases: Update of the diagnostic guidance document for Clostridium difficile infection. *Clin. Microbiol. Infect.* **2016**, *22*, S63–S81. [CrossRef]

7. Grześkowiak, M.; Pieper, R.; Huynh, H.A.; Cutting, S.M.; Vahjen, W.; Zentek, J. Impact of early-life events on the susceptibility to Clostridium difficile colonisation and infection in the offspring of the pig. *Gut Microbes* **2018**, *10*, 251–259. [CrossRef]
8. Gateau, C.; Couturier, J.; Coia, J.; Barbut, F. How to: Diagnose infection caused by Clostridium difficile. *Clin. Microbiol. Infect.* **2018**, *24*, 463–468. [CrossRef]
9. Carey-Ann, B.D.; Carroll, K.C. Diagnosis of Clostridium difficile Infection: An Ongoing Conundrum for Clinicians and for Clinical Laboratories. *Clin. Microbiol. Rev.* **2013**, *26*, 604–630. [CrossRef] [PubMed]
10. Terveer, E.M.; Crobach, M.J.T.; Sanders, I.M.J.G.; Vos, M.C.; Verduin, C.M.; Kuijper, E.J. Detection of Clostridium difficile in Feces of Asymptomatic Patients Admitted to the Hospital. *J. Clin. Microbiol.* **2017**, *55*, 403–411. [CrossRef] [PubMed]
11. Debast, S.; Bauer, M.; Kuijper, E. European Society of Clinical Microbiology and Infectious Diseases: Update of the Treatment Guidance Document for Clostridium difficile Infection. *Clin. Microbiol. Infect.* **2014**, *20*, 1–26. [CrossRef] [PubMed]
12. Origüen, J.; Corbella, L.; Orellana, M.D.L.A.; Fernández-Ruiz, M.; López-Medrano, F.; Juan, R.S.; Lizasoain, M.; Ruiz-Merlo, T.; Morales-Cartagena, A.; Maestro, G.; et al. Comparison of the clinical course of Clostridium difficile infection in glutamate dehydrogenase-positive toxin-negative patients diagnosed by PCR to those with a positive toxin test. *Clin. Microbiol. Infect.* **2018**, *24*, 414–421. [CrossRef]
13. Jarčuška, P.; Bátovský, M.; Drgoňa, L.; Lišková, A.; Holečková, K. *Odporúčaný Postup Diagnostiky a Liečby Kolitídy Spôsobenej Clostridium Difficile*; Slovenská Zdravotnícka Univerzita v Bratislave: Bratislava, Slovakia, 2015; Volume 12, p. S1. ISSN 1336-4790.
14. Brazier, J.S.; Borriello, S.P. Microbiology, Epidemiology and Diagnosis of Clostridium difficile Infection. *Curr. Top. Microbiol. Immunol.* **2000**, *250*, 1–33. [CrossRef] [PubMed]
15. Breznicky, J.; Novak, M. The most common etiological agents of prosthetic joint infections in orthopaedics. *Med. Glas.* **2019**, *16*, 185–189. [CrossRef]
16. Walk, S.T.; Micic, D.; Jain, R.; Lo, E.S.; Trivedi, I.; Liu, E.; Almassalha, L.M.; Ewing, S.A.; Ring, C.; Galecki, A.T.; et al. Clostridium difficile Ribotype Does Not Predict Severe Infection. *Clin. Infect. Dis.* **2012**, *55*, 1661–1668. [CrossRef] [PubMed]
17. Xpert® C.difficile/Epi 1 300-9680, Rev. J April 2020, Cepheid 904 Caribbean Drive Sunnyvale, CA 9408, USA. Avalaible online: https://www.cepheid.com/Package%20Insert%20Files/300-9680-Xpert-C.%20diff-Epi%20US-IVD%20PI%20Rev%20J.pdf (accessed on 7 August 2021).
18. McDonald, L.C.; Gerding, D.N.; Johnson, S.; Bakken, J.S.; Carroll, K.C.; Coffin, S.E.; Dubberke, E.R.; Garey, K.W.; Gould, C.V.; Kelly, C.; et al. Clinical Practice Guidelines for Clostridium difficile Infection in Adults and Children: 2017 Update by the Infectious Diseases Society of America (IDSA) and Society for Healthcare Epidemiology of America (SHEA). *Clin. Infect. Dis.* **2018**, *66*, e1–e48. [CrossRef] [PubMed]
19. Robotham, J.; Wilcox, M. Updated Guidance on the Diagnosis and Reporting of Clostridium Difficile. NHS, Advisory Committee on Antimicrobial Resistance and Healthcare Associated Infection (ARHAI). 2012. Available online: https://www.gov.uk/government/uploads/system/uploads/attachment.data/file/146808/dh_133016.pdf.pdf (accessed on 20 January 2020).
20. Zou, J.; Leung, V.; Champagne, S.; Hinch, M.; Wong, A.; Lloyd-Smith, E.; Nguyen, T.T.; Romney, M.G.; Sharma, A.; Payne, M.; et al. Clinical heterogeneity of patients with stool samples testing PCR+/Tox− from a two-step Clostridium difficile diagnostic algorithm. *Eur. J. Clin. Microbiol. Infect. Dis.* **2018**, *37*, 2355–2359. [CrossRef]
21. Freeman, J.; Vernon, J.; Pilling, S.; Morris, K.; Nicholson, S.; Shearman, S.; Longshaw, C.; Wilcox, M. The ClosER study: Results from a three-year pan-European longitudinal surveillance of antibiotic resistance among prevalent Clostridium difficile ribotypes, 2011–2014. *Clin. Microbiol. Infect.* **2017**, *24*, 724–731. [CrossRef]
22. Krehelova, M.; Nyč, O.; Sinajová, E.; Krutova, M. The predominance and clustering of *Clostridioides* (*Clostridium*) *difficile* PCR ribotype 001 isolates in three hospitals in Eastern Slovakia, 2017. *Folia Microbiol.* **2018**, *64*, 49–54. [CrossRef]
23. Nyc, O.; Krutova, M.; Liskova, A.; Matejkova, J.; Drabek, J.; Kuijper, E. The emergence of Clostridium difficile PCR-ribotype 001 in Slovakia. *Eur. J. Clin. Microbiol. Infect. Dis.* **2015**, *34*, 1701–1708. [CrossRef]
24. Kecerova, Z.; Cizek, A.; Nyc, O.; Krutova, M. Clostridium difficile isolates derived from Czech horses are resistant to enrofloxacin; cluster to clades 1 and 5 and ribotype 033 predominates. *Anaerobe* **2019**, *56*, 17–21. [CrossRef]
25. Novakova, E.; Kotlebova, N.; Gryndlerova, A.; Novak, M.; Vladarova, M.; Wilcox, M.; Kuijper, E.; Krutova, M. An Outbreak of *Clostridium* (*Clostridioides*) *difficile* Infections within an Acute and Long-Term Care Wards due to Moxifloxacin-Resistant PCR Ribotype 176 Genotyped as PCR Ribotype 027 by a Commercial Assay. *J. Clin. Med.* **2020**, *9*, 3738. [CrossRef]
26. Krutova, M.; Matejkova, J.; Kuijper, E.J.; Drevinek, P.; Nyc, O.; Czech Clostridium Difficile Study Group. Clostridium difficile PCR ribotypes 001 and 176—The common denominator of C. difficile infection epidemiology in the Czech Republic, 2014. *EuroSurveillance* **2016**, *21*, 29. [CrossRef]
27. Krutova, M.; Matejkova, J.; Tkadlec, J.; Nyc, O. Antibiotic profiling of Clostridium difficile ribotype 176—A multidrug resistant relative to C. difficile ribotype 027. *Anaerobe* **2015**, *36*, 88–90. [CrossRef] [PubMed]
28. Dresler, J.; Krutova, M.; Fucikova, A.; Klimentova, J.; Hruzova, V.; Duracova, M.; Houdkova, K.; Salovska, B.; Matejkova, J.; Hubalek, M.; et al. Analysis of proteomes released from in vitro cultured eight Clostridium difficile PCR ribotypes revealed specific expression in PCR ribotypes 027 and 176 confirming their genetic relatedness and clinical importance at the proteomic level. *Gut Pathog.* **2017**, *9*, 45. [CrossRef] [PubMed]
29. Reigadas, E.; Alcalá, L.; Valerio, M.; Marín, M.; Martin, A.; Bouza, E. Toxin B PCR cycle threshold as a predictor of poor outcome ofClostridium difficileinfection: A derivation and validation cohort study. *J. Antimicrob. Chemother.* **2016**, *71*, 1380–1385. [CrossRef]

30. Rao, K.; Micic, D.; Natarajan, M.; Winters, S.; Kiel, M.J.; Walk, S.T.; Santhosh, K.; Mogle, J.A.; Galecki, A.T.; Lebar, W.; et al. Clostridium difficileRibotype 027: Relationship to Age, Detectability of Toxins A or B in Stool with Rapid Testing, Severe Infection, and Mortality. *Clin. Infect. Dis.* **2015**, *61*, 233–241. [CrossRef]
31. Murad, Y.M.; Perez, J.; Ybazeta, G.; Mavin, S.; Lefebvre, S.; Weese, J.S.; Rousseau, J.; Diaz-Mitoma, F.; Nokhbeh, R. False Negative Results in Clostridium difficile Testing. *BMC Infect. Dis.* **2016**, *16*, 1–6. [CrossRef]
32. Fawley, W.N.; Knetsch, W.; MacCannell, D.R.; Harmanus, C.; Du, T.; Mulvey, M.R.; Paulick, A.; Anderson, L.; Kuijper, E.; Wilcox, M.H. Development and Validation of an Internationally-Standardized, High-Resolution Capillary Gel-Based Electrophoresis PCR-Ribotyping Protocol for Clostridium difficile. *PLoS ONE* **2015**, *10*, e0118150. [CrossRef]
33. Janežič, S.; Štrumbelj, I.; Rupnik, M. Use of Modified PCR Ribotyping for Direct Detection of Clostridium difficile Ribotypes in Stool Samples. *J. Clin. Microbiol.* **2011**, *49*, 3024–3025. [CrossRef] [PubMed]
34. Krutova, M.; Wilcox, M.; Kuijper, E. A two-step approach for the investigation of a Clostridium difficile outbreak by molecular methods. *Clin. Microbiol. Infect.* **2019**, *25*, 1300–1301. [CrossRef]

antibiotics

MDPI

Article

High Serum Levels of Toxin A Correlate with Disease Severity in Patients with *Clostridioides difficile* Infection

Guido Granata [1,†], Davide Mariotti [1,2,†], Paolo Ascenzi [2,3], Nicola Petrosillo [1,‡] and Alessandra di Masi [2,*,‡]

1 Clinical and Research Department for Infectious Diseases, National Institute for Infectious Diseases L. Spallanzani, IRCCS, 00149 Rome, Italy; guido.granata@inmi.it (G.G.); davide.mariotti16@gmail.com (D.M.); nicola.petrosillo@inmi.it (N.P.)
2 Department of Science, Section of Biomedical Sciences and Technologies, Roma Tre University, 00146 Rome, Italy; paolo.ascenzi@uniroma3.it
3 Accademia Nazionale dei Lincei, 00165 Rome, Italy
* Correspondence: alessandra.dimasi@uniroma3.it; Tel.: +39-06-57336363
† These authors contribute equally to this work.
‡ Co-last Authors.

Abstract: *Cloistridioides difficile* (CD) represents a major public healthcare-associated infection causing significant morbidity and mortality. The pathogenic effects of CD are mainly caused by the release of two exotoxins into the intestine: toxin A (TcdA) and toxin B (TcdB). CD infection (CDI) can also cause toxemia, explaining the systemic complications of life-threatening cases. Currently, there is a lack of sensitive assays to detect exotoxins circulating in the blood. Here, we report a new semi-quantitative diagnostic method to measure CD toxins serum levels. The dot-blot assay was modified to separately detect TcdA and TcdB in human serum with a limit of detection at the pg/mL levels. TcdA and TcdB concentrations in the plasma of 35 CDI patients were measured at the time of CDI diagnosis and at the fourth and tenth day after CDI diagnosis and initiation of anti-CDI treatment. TcdA and TcdB levels were compared to those determined in nine healthy blood donors. Toxemia was detected in the plasma of 33 out of the 35 CDI cases. We also assessed the relationship between TcdA serum levels and CDI severity, reporting that at the time of CDI diagnosis the proportion of severe CDI cases with a TcdA serum level > 60 pg/μL was higher than in mild CDI cases (29.4% versus 66.6%, $p = 0.04$). In conclusion, data reported here demonstrate for the first time that toxemia is much more frequent than expected in CDI patients, and specifically that high serum levels of TcdA correlate with disease severity in patients with CDI.

Keywords: *Clostridium difficile*; *Clostridioides difficile*; TcdA; TcdB; toxin; toxemia; plasma; method; quantification; CDI severity

Citation: Granata, G.; Mariotti, D.; Ascenzi, P.; Petrosillo, N.; di Masi, A. High Serum Levels of Toxin A Correlate with Disease Severity in Patients with *Clostridioides difficile* Infection. *Antibiotics* **2021**, *10*, 1093. https://doi.org/10.3390/antibiotics10091093

Academic Editor: Marc Maresca

Received: 19 July 2021
Accepted: 7 September 2021
Published: 10 September 2021

1. Introduction

The Gram-positive anaerobic bacterium *Clostridioides difficile* (CD) is a leading cause of nosocomial diarrhea worldwide, accounting for 15% of all such infections and resulting in significant morbidity, mortality, and prolonged hospital stay [1–3]. The clinical manifestations of CD infection (CDI) range from mild diarrhea to pseudomembranous colitis and toxic megacolon that is relatively uncommon but is associated with high morbidity and mortality [4]. A relevant issue during CDI is its high rate of recurrences (rCDI). Clinical studies show wide-ranging rCDI rates after the primary CDI, between 12% and 40% [5,6]. rCDI is associated with a higher risk of death and higher hospitalization costs [1].

The pathogenic effects of CD are mainly caused by the production of two exotoxins into the intestine: toxin A (TcdA) and toxin B (TcdB) [2,7]. TcdA and TcdB monoglucosylate and inactivate the Rho GTPases of host cells, causing several cytopathic effects, and ultimately colonocyte death and loss of intestinal barrier function [8,9]. Moreover, CD toxins induce an inflammatory response through the recruitment of neutrophils and mastocytes and the consequent release of cytokines [10].

CD toxins can reach the bloodstream of CDI patients, thus causing toxemia, which may explain the systemic complications of life-threatening cases [9,11]. To date, only three toxemia-positive cases (two adults and one child) have been reported in humans [12,13]. As the currently available tests for the detection of free toxins are in development and have low sensitivity [3,14,15], CDI-induced toxemia goes undetected in common clinical practice [9,11,15]. Therefore, the lack of a sensitive detection method to determine CD toxin levels in the blood or other body fluids makes it difficult to investigate the relationship between toxemia and systemic clinical manifestations of CDI [12].

Here, we performed a pilot study in which we report and validate a new diagnostic tool to measure serum levels of CD toxins and to define the relationship between the toxemia level and the degree of clinical severity in CDI patients. Setting up this sensitive method allowed us to also highlight that toxemia is much more frequent than expected in CDI patients, and specifically that high serum levels of TcdA correlate with disease severity in patients with CDI.

2. Results

2.1. Method Set-Up

With the aim of determining the levels of TcdA and TcdB in the serum of CDI patients, several preliminary tests were performed to set up all the parameters necessary to obtain the most sensitive results. In the beginning, a wide range of TcdA and TcdB concentrations were tested (i.e., 2000 pg/µL, 200 pg/µL, 20 pg/µL, 2 pg/µL, 0.2 pg/µL, 0.02 pg/µL, 0.002 pg/µL, 0.0002 pg/µL, and 0.00002 pg/µL (data not shown). Given the different sensitivities of the two primary anti-TcdA and anti-TcdB antibodies used, the scales of the standard curves were adapted to the single toxin, reaching the optimal conditions of 200, 500, 1000, 1500, and 2000 pg/µL for TcdA, and 2, 5, 10, 20, 50, and 100 pg/µL for TcdB (Figure 1). Toxin concentrations below which it was not possible to obtain a quantifiable signal and above which the signal was saturated were excluded.

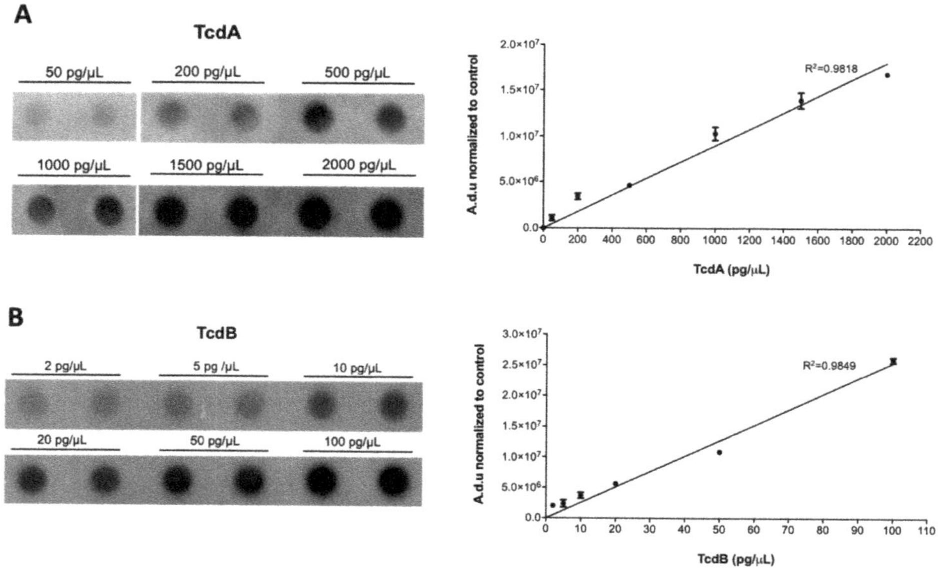

Figure 1. Representative images and the standard curve of (**A**) TcdA and (**B**) TcdB dot plots necessary for determining the concentration of the toxins in the blood of CDI patients. Toxin concentrations are reported as the mean value of triplicate dots ± standard deviation (SD) normalized to control (i.e., 0 pg/mL); a.d.u., arbitrary densitometric unit.

Besides the definition of the optimal TcdA and TcdB concentrations required to set up the standard curve, we also verified that the resuspension of *C. difficile* toxins in PBS prior to the dot-blot caused the complete loss of the signal. Toxin resuspension in TBS allowed for the restoration of the required sensitivity (Supplementary Materials: Figure S1). Indeed, as Tris-HCl allows lipids to be resuspended [16,17], the results obtained demonstrated that the choice of the buffer is critical to allow the solubilization of the serum lipid fraction (e.g., albumin, lipoproteins, and chylomicrons) present in the samples.

We also demonstrated the absence of antibody cross-reactivity events, supporting the specificity of the assay for the detection of TcdA and TcdB (Figure S2).

2.2. Clinical Features of CDI Patients

The demographic and epidemiological data, comorbidities, clinical characteristics, and outcome of the 35 CDI patients enrolled in this study are reported in Table S1. Among them, 18 (51.4%) patients were female. The mean age of the 35 CDI patients was 60 years, ranging between 19 and 86 years. The mean age-adjusted Charlson co-morbidity index (CCI) at admission was 3.6, ranging between 0 and 8. Among the 35 CDI patients, 30/35 (85.7%) cases had a primary CDI and 5/35 (14.3%) had an rCDI. Regarding CDI severity, 17/35 (48.6%) and 18/35 (51.4%) cases had mild and severe CDI, respectively.

At admission, 25/35 (71.4%) patients reported at least one comorbidity, including cardiovascular disease, chronic obstructive pulmonary disease (COPD), diabetes, and immunodeficiency in 13/35 (37.1%), 9/35 (25.7%), 7/35 (20.0%), and 7/35 (20.0%), respectively. Regarding patient outcomes, 34/35 (97.1%) CDI cases were discharged without complications; one patient (2.8%) died in the hospital. Therefore, 34 patients were followed up for 30 days from the hospital discharge. Of these 34 patients, 28/34 (82.4%) fully recovered at home, presenting no subsequent rCDI. Five patients (14.7%) developed rCDI and were readmitted to the hospital. One other patient (2.9%) was readmitted to the hospital for reasons other than CDI and died during the hospital stay (Table S1).

2.3. TcdA and TcdB Serum Levels and CDI Severity

The definitions of CDI, microbiological evidence of CD, CDI recurrence, mild CDI, severe CDI, and complicated CDI are reported in Table S2. The mean laboratory findings, total toxemia, and TcdA and TcdB serum levels at CDI diagnosis (T0), as well as at 4 (T4) and 10 days (T10) after CDI diagnosis of the 35 CDI patients included in this study are reported in Table 1.

Table 1. Mean laboratory findings and mean toxemia at CDI diagnosis (T0), and at 4 (T4) and 10 days (T10) after CDI diagnosis of the 35 CDI patients included in the study. SD: standard deviation.

Laboratory Findings	T0	T4	T10
Total white blood cells peripheral count (10^3 cells/μL ± SD)	11.04 ± 5.99	7.03 ± 2.59	6.33 ± 2.64
Neutrophils peripheral count (10^3 cells/μL ± SD)	8.18 ± 5.45	4.41 ± 2.25	4.11 ± 2.46
Blood creatinine value (mg/dL ± SD)	1.0 ± 0.6	0.8 ± 0.3	0.8 ± 0.2
Blood albumin value (g/dL ± SD)	3.3 ± 0.5	3.4 ± 0.6	3.6 ± 0.7
Total toxemia (TcdA + TcdB, pg/μL ± SD)	99.24 ± 103.24	89.74 ± 78.18	57.70 ± 72.70
TcdA (pg/μL ± SD)	92.28 ± 96.08	83.75 ± 74.81	49.96 ± 70.96
TcdB (pg/μL ± SD)	6.96 ± 25.71	5.99 ± 22.2	7.74 ± 22.6

Serum levels of TcdA and TcdB in the 35 CDI patients serum enrolled in this study, as well as in the 9 healthy donors, were assessed using the standard curve set up for each CD toxin. Notably, neither TcdA nor TcdB was detected in the serum of the 9 healthy donors. Toxemia was detected at least at one time point in 33 out of the 35 CDI patients and was mainly referable to TcdA (Table S3). The mean total toxemia serum levels ± standard deviation (SD) was 99.24 ± 103.24 pg/μL, 89.74 ± 78.18 pg/μL, and 57.70 ± 72.70 pg/μL at T0, T4, and T10 (Table 1), respectively. TcdA contributed significantly to toxemia, as the mean value of TcdA serum levels were 92.28 ± 96.08 pg/μL, 83.75 ± 74.81 pg/μL, and 49.96 ± 70.96 pg/µL, at T0, T4, and T10, respectively. On the contrary, the mean value of TcdB serum levels was significantly lower compared to those of TcdA (i.e., 6.96 ± 25.71 pg/µL, 5.99 ± 22.2 pg/µL, and 7.74 ± 22.6 pg/µL at T0, T4, and T10, respectively) and no significant variations were detected over time and with respect to CDI severity (Table 1 and Table S3).

When the 35 CDI cases were grouped according to CDI severity, we found that at CDI diagnosis (i.e., T0), mild and severe CDI cases had a mean TcdA serum level of 64.68 ± 92.22 pg/µL and 116.81 ± 95.19 pg/µL, respectively, and a mean TcdB serum level of 5.95 ± 16.31 pg/µL and 7.86 ± 32.34 pg/µL, respectively (Table 2). At T4, mild and severe CDI cases had a mean TcdA serum level of 51.76 ± 58.48 pg/µL and 115.74 ± 77.14 pg/µL, respectively ($p = 0.01$), and a mean TcdB serum level of 4.21 ± 12.85 pg/µL and 7.76 ± 29.07 pg/µL, respectively. At T10, mild and severe CDI cases had a mean TcdA serum level of 30.80 ± 52.92 pg/µL and 66.73 ± 81.65 pg/µL and a mean TcdB serum level of 4.59 ± 12.74 pg/µL and 10.50 ± 28.79 pg/µL, respectively (Table 2).

Table 2. Clinical features, comorbidities, laboratory findings, and outcome of the 18 cases with mild CDI and the 17 cases with severe CDI before diagnosis, at T0, T4, and T10. RR: Risk ratio. CI: Confidence interval. SD: Standard deviation. CCI: Charlson Co-morbidity Index.

	Mild CDI ($N = 17$)	Severe CDI ($N = 18$)	RR (95% CI)	Fisher's Test *
Female gender	11 (64.7%)	7 (38.8%)	0.5 (0.2–1.2)	$p = 0.1$
Mean age (years)	55.7	63.5	-	$p = 0.2$
Mean age-adjusted CCI at admission ± SD	2.4 ± 2.3	4.7 ± 2.9	-	$p = 0.01$
Comorbidities				
No comorbidities	7 (41.1%)	3 (16.6%)	1.7 (0.9–3.2)	$p = 0.1$
Cardiovascular disease	4 (23.5%)	9 (50.0%)	1.9 (0.7–4.6)	$p = 0.1$
Heart failure	1 (5.9%)	3 (16.6%)	2.0 (0.3–11.6)	$p = 0.3$
Diabetes	2 (11.7%)	5 (27.7%)	1.8 (0.5–6.3)	$p = 0.4$
Renal failure	0 (0%)	3 (16.6%)	-	$p = 0.2$
Inflammatory bowel disease	1 (5.8%)	1 (5.5%)	0.9 (0.2–4.0)	$p = 1$
Chronic liver failure	1 (5.8%)	1 (5.5%)	0.9 (0.2–4.0)	$p = 1$
Neurological disease	0 (0%)	4 (22.2%)	-	$p = 0.1$
Vasculitis	0 (0%)	2 (11.1%)	-	$p = 0.4$
COPD	6 (35.3%)	3 (16.6%)	0.6 (0.3–1.2)	$p = 0.2$
Solid cancer	1 (5.8%)	2 (11.1%)	1.5 (0.2–7)	$p = 1$
Blood cancer	1 (5.8%)	2 (11.1%)	1.5 (0.2–7.7)	$p = 1$
Transplant, immunodeficiency, immunosuppression	1 (5.8%)	6 (33.3%)	4 (0.6–25.2)	$p = 0.08$
Other bacteria infections at admission	6 (35.3%)	7 (38.8%)	1.0 (0.5–2.2)	$p = 1$
Laboratory findings before CDI diagnosis				
Basal Albumin (g/dL ± SD)	3.7 ± 0.6	3.5 ± 0.6	-	$p = 0.5$
Basal Creatinine (mg/dL ± SD)	0.70 ± 0.1	0.8 ± 0.3	-	$p = 0.2$
Laboratory findings at CDI diagnosis (T0)				
White blood cell peripheral count (10^3 cells/µL ± SD)	8.81 ± 3.52	13.15 ± 7.10	-	$p = 0.02$
Neutrophils peripheral count (10^3 cells/µL ± SD)	5.70 ± 3.14	10.52 ± 6.18	-	$p = 0.007$
Creatinine (mg/dL ± SD)	0.8 ± 0.3	1.2 ± 0.7	-	$p = 0.02$
Albumin (g/dL ± SD)	3.5 ± 0.5	3.2 ± 0.5	-	$p = 0.2$
TcdA (pg/µL ± SD)	64.68 ± 92.22	116.81 ± 95.19	-	$p = 0.1$
TcdB (pg/µL ± SD)	5.95 ± 16.31	7.86 ± 32.34	-	$p = 0.8$
TcdA + TcdB (pg/µL ± SD)	70.63 ± 71.65	124.67 ± 89.23	-	$p = 0.1$
TcdA > 60 pg/µL	5 (29.4%)	12 (66.6%)	2.0 (1.0–4.2)	$p = 0.04$
Laboratory findings at T4				
White blood cell peripheral count (10^3 cells/µL ± SD)	6.95 ± 2.38	7.09 ± 2.84	-	$p = 0.8$
Neutrophils peripheral count (10^3 cells/µL ± SD)	4.25 ± 2.18	4.56 ± 2.37	-	$p = 0.6$
Creatinine (mg/dL ± SD)	0.7 ± 0.2	0.9 ± 0.3	-	$p = 0.1$
Albumin (g/dL ± SD)	3.6 ± 0.5	3.2 ± 0.6	-	$p = 0.09$
TcdA (pg/µL ± SD)	51.76 ± 58.48	115.74 ± 77.14	-	$p = 0.01$
TcdB (pg/µL ± SD)	4.21 ± 12.85	7.76 ± 29.07	-	$p = 0.7$
TcdA + TcdB (pg/µL ± SD)	55.98 ± 48.17	123.51 ± 79.36	-	$p = 0.01$
TcdA > 60 pg/µL	5 (29.4%)	12 (66.6%)	2.4 (1.08–5.3)	$p = 0.03$

Table 2. *Cont.*

	Mild CDI (N = 17)	Severe CDI (N = 18)	RR (95% CI)	Fisher's Test *
Laboratory findings at T10				
White blood cell peripheral count (10^3 cells/μL ± SD)	6.14 ± 1.81	6.49 ± 3.36	-	$p = 0.7$
Neutrophils peripheral count (10^3 cells/μL ± SD)	4.06 ± 1.66	4.15 ± 3.05	-	$p = 0.9$
Creatinine (mg/dL ± SD)	0.7 ± 0.2	0.8 ± 0.2	-	$p = 0.2$
Albumin (g/dL ± SD)	3.7 ± 0.7	3.5 ± 0.7	-	$p = 0.4$
TcdA (pg/μL ± SD)	30.80 ± 52.92	66.73 ± 81.65	-	$p = 0.1$
TcdB (pg/μL ± SD)	4.59 ± 12.74	10.50 ± 28.79	-	$p = 0.4$
TcdA + TcdB (pg/μL ± SD)	35.39 ± 40.06	77.23 ± 66.65	-	$p = 0.1$
TcdA > 60 pg/μL	3 (17.6%)	4 (22.2%)	1.1 (0.4–2.9)	$p = 1$
Patients outcome				
Deceased	0 (0%)	1 (5.5%)	0.5 (0.3–0.7)	$p = 1$
rCDI	3 (17.6%)	2 (11.1%)	1.5 (0.2–10.3)	$p = 1$

* Paired *t*-test for non-categorical variables.

The limited number of patients enrolled in this pilot study and the high variability of CD toxins concentration among CDI patients serum may be responsible for the large SD values determined. To reduce this noise, we performed a separate analysis of TcdA plasma concentration over time in mild and severe CDI cases. As reported in Figure 2, TcdA levels significantly decreased at T10 compared to T0 ($p = 0.0287$) and T4 ($p = 0.0452$) in mild but not in severe CDI. This might suggest that the severity of the symptoms is correlated to the persistence of TcdA in patients' serum.

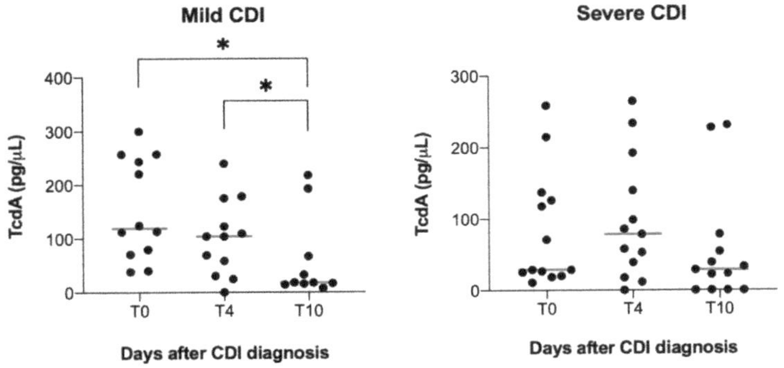

Figure 2. Changes of TcdA plasma levels in mild and severe CDI cases. TcdA levels significantly decreased at 10 days (T10) after CDI diagnosis in mild cases compared to levels measured at T0 and T4. Patients whose TcdA levels at T0 were 0 pg/μL were not included in these graphs. One way-ANOVA test, * $p < 0.05$.

To assess the relationship between TcdA serum concentration and CDI severity, CDI cases were divided into two groups according to their TcdA serum levels. We set a cut-off, i.e., serum TcdA ≤ 60 pg/μL and serum TcdA > 60 pg/μL (Table 2). At T0 and T4, the proportion of severe CDI cases with a TcdA serum level > 60 pg/μL was higher than among mild CDI cases (at T0: 29.4% versus 66.6%, $p = 0.04$; at T4: 29.4% versus 66.6%; RR: 1.1, 95% CI: 0.4–2.9; $p = 0.01$) (Table 2). The risk factors for TcdA serum levels > 60 pg/μL and for TcdB detectable levels (>4 pg/μL) at the CDI diagnosis are shown in Tables S4 and S5, respectively.

3. Discussion

CD represents a major public healthcare-associated infection, causing significant morbidity, mortality, and economic burden [18]. Over the past two decades, CDI diagnostic techniques have changed in line with a greater understanding of CDI physiopathology [18]. However, currently, there is relevant under-diagnosis and misdiagnosis of CDI.

Until recently, the phenomenon of the extra-intestinal damage caused by CD toxins has been undervalued [13]. It has been hypothesized that such a low number of toxemia-positive cases is due to the lack of sensitive toxin detection methods and possibly to the presence in human serum of anti-toxin antibodies [13,15]. To date, assays that allow detection of toxemia are (i) the tissue culture cytotoxicity assay, which displays a limit of detection (LOD) of 1–10 ng/mL for TcdA and 10–100 pg/mL for TcdB [12] and (ii) the ultrasensitive immunocytotoxicity assay, characterized by a LOD of 0.1–1.0 pg/mL for TcdA (when used with enhancing antibody A1H3) and 10.0 pg/mL for TcdB [13,19]. Very recently, an ultrasensitive single molecule array able to detect serum concentrations of TcdA and TcdB separately in the range of pg/mL was developed. However, this method was unable to detect TcdA or TcdB in a large panel of serum samples from CDI patients, including the severe forms [20].

Although circulating neutralizing antibodies could reduce the sensitivity of CD toxins detection in human plasma [13,15], we set up a semi-quantitative method that allows to separately detect TcdA and TcdB plasma levels in the range of pg/μL in CDI patients. Results obtained indicated that TcdA contributed significantly to toxemia. Indeed, TcdA serum levels > 60 pg/μL were measured in the plasma of severe CDI cases, and a statistically significant association between TcdA serum levels higher than 60 pg/μL and CDI severity was found, while no association was observed between TcdB toxemia and CDI severity. Remarkably, no detectable TcdB levels were found in the five rCDI patients. As previously reported, specific blockers present in the serum, such as antibodies or serum proteins, may be responsible for reducing the sensitivity of toxins detection in plasma [7,9,13,15]. Therefore, it cannot be excluded that the complete elimination of these blockers from CDI patients' serum would further increase the sensitivity of our method.

Other plasma blockers such as serum proteins may cause reduced sensitivity of methods that aim at detecting CDI toxins in plasma. Albumin, which is the most abundant protein in human plasma, is able to bind both TcdA and TcdB with high affinity [21,22]. Indeed, low albumin levels indicate a higher risk of acquiring and developing severe CDI and are associated with recurrent and fatal disease [22,23]. Here, we report higher basal albumin levels in patients with TcdA levels > 60 pg/μL at CDI onset (3.3 versus 3.9 g/dL, $p = 0.02$). This indicates that the semi-quantitative method reported here allows for overcoming the limitations due to albumin. This was possible thanks to the use of a resuspension buffer containing Tris-HCl, which solubilizes lipophilic molecules (e.g., albumin, lipoproteins, and chylomicrons) typically present in serum [16,17]. So, while CD toxins and CDI sera suspended in PBS were not detectable with our semi-quantitative dot-blot method, toxins resuspension in the TBS buffer allowed us to overcome this limitation. Notably, both immunoglobulins and albumin are part of humoral immunity, which plays a crucial role in protecting individuals from severe and/or rCDI [9,24–27].

To date, the role of TcdA in the pathogenesis of CDI is controversial. One paper suggests that CD mutants lacking TcdB, but expressing TcdA, do not cause colitis [19], whereas two other papers highlighted a key role played by TcdA in the disease [7,28]. These different findings possibly reflect differences in CD strains and in the experimental models of the studies [29]. A possible explanation for our findings is that TcdB tends to bind and concentrate more efficiently in the human gut cells than TcdA, leading to relatively higher TcdB intracellular concentrations and higher TcdA concentrations in the gut lumen. This agrees with histopathological analysis of cecal and colonic tissues collected from infected mice showing that TcdB is responsible for the majority of intestinal damage arising during infection, with TcdA causing more superficial and localized damage [24]. Therefore, the two CD toxins may exert different activities and subsequent pathological effects. Moreover, TcdB has been reported as a more potent enterotoxin than TcdA in human intestinal explants [30]. Therefore, our data highlighting the presence of TcdA in CDI patients serum may be an epiphenomenon of the increased endothelial gut permeability in severe CDI patients. Notably, although higher levels of TcdA than TcdB were detected in the sera of CDI patients with a severe form of CDI, these do not specifically indicate that TcdA is the major toxin in CDI.

The CD binary toxin (CDT) is considered an important additional toxin that plays a role in CDI pathogenesis, as strains producing only CDT have been isolated from patients with colitis [31]. However, only a few strains of CD synthesize CDT in the absence of TcdA and TcdB, and the role of CDT in CDI is still unclear [9,30–33]. Although we did not quantify CDT plasma levels in the patients enrolled in the present study, we assessed via PCR the presence of the binary toxin encoding gene (i.e., *tcdC*) in the CD strains responsible for CDI. No significant association was found between the presence of the *tcdC* gene and CDI severity (Table S3).

Among the limitations of this study, the relatively low number of patients enrolled should be mentioned. However, it should be also noted that this was intended as a pilot study providing the means to evaluate the technical aspects of the new sensitive method we have set up while serving as a platform to generate preliminary data and foster investigator development. The possibility to determine CD toxin levels in serum will allow for better evaluation of the patient's prognosis and to address the clinical efforts towards the management of CDI. For the future, a larger study including a higher number of CDI patients with different levels of disease severity will be necessary to support our data which indicate that the presence of TcdA in the blood of CDI patients may be a more sensitive predictor of the disease severity than TcdB.

4. Materials and Methods

This study was performed at the Infection Disease Unit of the National Institute for Infectious Diseases "L. Spallanzani" (Rome, Italy) between January 2019 and August 2020. The study was approved by the Ethic Committee of the hospital (National Institute for Infectious Diseases "L. Spallanzani", IRCCS, Rome; Ethics Committee registry number: 22/2018). Informed consent was obtained from each enrolled patient.

4.1. Study Design

4.1.1. Healthy Blood Donors Enrolment

Nine adult (>18 years old) healthy individuals were voluntarily included in the study as a control group. For each healthy control, a single blood collection and determination of CD serum toxins was performed. To exclude CD colonization, all the controls included in the study underwent CD screening using an enzyme immunoassay test on the same day as the blood collection and CD toxins' serum level determination. Rectal swabs were obtained when the healthy donors were not able to produce stool samples.

4.1.2. CDI Patient Enrolment

Between January 2019 and August 2020, all the adult patients (age $\geq$ 18 years) admitted to our Infection Disease Unit with a diagnosis of CDI were prospectively enrolled in this study. CDI diagnosis was made in the presence of a clinical picture characterized by diarrhea or ileum or toxic megacolon and microbiological evidence of CDI (Table S5). Demographic, epidemiological, and clinical data (age and gender, date of hospital admission, patient comorbidities, CDI onset, and clinical characteristics, medications given for CDI, antimicrobial treatments before and after the diagnosis of CDI, laboratory findings, and patient outcome) were collected in clinical record forms (CRF) by trained healthcare personnel. All the CDI cases were followed up to thirty days after the end of the anti-CDI treatment for the CDI episode to assess for new onset of diarrhea, recurrence of CDI, and mortality. In the case of hospital discharge before the end of follow-up, patients were contacted by phone call.

In order to assess the relationship between CD toxin serum level and the severity and recurrence rate of CDI, for each CDI case, three determinations of serum toxins were performed: (i) T0, which corresponds to the time of CDI diagnosis, before the initiation of the anti-CDI treatment; (ii) T4, which corresponds to the fourth day after CDI diagnosis and initiation of the anti-CDI treatment; and (iii) T10, which corresponds to the tenth day after CDI diagnosis and initiation of the anti-CDI treatment.

4.2. *Experimental Methodology*

4.2.1. Preparation of Serum Samples from Healthy Controls and CDI Patients

Blood samples were collected from healthy controls and CDI patients. CDI patients were diagnosed by enzyme immunoassay. The isolation of the plasma component from serum was performed by centrifuging samples at 700× *g* for 5 min. Samples were immediately stored at −20 °C until dot-blot analysis.

4.2.2. Reagents and Antibodies

All the reagents were purchased from Merck KGaA (Darmstadt, Germany). Recombinant TcdA (BML-G140) and TcdB (BML-G150) were obtained from Enzo Life Sciences (Farmingdale, NY, USA). Toxins were reconstituted in 250 µL of distilled H_2O to reach a final concentration of 200 ng/µL.

4.2.3. Dot-Blot Analysis

Standard Reference

The sensitivity of the method has been assessed using toxemia-negative spiked commercial human serum (Merck KGaA, Darmstadt, Germany). Serial dilutions of TcdA and TcdB were obtained by diluting the 200 ng/mL working solution of each toxin in a mixture composed of 1 µL commercial human serum and 49 µL TBS (100 mM NaCl, 10 mM Tris-HCl pH 7.5, 1 mM EDTA). The following final concentrations, determined specifically for each toxin depending on the sensitivity of the primary anti-TcdA and anti-TcdB antibody, were used to set up the standard curve: 200, 500, 1000, 1500, and 2000 pg/µL for TcdA, and 2, 5, 10, 20, 50, and 100 pg/µL for TcdB. Fifty microliters of each toxin dilution were spotted in triplicate onto a polyvinildiene difluoride (PVDF) membrane. The membrane was then placed into the BioDotTM Microfiltration apparatus (Bio-Rad, Hercules, CA, USA) and subjected to moderate suction for 5 s by vacuum pumping (HydroTechTM Vacuum Pump; Bio-Rad, Hercules, CA, USA). Following aspiration, the membrane was blocked in 5% non-fat dry milk dissolved in TBS/0.1% Tween-20 (TTBS) (*w*/*v*) for 1 h at room temperature (RT). The membrane was hybridized overnight at 4 °C with the anti-*Clostridioides difficile* TcdA (MCA2597; Bio-Rad, Hercules, CA, USA) or the anti-*Clostridioides difficile* TcdB (MCA4737; Bio-Rad, Hercules, CA, USA) primary antibodies diluted 1:20 in 5% non-fat dry milk dissolved in TTBS (*w*/*v*). After membrane washing, filters were incubated for 1 h at RT with the horseradish peroxidase-conjugated goat anti-mouse secondary antibody (#1706516; Bio-Rad, Hercules, CA, USA) diluted 1:1000 in PBS/0.01% Tween-20 (*v*/*v*). After membrane washing, dot signals were visualized using the Clarity™ Western ECL substrate (Bio-Rad, Hercules, CA, USA). Images were acquired using the ChemiDoc™ Imaging system (Bio-Rad, Hercules, CA, USA). Toxin levels were quantified using the Image Lab software (version 2.1.0.35.deb, Bio-Rad, Hercules, CA, USA).

Determination of Toxins Concentration in Serum Samples Derived from CDI Patients and Healthy Controls

One microliter of human sera derived from the 9 healthy donors and the 35 CDI patients was diluted in 49 µL TBS (dilution 1:50). The 50 µL solution was spotted in triplicate onto a PVDF membrane, then placed into the BioDotTM Microfiltration apparatus. The next experimental procedure was the same as reported in Section Standard Reference.

4.3. *Data Analysis*

Toxin concentrations are reported as the mean value of triplicate dots ± SD. Quantitative variables were tested for normal distribution and compared by means of paired Student's *t*-test. Comparisons between CD toxin concentrations in mild and severe CDI cases were performed by One way-ANOVA test. Qualitative differences between groups were assessed by use of Fisher's exact test. The precision of the risk ratio was determined by calculating a 95% confidence interval. The relationship between categorical variables and CDI severity was assessed by Pearson Chi-Square analysis. The risk ratio and 95% confidence interval were calculated. Statistical analysis was performed using the software programs GraphPad InStat 3.1 Software Inc. (San Diego, CA, USA) and IBM SPSS Statistics for Windows version 24.0 (IBM Corp. Released 2016; Armonk, NY, USA). Results were considered significant when p values were ≤ 0.05.

5. Conclusions

In conclusion, setting up this sensitive method allowed us to highlight that toxemia is much more frequent than expected in CDI patients, and more specifically, that high serum levels of TcdA correlate with disease severity in patients with CDI.

Supplementary Materials: The following are available online at https://www.mdpi.com/article/10.3390/antibiotics10091093/s1, Figure S1: Representative images of dot-blot experiment using the commercial TcdA and TcdB resuspended in either PBS or TBS. Figure S2: Cross-reactivity experiments to evaluate the specificity of the dot-blot assay. Table S1: Demographic and epidemiological data, comorbidities, clinical characteristics, and outcome of the 35 CDI cases included in the study. Table S2: Definitions of CDI, microbiological evidence of CDI, CDI recurrence, mild CDI, and severe CDI adopted in the study. Table S3: TcdA and TcdB plasma levels determined in the 35 CDI patients. Table S4: Risk factors for a high level of TcdA toxemia (TcdA > 3 ng/mL) at the CDI onset. Table S5: Risk factors for a detectable level of TcdB toxemia (TcdB > 0.2 ng/mL) at the CDI onset.

Author Contributions: Conceptualization, A.d.M. and N.P.; design of the methodology, A.d.M., D.M., P.A. and G.G.; performed investigation, A.d.M., D.M. and G.G.; performed formal analysis, A.d.M., D.M. and G.G.; resources, A.d.M. and N.P.; project administration, A.d.M. and N.P.; funding acquisition, A.d.M.; drafted manuscript, A.d.M. and G.G. All authors have read and agreed to the published version of the manuscript.

Funding: This work was supported by a grant to A.d.M. from Merck Sharp & Dohme Corp in the framework of Merck Trial Research Program. The results reported in this paper come from the authors and do not necessarily represent those of Merck Sharp & Dohme Corp. This study was also supported by grants from Ateneo Roma Tre to A.d.M. The Grant of Excellence Departments, MIUR (ARTICOLO 1, COMMI 314–337 LEGGE 232/2016) to Department of Science, University Roma Tre is also gratefully acknowledged.

Institutional Review Board Statement: The study was conducted according to the guidelines of the Declaration of Helsinki and approved by the Ethics Committee of the National Institute for Infectious Diseases "L. Spallanzani", IRCCS, Rome; Ethics Committee registry number: 22/2018.

Informed Consent Statement: Informed consent was obtained from all subjects involved in the study.

Data Availability Statement: The data presented in this study are available on request from the corresponding author. The data are not publicly available due to privacy and ethical restrictions.

Conflicts of Interest: N.P. received an honorary fee as a speaker from MSD, Pfizer, Shionogi, Becton & Dickinson, Johnson & Johnson. G.G., A.d.M., D.M. and P.A. declare no conflict of interest.

References

1. Evans, C.T.; Safdar, N. Current trends in the epidemiology and outcomes of *Clostridium difficile* infection. *Clin. Inf. Dis.* **2015**, *60*, S66–S71. [CrossRef]
2. Leffler, D.A.; Lamont, J.T. *Clostridium difficile* infection. *N. Engl. J. Med.* **2015**, *373*, 287–288. [CrossRef] [PubMed]
3. Guery, B.; Galperine, T.; Barbut, F. *Clostridioides difficile*: Diagnosis and treatments. *BMJ* **2019**, *366*, l4609. [CrossRef] [PubMed]
4. Shellito, A.D.; Russell, M.M. Diverting loop ileostomy for *Clostridium Difficile* colitis: A systematic review and meta-analysis. *Am. Surg.* **2020**, *86*, 1269–1276. [CrossRef] [PubMed]
5. Abou Chakra, C.N.; Pépin, J.; Sirard, S.; Valiquette, L. Risk factors for recurrence, complications and mortality in *Clostridium difficile* infection: A systematic review. *PLoS ONE* **2014**, *9*, e98400. [CrossRef] [PubMed]
6. Sheitoyan-Pesant, C.; Abou Chakra, C.N.; Pepin, J.; Marcil-Heguy, A.; Nault, V.; Valiquette, L. Clinical and healthcare burden of multiple recurrences of *Clostridium difficile* infection. *Clin. Infect. Dis.* **2016**, *62*, 574–580. [CrossRef]

7. Kuehne, S.A.; Cartman, S.T.; Heap, J.T.; Kelly, M.L.; Cockayne, A.; Minton, N.P. The role of toxin A and toxin B in *Clostridium difficile* infection. *Nature* **2010**, *467*, 711–713. [CrossRef] [PubMed]
8. Rupnik, M.; Wilcox, M.H.; Gerding, D.N. *Clostridium difficile* infection: New developments in epidemiology and pathogenesis. *Nat. Rev. Microbiol.* **2009**, *7*, 526–536. [CrossRef]
9. Di Bella, S.; Ascenzi, P.; Siarakas, S.; Petrosillo, N.; di Masi, A. *Clostridium difficile* toxins A and B: Insights into pathogenic properties and extraintestinal effects. *Toxins* **2016**, *8*, 134. [CrossRef]
10. Kelly, C.P. Can we identify patients at high risk of recurrent *Clostridium difficile* infection? *Clin. Microbiol. Infect.* **2012**, *18*, 21–27. [CrossRef]
11. Steele, J.; Chen, K.; Sun, X.; Zhang, Y.; Wang, H.; Tzipori, S.; Feng, H. Systemic dissemination of *Clostridium difficile* toxins A and B is associated with severe, fatal disease in animal models. *J. Infect. Dis.* **2011**, *205*, 384–391. [CrossRef]
12. Qualman, S.J.; Petric, M.; Karmali, M.A.; Smith, C.R.; Hamilton, S.R. *Clostridium difficile* invasion and toxin circulation in fatal pediatric pseudomembranous colitis. *Am. J. Clin. Pathol.* **1990**, *94*, 410–416. [CrossRef] [PubMed]
13. Yu, H.; Chen, K.; Wu, J.; Yang, Z.; Shi, L.; Barlow, L.L.; Aronoff, D.M.; Garey, K.W.; Savidge, T.C.; von Rosenvinge, E.C.; et al. Identification of toxemia in patients with *Clostridium difficile* infection. *PLoS ONE* **2015**, *10*, e0124235. [CrossRef] [PubMed]
14. Burnham, C.-A.D.; Carroll, K.C. Diagnosis of *Clostridium difficile* infection: An ongoing conundrum for clinicians and for clinical laboratories. *Clin. Microbiol. Rev.* **2013**, *26*, 604–630. [CrossRef] [PubMed]
15. Sprague, R.; Warny, K.; Pollock, N.; Daugherty, K.; Lin, Q.; Xu, H.; Cuddemi, C.; Barrett, C.; Chen, X.; Banz, A.; et al. Absence of toxemia in *Clostridioides difficile* infection: Results from ultrasensitive toxin assay of serum. *Dig. Dis. Sci.* **2020**, *810*, 1–4. [CrossRef]
16. Graff, G.; Anderson, L.A.; Jaques, L.W. Preparation and purification of soybean lipoxygenase-derived unsaturated hydroperoxy and hydroxy fatty acids and determination of molar absorptivities of hydroxy fatty acids. *Anal. Biochem.* **1990**, *188*, 38–47. [CrossRef]
17. Jin, L.; Engelhart, A.E.; Adamala, K.; Szostak, J.W. Preparation, purification, and use of fatty acid-containing liposomes. *JoVE* **2018**, *132*, e57324. [CrossRef] [PubMed]
18. Rao, K.; Malani, P.N. Diagnosis and treatment of *Clostridioides (Clostridium) difficile* infection in adults in 2020. *JAMA* **2020**, *323*, 1403–1404. [CrossRef]
19. Lyras, D.; O'Connor, J.R.; Howarth, P.M.; Sambol, S.P.; Carter, G.P.; Phumoonna, T.; Poon, R.; Adams, V.; Vedantam, G.; Johnson, S.; et al. Toxin B is essential for virulence of *Clostridium difficile*. *Nature* **2009**, *458*, 1176–1179. [CrossRef]
20. Pollock, N.R.; Banz, A.; Chen, X.; Williams, D.; Xu, H.; Cuddemi, C.A.; Cui, A.X.; Perrotta, M.; Alhassan, E.; Riou, B.; et al. Comparison of *Clostridioides difficile* stool toxin concentrations in adults with symptomatic infection and asymptomatic carriage using an ultrasensitive quantitative immunoassay. *Clin. Infect. Dis.* **2019**, *68*, 78–86. [CrossRef]
21. Di Masi, A.; Leboffe, L.; Polticelli, F.; Tonon, F.; Zennaro, C.; Caterino, M.; Stano, P.; Fischer, S.; Hägele, M.; Müller, M.; et al. Human serum albumin is an essential component of the host defense mechanism against *Clostridium difficile* intoxication. *J. Infect. Dis.* **2018**, *218*, 1424–1435. [CrossRef]
22. Di Bella, S.; di Masi, A.; Turla, S.; Ascenzi, P.; Gouliouris, T.; Petrosillo, N. The protective role of albumin in *Clostridium difficile* infection: A step toward solving the puzzle. *Infect. Control. Hosp. Epidemiol.* **2015**, *36*, 1478–1479. [CrossRef]
23. Kumarappa, V.S.; Patel, H.; Shah, A.; Baddoura, W.; DeBari, V.A. Temporal changes in serum albumin and total protein in patients with hospital-acquired Clostridium difficile infection. *Ann. Clin. Lab. Sci.* **2014**, *44*, 32–37.
24. Carter, G.P.; Chakravorty, A.; Pham Nguyen, T.A.; Mileto, S.; Schreiber, F.; Li, L.; Howarth, P.; Clare, S.; Cunningham, B.; Sambol, S.P.; et al. Defining the roles of TcdA and TcdB in localized gastrointestinal disease, systemic organ damage, and the host response during *Clostridium difficile* infections. *mBio* **2015**, *6*, e00551. [CrossRef]
25. Tonon, F.; Di Bella, S.; Grassi, G.; Luzzati, R.; Ascenzi, P.; di Masi, A.; Zennaro, C. Extra-intestinal Effects of *C.difficile* toxin A and B: An in vivo study using the Zebrafish embryo model. *Cells* **2020**, *9*, 2575. [CrossRef]
26. Solomon, K.; Martin, A.J.; O'Donoghue, C.; Chen, X.; Fenelon, L.; Fanning, S.; Kelly, C.P.; Kyne, L. Mortality in patients with *Clostridium difficile* infection correlates with host pro-inflammatory and humoral immune responses. *J. Med. Microbiol.* **2013**, *62*, 1453–1460. [CrossRef]
27. Vita, G.M.; De Simone, G.; Leboffe, L.; Montagnani, F.; Mariotti, D.; Di Bella, S.; Luzzati, R.; Gori, A.; Ascenzi, P.; di Masi, A. Human serum albumin binds Streptolysin O (SLO) toxin produced by Group a Streptococcus and inhibits its cytotoxic and hemolytic effects. *Front. Immunol.* **2020**, *11*, 2969. [CrossRef]
28. Kuehne, S.A.; Collery, M.M.; Kelly, M.L.; Cartman, S.T.; Cockayne, A.; Minton, N.P. Importance of toxin A, toxin B, and CDT in virulence of an epidemic *Clostridium difficile* strain. *J. Infect. Dis.* **2014**, *209*, 83–86. [CrossRef] [PubMed]
29. Abt, M.C.; McKenney, P.T.; Pamer, E.G. *Clostridium difficile* colitis: Pathogenesis and host defence. *Nat. Rev. Microbiol.* **2016**, *14*, 609–620. [CrossRef] [PubMed]
30. Savidge, T.C.; Pan, W.H.; Newman, P.; O'brien, M.; Anton, P.M.; Pothoulakis, C. *Clostridium difficile* toxin B is an inflammatory enterotoxin in human intestine. *Gastroenterology* **2003**, *125*, 413–420. [CrossRef]
31. Carman, R.J.; Stevens, A.L.; Lyerly, M.W.; Hiltonsmith, M.F.; Stiles, B.G.; Wilkins, T.D. *Clostridium difficile* binary toxin (CDT) and diarrhea. *Anaerobe* **2011**, *17*, 161–165. [CrossRef] [PubMed]

32. Gerding, D.N.; Johnson, S.; Rupnik, M.; Aktories, K. *Clostridium difficile* binary toxin CDT: Mechanism, epidemiology, and potential clinical importance. *Gut Microbes* **2014**, *5*, 15–27. [CrossRef] [PubMed]
33. Knapp, O.; Benz, R.; Popoff, M.R. Pore-forming activity of clostridial binary toxins. *Biochim. Biophys. Acta* **2016**, *1858*, 512–525. [CrossRef] [PubMed]

antibiotics

Article

Mortality Following *Clostridioides difficile* Infection in Europe: A Retrospective Multicenter Case-Control Study

Jacek Czepiel [1,*], Marcela Krutova [2,3], Assaf Mizrahi [3,4,5], Nagham Khanafer [3,6,7], David A. Enoch [8], Márta Patyi [9], Aleksander Deptuła [10], Antonella Agodi [11], Xavier Nuvials [12], Hanna Pituch [3,13], Małgorzata Wójcik-Bugajska [14], Iwona Filipczak-Bryniarska [15], Bartosz Brzozowski [16], Marcin Krzanowski [17], Katarzyna Konturek [18], Marcin Fedewicz [19], Mateusz Michalak [20], Lorra Monpierre [4], Philippe Vanhems [6,7], Theodore Gouliouris [8], Artur Jurczyszyn [21], Sarah Goldman-Mazur [21], Dorota Wultańska [13], Ed J. Kuijper [3,22,23], Jan Skupień [24], Grażyna Biesiada [1] and Aleksander Garlicki [1]

1 Department of Infectious and Tropical Diseases, Jagiellonian University Medical College, 30-688 Krakow, Poland; gbiesiada@op.pl (G.B.); agarlicki@gmail.com (A.G.)
2 Department of Medical Microbiology, Charles University, 2nd Faculty of Medicine and Motol University Hospital, 15006 Prague, Czech Republic; marcela.krutova@lfmotol.cuni.cz or marcela.krutova@seznam.cz
3 ESCMID Study Group for Clostridioides Difficile (ESGCD), 4001 Basel, Switzerland; amizrahi@hpsj.fr (A.M.); nagham.khanafer@chu-lyon.fr (N.K.); hanna.pituch@wum.edu.pl (H.P.); e.j.kuijper@lumc.nl (E.J.K.)
4 Service de Microbiologie Clinique, Groupe Hospitalier Paris Saint-Joseph, 75014 Paris, France; lorra.monpierre@hotmail.fr
5 Institut Micalis UMR 1319, Université Paris-Saclay, INRAe, AgroParisTech, 92290 Châtenay Malabry, France
6 Unité d'Hygiène, Epidémiologie et Prévention, Groupement Hospitalier Centre, Hospices Civils de Lyon, 69002 Lyon, France; philippe.vanhems@chu-lyon.fr
7 Centre International de Recherche en Infectiologie (CIRI), Public Health, Epidemiology and Evolutionary Ecology of Infectious Diseases (PHE3ID), Université de Lyon, 69372 Lyon, France
8 Clinical Microbiology & Public Health Laboratory, Public Health England, Addenbrooke's Hospital, Hills Road, Cambridge CB2 0QQ, UK; david.enoch@addenbrookes.nhs.uk (D.A.E.); theodore.gouliouris@addenbrookes.nhs.uk (T.G.)
9 Hygienic Department, Bács-Kiskun County Teaching Hospital, 6000 Bács-Kiskun, Hungary; patyim@kmk.hu
10 Department of Propaedeutics of Medicine and Infection Prevention, Ludwik Rydygier Collegium Medicum in Bydgoszcz, Nicolaus Copernicus University, 85-094 Bydgoszcz, Poland; deptula.aleksander@gmail.com
11 Department of Medical and Surgical Sciences and Advanced Technologies "GF Ingrassia", University of Catania, 95123 Catania, Italy; agodia@unict.it
12 Critical Care Department, Vall d'Hebron Hospital, Vall d'Hebron Institut de Recerca (VHIR), SODIR Group, Universitat Autònoma de Barcelona, 08035 Barcelona, Spain; fxnuvials@vhebron.net
13 Department of Medical Microbiology, Medical University of Warsaw, 02-004 Warsaw, Poland; dorota.wultanska@wum.edu.pl
14 Department of Internal and Geriatric Diseases, Jagiellonian University Medical College, 30-688 Krakow, Poland; mwojcik@su.krakow.pl
15 Department of Pain Treatment and Palliative Care, Jagiellonian University Medical College, 30-688 Krakow, Poland; inusia_bryniarska@yahoo.pl
16 Department of Gastroenterology and Hepatology, Jagiellonian University Medical College, 30-688 Krakow, Poland; bartek.brzozowski@op.pl
17 Department of Nephrology and Dialysis Unit, Jagiellonian University Medical College, 30-688 Krakow, Poland; mkrzanowski@op.pl
18 Intensive Care Unit, University Hospital, 30-688 Krakow, Poland; kliber@su.krakow.pl
19 Józef Babiński Hospital, 30-393 Krakow, Poland; marcin.fedewicz@gmail.com
20 Ludwik Rydygier Hospital, 31-826 Krakow, Poland; michalakcontact@gmail.com
21 Department of Hematology, Jagiellonian University Medical College, 30-688 Krakow, Poland; mmjurczy@cyf-kr.edu.pl (A.J.); senoritagoldman@gmail.com (S.G.M.)
22 Department of Medical Microbiology, Centre for Infectious Diseases, Leiden University Medical Center, 2333 Leiden, The Netherlands
23 Centre for Infectious Diseases Research, Diagnostics and Laboratory, Surveillance, Rijksinstituut voor Volksgezondheid en Milieu, 2333 Bilthoven, The Netherlands
24 Department of Metabolic Diseases, Jagiellonian University Medical College, 30-688 Krakow, Poland; jan.skupien@gmail.com
* Correspondence: jacek.czepiel@uj.edu.pl; Tel./Fax: +48-124002022/17

Citation: Czepiel, J.; Krutova, M.; Mizrahi, A.; Khanafer, N.; Enoch, D.A.; Patyi, M.; Deptuła, A.; Agodi, A.; Nuvials, X.; Pituch, H.; et al. Mortality Following *Clostridioides difficile* Infection in Europe: A Retrospective Multicenter Case-Control Study. *Antibiotics* **2021**, *10*, 299. https://doi.org/10.3390/antibiotics10030299

Academic Editor: Guido Granata

Received: 15 February 2021
Accepted: 10 March 2021
Published: 13 March 2021

Abstract: We aimed to describe the clinical presentation, treatment, outcome and report on factors associated with mortality over a 90-day period in *Clostridioides difficile* infection (CDI). Descriptive, univariate, and multivariate regression analyses were performed on data collected in a retrospective case-control study conducted in nine hospitals from seven European countries. A total of 624 patients were included, of which 415 were deceased (cases) and 209 were still alive 90 days after a CDI diagnosis (controls). The most common antibiotics used previously in both groups were β-lactams; previous exposure to fluoroquinolones was significantly ($p = 0.0004$) greater in deceased patients. Multivariate logistic regression showed that the factors independently related with death during CDI were older age, inadequate CDI therapy, cachexia, malignancy, Charlson Index, long-term care, elevated white blood cell count (WBC), C-reactive protein (CRP), bacteraemia, complications, and cognitive impairment. In addition, older age, higher levels of WBC, neutrophil, CRP or creatinine, the presence of malignancy, cognitive impairment, and complications were strongly correlated with shortening the time from CDI diagnosis to death. CDI prevention should be primarily focused on hospitalised elderly people receiving antibiotics. WBC, neutrophil count, CRP, creatinine, albumin and lactate levels should be tested in every hospitalised patient treated for CDI to assess the risk of a fatal outcome.

Keywords: *Clostridioides difficile* infection; co–morbidities; mortality; malignancy; outcome; risk factors

1. Introduction

Clostridioides difficile (*C. difficile*), formerly known as *Clostridium difficile*, is the most common cause of healthcare-associated infectious diarrhoea in the developed world. The incidence and severity of *C. difficile* infections (CDI) have risen in recent years with a considerable impact in terms of morbidity, mortality, and financial cost [1]. The burden of healthcare-associated CDIs in acute care hospitals in the European Economic Area was estimated at 123,997 cases annually [2]. In the United States, *C. difficile* is the most common cause of healthcare–associated infections, accounting for approximately 15% of them [3]. According to data from 2012, *C. difficile* caused approximately half a million infections and 29,000 deaths in the US [4]. The pooled incidence rate of CDI in Asia was calculated by meta-analysis at 5.3/10,000 patient days (95% CI 4.0–6.7) [5].

Increasing antibiotic use, improved life expectancy, increasing numbers of at-risk patients and the emergence of hypervirulent epidemic strains (e.g., ribotype PCR 027) may explain the increased incidence of CDI and these factors, in addition to hospitalisation, are key factors in the development of CDI [6,7]. Inflammatory bowel disease, gastrointestinal surgery, and conditions impairing the immune system (e.g., malignant neoplasms, transplantation, chronic kidney disease, and immunosuppressant use) also predispose towards CDI [8,9]. The clinical spectrum of CDI varies in severity from asymptomatic carriage and self-limited, mild diarrhoea to severe colitis, intestinal perforation, toxic megacolon, and death [7,10]. Mortality rates in CDI vary widely between studies. Before 2000, mortality associated with CDI was <2%, whereas mortality in studies since 2000 averaged 5% in endemic case and 7–17% in epidemic cases [11–15]. The mortality has been twice as high in Intensive Care Unit (ICU) patients with CDI compared to ICU patients without CDI [16,17].

We aimed to describe the risk factors, clinical presentation, and management of patients with CDI as well as reported factors associated with mortality in the 90-day period after diagnosis.

2. Materials and Methods

2.1. Study Population

Using the European Society of Clinical Microbiology and Infectious Diseases (ESCMID) Study Group for C. difficile members, 17 hospitals were selected for this study. Nine hospitals from seven European countries (Czech Republic, France, Hungary, Italy, Poland, Spain, and United Kingdom) participated in this retrospective case-control study.

Patients hospitalised between January 2011 and December 2019 with a diagnosis of CDI who died within 90 days following a CDI diagnosis formed the case group that was compared in a 2:1 ratio to a group of control patients with a CDI diagnosis hospitalised in the same wards over the same time period who survived.

2.2. Data Collection

Electronic hospital databases were used to collect patient data on: sex, age, body mass index (BMI), prior hospitalisations, dwelling in a long-term care (LTC) facility, recent surgery, parenteral nutrition, previous use (in last 3 months) of antibiotics, probiotics, proton pump inhibitors (PPIs), H2 blockers (H2b), immunosuppressants (defined as agents that can suppress or prevent the immune response), information on comorbidities needed to calculate the Charlson Index and dates of admission, CDI diagnosis, and deaths. The following data on the CDI episode were gathered: episode number, blood parameters at the time of diagnosis [white blood cell count (WBC), neutrophil count, C-reactive protein (CRP), creatinine, albumin, and lactate levels], associated bacteraemia, imaging procedures performed (abdominal ultrasound, computed tomography), colonoscopy and CDI therapy, as well as outcomes and complications (i.e., failure of any organ, infection, ileus, colon perforation, toxic megacolon, and bleeding from the digestive tract).

2.3. Definitions

A CDI case was defined as a patient with the symptoms of CDI and positive laboratory test(s) according to ESCMID guidelines [18]. Healthcare–associated CDI (HA–CDI) was defined as a patient who developed the symptoms of CDI in a healthcare facility on day three or later, following admission to a healthcare facility on day one, or who had onset in the community within four weeks after being discharged from a healthcare facility. Community-associated CDI (CA–CDI) was defined as a patient who had the onset of symptoms either outside of the healthcare facilities, or whose symptoms appeared in a healthcare facility within 48 h after admission but who had not been discharged from a healthcare facility within a 12 week period prior to the onset of symptoms [19]. Cases that did not fit any of these criteria were classified as unknown.

2.4. Statistical Analysis

For descriptive purposes continuous variables are presented as medians, lower (1 st) and upper (3 rd) quartiles. Categorical variables are presented as counts and percentages. Summary statistics were computed for the group of deceased patients and the control group of patients, who recovered from CDI. The frequencies of categorical variables were compared with the χ^2 test or Fisher's exact test, where applicable. Spearman correlation coefficients with appropriate asymptotic tests were calculated for select continuous variables and time to death. For categorical variables (including binary and ordinal ones), we used Kendall's correlation. To identify a set of statistically independent predictors of CDI mortality, we used logistic regression models. Variable selection was performed using the LASSO (least absolute shrinkage and selection operator) method with 10-fold cross-validation. A one standard deviation rule was used to select a parsimonious set of candidate variables. In the final multivariate logistic model, we retained only statistically significant predictors, and their joint predictive performance was evaluated with C-statistic. p-values <0.05 were considered to be significant. Data processing and statistical calculations were performed with R 3.6.3 (The R Foundation for Statistical Computing, Vienna, Austria).

3. Results

3.1. Descriptive Analysis of Included Patients

Data were collected from 624 hospitalised patients with CDI; 415 patients died (cases) and 209 patients were still alive 90 days after a CDI diagnosis (controls). The gender distribution was similar in both groups but slightly skewed toward women, (210; 51% in the deceased group), versus 118 (57%) in the controls ($p = 0.17$). The median age was 80 years in the deceased group and 72 years in the control group ($p < 0.001$). People ≥ 65 years-old constituted 86% (n = 357) of the deceased group and 67% (n = 140) in the control group ($p < 0.001$). People ≥80 years-old constituted 50% (n = 208) of the deceased group and 28% (n = 59) in the control group ($p < 0.001$). The patients' median age in the deceased group was, on average, 8 years higher and their Charlson Index was twice as high as in the control group ($p < 0.001$). The comparison of data on previous hospitalisations, surgeries, LTC stays, parenteral nutrition, use of probiotics, PPI, and H2b between the two groups of patients are shown in Table 1.

Table 1. Comparison of demographic and clinical data in the study groups.

Characteristic	CDI–Deceased Group (N = 415)	CDI–Control Group (N = 209)	*p* Value
	N (%) or Median (1st, 3rd Quartile)	N (%) or Median (1st, 3rd Quartile)	
Age (years)	80 (70, 86)	72 (59, 82)	<0.0001
Sex (male)	205 (49.4%)	91 (43.5%)	0.17
BMI (kg/m^2) *	24.2 (21.1, 27.7)	25.0 (22.1, 27.8)	0.39
Charlson Index	4 (3, 6)	2 (1, 4)	<0.0001
Previous hospitalisations	313 (75.4%)	132 (63.2%)	0.001
Previous parenteral nutrition	33 (8.0%)	17 (8.1%)	0.94
Previous surgery	77 (18.6%)	47 (22.5%)	0.24
Previous LTC facility	56 (13.5%)	10 (4.8%)	0.0008
Previous probiotics use	61 (14.7%)	21 (10.0%)	0.11
Previous PPI use *	219 (56.4%)	104 (50.2%)	0.15
Previous H2b use *	22 (5.3%)	9 (4.3%)	0.59

BMI, body mass index; CDI, *Clostridioides difficile* infection; H2b, H2 blockers; LTC, long term care; PPI proton pomp inhibitors.* Missing data: BMI: 186 cases in the deceased group and 49 cases in the control group; PPI use: 27 cases in the deceased group and 2 cases in the control group; H2b use: 2 cases in the deceased group and 1 case in the control group.

The number of patients who had HA-CDI was 280 (68%) among the deceased patients and 131 (63%) in the control group with CA-CDI. Fourteen (3%) in the deceased group and 20 (10%) in the control group ($p = 0.006$) were classed as CA–CDI. The origin of the CDI was unknown in 121 patients (29%) from the deceased group and in 58 patients (28%) from the control group.

Table 2 lists the most commonly used antibiotics (or antibiotic class) in the preceding 3 months. The use of β-lactams was most prevalent in both groups. The administration of fluoroquinolones was more frequent in the deceased group than in the control group.

Table 2. Antibiotics used in the 3 months prior to the episode of CDI.

Antibiotic	CDI–Deceased Group N (%)	CDI–Control Group N (%)	*p* Value
No antibiotic	35 (8.4%)	25 (12.0%)	0.16
Fluoroquinolones	160 (38.6%)	51 (24.4%)	0.0004
BLBLI	152 (36.6%)	60 (28.7%)	0.049
Third generation cephalosporins	147 (35.4%)	60 (28.7%)	0.09
Carbapenems	68 (16.4%)	31 (14.8%)	0.62
Aminoglycosides	45 (10.8%)	14 (6.7%)	0.09
Metronidazole	27 (6.5%)	27 (12.9%)	0.007

BLBLI, β-lactam/β-lactamase inhibitor; CDI, *Clostridioides difficile* infection; Some patients used more than one antibiotic, therefore the percentage sum does not equal 100%.

The incidence of co-morbidities as possible risk factors for CDI mortality is shown in Table 3. At least one co-morbidity was recorded in 76% of patients in the deceased group and 53% in the control group ($p < 0.001$). In the deceased group, a malignancy was the most prevalent comorbidity. Diabetes, chronic kidney disease, cachexia, and liver cirrhosis were also more common in deceased patients compared to controls.

Table 3. The frequency of co-morbidities regarded as possible risk factors for CDI mortality.

Comorbidity	CDI–Deceased Group N (%)	CDI–Control Group N (%)	*p* Value
At least one comorbidity	316 (76.1%)	111 (53.1%)	<0.0001
Malignancy	155 (37.3%)	40 (19.1%)	<0.0001
Diabetes mellitus	120 (28.9%)	38 (18.2%)	0.004
Chronic kidney disease	112 (27.0%)	32 (15.3%)	0.001
Immunosuppressive therapy	73 (17.6%)	39 (18.7%)	0.74
Cachexia	47(11.3%)	5 (2.4%)	0.0001
Immunosuppressive disease	17 (4.1%)	6 (2.9%)	0.44
Liver cirrhosis	14 (3.4%)	0 (0%)	0.004
IBD	5 (1.2%)	4 (1.9%)	0.49

CDI, *Clostridioides difficile* infection; IBD, inflammatory bowel disease. Some patients had more than one factor, therefore the percentage sum does not always equal 100%.

3.2. The Clinical Course of CDI

Data pertaining to the course of CDI are shown in Table 4. An increased WBC, neutrophils, CRP, creatinine, and lactate, and a lower serum albumin concentration were found to be significantly more frequent in patients with a fatal outcome of CDI compared to the control group. Complications during the course of CDI and cognitive impairment were more common in the deceased group compared to controls. The time between admission of patients and a CDI diagnosis was longer in the deceased group of patients compared to the controls.

Table 4. Data pertaining to the clinical course of CDI.

Characteristic	CDI–Deceased Group		CDI–Control Group		*p* Value
	N (%) or Median (1st, 3rd Quartile)	N Missing	N (%) or Median (1st, 3rd quartile)	N Missing	
Body temperature (°C)	36.6 (36.5, 37.1)	127	36.8 (36.6, 37.6)	74	0.005
WBC count (×1000/μL)	13.7 (8.8, 22.3)	14	9.6 (7.2, 14.0)	1	<0.0001
Neutrophil count (×1000/μL)	10.4 (6.1, 18.0)	186	7.2 (4.7, 10.9)	51	<0.0001
CRP (mg/L)	116 (70, 198)	67	65 (23, 120)	17	<0.0001
Serum creatinine (μmol/L)	107 (67, 192)	34	75 (60, 113)	5	<0.0001
Serum albumin (g/L)	24 (20, 28)	173	28 (23, 32)	99	<0.0001
Serum lactate (mmol/L)	1,8 (1.4, 3.3)	356	1.0 (0.8, 1.7)	187	0.0002
Bacteremia	45 (10.8%)	0	6 (2.9%)	0	0.0006
Episode number		0		0	0.18
1	365 (88.0%)		177 (84.7%)		
2	41 (9.9%)		22 (10.5%)		
3	6 (1.4%)	0	5 (2.4%)	0	0.18
4	2 (0.5%)		5 (2.4%)		
5	1 (0.2%)		0 (0%)		
Complications (without deaths)	101 (24.3%)	0	21 (10.0%)	0	<0.0001
Cognitive impairment	92 (22.2%)	0	6 (2.9%)	0	<0.0001
Surgery after CDI diagnosis	10 (2.4%)	0	4 (1.9%)	0	0.78
Days from admission to diagnosis	7 (1, 18)	1	5 (1, 13)	0	0.01
Days from diagnosis to death	12 (4, 25)	0	NA	NA	NA

CDI, *Clostridioides difficile* infection; CRP, C-reactive protein; NA, not applicable; WBC, white blood cells.

Abdominal ultrasound was performed in 36 cases in the deceased group (9%) and 37 cases (18%) in the control group ($p < 0.001$). Findings of importance in CDI (ascites, thickening of the intestinal wall of the colon, and/or increase in the lumen diameter of the colon) were discovered in 29 cases (81%) of the deceased group, compared to 14 (38%) in tests performed on the control group ($p < 0.001$). CT imaging was performed in 54 cases in the deceased group (13%) and in 15 cases in the control group (7%), $p = 0.03$. Important findings on CT (same as in ultrasonography) were discovered in 76% of procedures performed on the deceased group, compared to 67% in the control group ($p = 0.51$). Colonoscopy was performed on 7 patients in the deceased group (1.7%) and on 5 patients in the control group (2.4%), $p = 0.55$.

Fourteen different CDI treatment regimens were employed in the deceased group and eight in the control group. The chosen therapy was changed due to side effects in 3 cases (1%) in the deceased group, and in 3 cases (1%) in controls. Oral metronidazole was the most common treatment in both groups, n = 179, at 43% in the deceased group, and n = 100, as well as 48% in the control group. This treatment was unchanged in 131 and 86 patients from the respective groups. Thirteen people (3.1%) in the deceased group and 5 patients (2.4%) in the control group did not receive any antibiotic treatment for CDI.

The most common complications in the deceased group were failure of at least one vital organ (n = 36; 9%), pneumonia (n = 32; 8%), and sepsis (n = 14; 3%). Blood cultures were positive in five patients in the deceased group; the confirmed pathogens were: *Acinetobacter baumannii, Citrobacter koseri, Enterobacter cloacae, Candida albicans* and a mixture from one patient (*Staphylococcus epidermidis, Staphylococcus haemolyticus,* and *Enterococcus faecium*). Complications involving the gastrointestinal tract included ileus (n = 7; 2%), toxic megacolon (n = 3; 1%), bleeding (n = 3; 1%), intestinal ischaemia (n = 2; 0.5%), and gastrointestinal perforation (n = 1; 0.2%). The most commonly occurring complications in the control group were secondary infections: pneumonia (n = 10; 5%), urinary tract infections (n = 6; 3%), and sepsis (n = 4; 2%).

3.3. Predictors of Death in CDI

Multivariate logistic regression identified 11 factors that together discriminated CDI deaths from controls. The most important were advanced age, the presence of malignancy, a higher Charlson Index, WBC (1000/µL increase), CRP (100 mg/L increase), the presence of complications, and the presence of cognitive impairment (Table 5). The discriminative accuracy of this model was considerably high, as the C–statistic was 0.864.

Table 5. List of independent death predictors in a multivariate logistic regression model.

Covariate	Odds Ratio (95% Confidence Interval)	*p* Value
Age (10–year increase)	1.57 (1.31, 1.89)	<0.001
inadequate antibiotics *	3.70 (1.08, 12.69)	0.04
Cachexia	5.00 (1.34, 18.57)	0.02
Malignancy	2.62 (1.43, 4.81)	0.002
Charlson Index (1 unit increase)	1.24 (1.11, 1.39)	0.0001
long term care	2.42 (1.05, 5.58)	0.04
WBC (1000/µL increase)	1.03 (1.01, 1.06)	0.005
CRP (100 mg/l increase)	1.80 (1.34, 2.43)	0.0001
Bacteremia	3.35 (1.06, 9.93)	0.04
Complications (without deaths)	3.95 (2.08, 7.50)	<0.001
Cognitive impairment	7.50 (2.73, 20.66)	<0.001

Model C-statistic = 0.864; CRP C-reactive protein; WBC white blood cell; *- use of ineffective treatment such as intravenous metronidazole or vancomycin in monotherapy, or ineffective antibiotics, such as tigecycline.

Correlation was assessed between selected parameters and the time from CDI diagnosis to death. Advanced age, higher levels of WBC, neutrophil, CRP or creatinine, the presence of malignancy, cognitive impairment, and complications were strongly correlated with hastening death (Table 6).

Table 6. Spearman or Kendall (for categorical, binary or ordinal variables) correlations between select characteristics and days from CDI diagnosis to death.

Variable	ρ/τ	*p* Value
Age	−0.15	0.0024
Malignancy	0.08	0.038
WBC count	−0.17	0.0005

Table 6. *Cont.*

Variable	ρ/τ	*p* Value
Neutrophil count	−0.30	<0.0001
CRP	−0.27	<0.0001
Serum creatinine	−0.18	0.0005
Complications (without deaths)	0.11	0.0093
Cognitive impairment	−0.14	0.0008

CRP C–reactive protein; WBC white blood cell, included only variables with $p < 0.05$.

Research data are available as Supplementary Materials.

4. Discussion

To the best of our knowledge, this study is the largest analysis of patients with a fatal outcome of CDI in multiple sites across Europe.

We confirm that increasing age is an important risk factor for a fatal outcome of CDI, as described previously [20,21]. A systematic review which included 30 studies showed that increasing age is among the most reported risk factor for mortality in patients with CDI [22]. This is most likely due to the weaker immune response to the *C. difficile* toxin. Moreover, the elderly are characterized by a greater number of chronic diseases, including those that contribute to a worse course of CDI, such as chronic kidney disease, diabetes, or malignancy [23]. Gender is not an important factor since the risk was similar for both males and females, as described in other studies [21,24,25].

The presence of any comorbidity ($p < 0.0001$) and increasing Charlson Index ($p = <0.0001$) were also associated with increased mortality. This has been described elsewhere [20,21,26], but some studies did not confirm such observations [27]. This may be the result of the different characteristics of the population or study design. Oncology patients face a number of risk factors that are predisposed to CDI acquisition, including frequent and prolonged hospitalisations, increased antibiotic use (both prophylactic and therapeutic), and chemotherapy [28]. We found malignancy to be an independent factor of mortality risk. The pathogenesis of CDI, during and after chemotherapy, is not yet fully understood but suggestions include a negative impact on the gastrointestinal microbiota, direct damage to intestinal mucosa, and immunological mechanisms in the neoplastic process predisposing to CDI [29–31]. In a large analysis of outcomes of 30,000 patients with cancer, those with CDI had a significantly higher mortality rate (9.4% vs. 7.5%, $p < 0.0001$) [32]. Among other comorbidities, liver cirrhosis and cachexia were more prevalent in the deceased group but only cachexia was independent death risk predictor. Patients with liver cirrhosis and cachexia are typically characterised by low levels of albumin, a recognised risk factor for severe CDI [7], and in our study, low albumin levels were strongly correlated with the risk of death. Surprisingly IBD was not related with 90-days mortality; however, the total number of patients with IBD in both groups was low. IBD is a known risk factor both for development of CDI and mortality [24,33]. We also noted an association with chronic kidney disease and increased mortality which has also been reported previously, particularly in patients with end-stage renal disease and patients on dialysis, compared to the general population [34,35]. Diabetes is also a predisposing factor for CDI development and recurrence [36,37], but it was not shown to be a mortality-related factor [20,25,27]. In our study diabetes was more prevalent in the deceased group, but it was not independent death predictor, when assessed in the multivariate logistic regression model.

CDI is a recognised problem in LTC facilities; residents are often elderly with multiple co-morbidities. LTC admission 90 days before CDI was related with 30-day all-cause mortality in one study [27]. We also found that previous LTC residency was more prevalent in the deceased group and was independently associated with a fatal outcome.

It is suggested that a patients' weight has an impact on outcome from CDI. One study suggested that being underweight (BMI < 19) or morbidly obese (BMI > 40) was associated with an increased in-hospital mortality in patients with CDI [38], while another reported that underweight patients with CDI are at higher risk of poor outcome than normal, overweight, and obese patients [39]. Therefore, one of our aims was to establish if there was any association between a patient's BMI and its impact on the course of CDI. Calculating BMI sometimes poses a challenge, since the most severely ill, often bedridden patients cannot be weighed properly. BMI data were only available in 55% of our cases; however, considering the large population of patients in our study, their number was sufficient to conclude that BMI did not increase mortality in CDI.

Previous hospitalisation was more prevalent in the deceased group but was not independent risk factor of death, which confirmed the findings of Morrison et al. study [24].

In our study, the previous use of PPIs and/or H2b before a CDI episode was not associated with a fatal outcome; these findings are contrary to a study by Morrison et al. [24]. In another report, the use of PPIs, but not H2b, was a predictor of mortality within 30 days after the end of treatment for a CDI recurrence; however, there are some differences in the methodology compared to our study [27].

Antibiotic use alters gut microbiota that physiologically protects the gastrointestinal tract from colonisation by pathogens, including *C. difficile*. In our study, we demonstrated that antibiotic treatment was the most common risk factor for CDI mortality (92% in the deceased group and 88% in the control group). The most frequently used antimicrobials were β-lactams and fluoroquinolones, two of the "4C" antibiotics in which stewardship intervention can lead to a decline in prevalence of epidemic *C. difficile* ribotypes [40].

In our population of 624 study participants, every patient had at least one risk factor for the development of CDI. It is also notable that only 7 patients (1.1%) did not have any of the 3 main CDI risk factors (age > 65; previous hospitalisation or antibiotic use). This is of importance, since it suggests that patients with no risk factors are less likely to develop CDI.

We analysed blood parameters which are known risk markers for poor outcomes in CDI [41–43]. These parameters are very useful in clinical practice, as they can be assessed cheaply, objectively, and early in the course of CDI. The differences in their values between both groups are pronounced. It is worth noting, however, that although the WBC count was almost always tested, this was not always the case for other parameters and the percentage of tests performed (creatinine, CRP, neutrophil count, albumin and lactate) was low. We found that WBC and neutrophil counts, CRP, and creatinine were strongly correlated with shortening the time from CDI diagnosis to death. Moreover, WBC and CRP were independent predictors of death.

In the deceased group, 88% of patients died during the first episode which is consistent with the notion that the highest risk of death is associated with the first episode of CDI [44]. Colonoscopies were rarely performed in our study. Endoscopic evaluation can be useful; however, it is indicated only if diagnostic problems occur, e.g., when an alternative diagnosis is suspected and direct visualisation and/or biopsy of the bowel mucosa is needed [7]. Computed tomography and ultrasounds are useful among patients with severe CDI helping to evaluate for presence of complications like toxic megacolon or bowel perforation [45]. The number of these examinations in our study was relatively small, and it is especially surprising that ultrasound examinations were performed much less frequently in the deceased group.

Oral metronidazole was the most frequently used drug in CDI treatment in our study. This is despite recent guidance suggesting vancomycin and/or fidaxomicin be used as first line in CDI [10]; however, the majority of patients in our study were hospitalised before this guideline could be implemented. Nevertheless, most patients did not receive the correct treatment choice according to the guidelines [10,18]. This indicates the need for hospitals' infection prevention and control teams to organise dedicated seminars on CDI for medical personnel. The knowledge about correct antibiotic prescriptions and antimicrobial resistance is one of the main important threats identified by the World Health Organisation [46]. One study involving 1179 junior doctors found that questions on antimicrobial use were poorly answered, whilst 81% of participants stated that teaching about appropriate antimicrobial use was inadequate during their medical training and 71% disagreed that they received the right examples from their tutors [47].

Our study shows that CDI therapy was well tolerated, since the percentage of patients whose therapy was altered due to side effects was very small. As it can be seen in Supplementary Materials, almost all patients were treated with the use of well-known conventional drugs. Only one patient was a participant of a cadazolid trial. Cadazolid is a novel quinoxolidinone antibiotic developed for treating CDI, which was safe and well tolerated but did not achieve its primary endpoint of non-inferiority to vancomycin for clinical cure in one of two phase 3 CDI trials [48]. Three patients were treated with the use of intravenous immunoglobulin (IVIG) which sometimes is used in CDI treatment, but reports as to its effectiveness are ambiguous [49,50]. None were treated with Bezlotoxumab, a monoclonal antibody that binds to *C. difficile* toxin B, which was approved by the FDA in 2016 for prevention of recurrent CDI in patients at high risk of CDI recurrence [51].

Our study has several limitations. It was a retrospective study and some data were unavailable. In addition, there are substantial differences in the numbers of patients included by each centre. However, we did not want to refuse any centre that wished to participate. We were unable to distinguish between cases when CDI was the primary cause of death and when it was not, and there was no ribotyping / sequencing data.

5. Conclusions

In our multicentre study, the independent risk factors for mortality at day 90 were older age, inadequate CDI therapy, cachexia, malignancy, Charlson Index, LTC facility care, elevated WBC, elevated CRP, bacteraemia, complications, and cognitive impairment. CDI prevention should be primarily focused on hospitalised elderly people receiving antibiotics, especially fluoroquinolones or β-lactam/β-lactamase inhibitors. For this group, we suggest using available preventive measures all the time, instead of, as is presently often done, after CDI diagnosis.

Supplementary Materials: The following are available online at https://www.mdpi.com/2079-6382/10/3/299/s1 Research data.

Author Contributions: Conceptualization, J.C., M.K. (Marcela Krutova), A.M., N.K., D.A.E., M.P., A.A., and X.N.; Formal analysis, J.S.; Investigation, J.C., M.K. (Marcela Krutova), A.M., N.K., D.A.E., M.P., A.A. and X.N.; Visualisation, J.S.; Writing—original draft, J.C., M.K. (Marcela Krutova), A.M., N.K., D.A.E., M.P., A.A. and X.N.; Writing—review & editing, J.C., M.K. (Marcela Krutova), A.M., N.K., D.A.E., M.P., A.D., A.A., X.N., H.P., M.W.-B., I.F.-B., B.B., M.K. (Marcin Krzanowski), K.K., M.F., M.M., L.M., P.V., T.G., A.J., S.G.-M., D.W., E.J.K., J.S., G.B. and A.G. All authors have read and agreed to the published version of the manuscript.

Funding: This research did not receive any specific grant from funding agencies in the public, commercial, or not-for-profit sectors.

Institutional Review Board Statement: The study was conducted according to the guidelines of the Declaration of Helsinki (as revised in Brazil 2013). Since it was a retrospective study, based on standard data gathered at the hospitals (data that were sent anonymously and with no identifying personal information), informed consent was not required.

Informed Consent Statement: Informed consent was not required.

Data Availability Statement: Research data are available as Supplementary Materials.

Acknowledgments: We would like to express our appreciation for help in data acquisition to: Martina Barchitta and Claudia La Mastra from Department of Medical and Surgical Sciences and Advanced Technologies "GF Ingrassia", University of Catania, Catania, Italy; Graziella Manciagli, Giuseppe Giammanco, Angela Privitera, and Nunzio Sciacca from ARNAS Garibaldi Nesima Hospital, Catania, Italy.

Conflicts of Interest: The authors declare no conflict of interest.

References

1. Elliott, B.; Androga, G.O.; Knight, D.R.; Riley, T.V. *Clostridium difficile* infection: Evolution, phylogeny and molecular epidemiology. *Infect. Genet. Evol.* **2017**, *49*, 1–11. [CrossRef] [PubMed]
2. European Surveillance of *Clostridium difficile* infections. In *Surveillance Protocol Version 2.2*; European Centre for Disease Prevention and Control (ECDC): Stockholm, Sweden, 2015. [CrossRef]
3. Magill, S.S.; O'Leary, E.; Janelle, S.J.; Thompson, D.L.; Dumyati, G.; Nadle, J.; Wilson, L.E.; Kainer, M.A.; Lynfield, R.; Greissman, S.; et al. Emerging Infections Program Hospital Prevalence Survey Team. Changes in prevalence of health care-associated infections in U.S. hospitals. *N. Engl. J. Med.* **2018**, *379*, 1732–1744. [CrossRef] [PubMed]
4. Lessa, F.C.; Mu, Y.; Bamberg, W.M.; Beldavs, Z.G.; Dumyati, G.K.; Dunn, J.R.; Farley, M.M.; Holzbauer, S.M.; Meek, J.I.; Phipps, E.C.; et al. Burden of *Clostridium difficile* infection in the United States. *N. Engl. J. Med.* **2015**, *372*, 825–834. [CrossRef]
5. Borren, N.Z.; Ghadermarzi, S.; Hutfless, S.; Ananthakrishnan, A.N. The emergence of *Clostridium difficile* infection in Asia: A systematic review and meta-analysis of incidence and impact. *PLoS ONE* **2017**, *12*, e0176797. [CrossRef] [PubMed]
6. He, M.; Miyajima, F.; Roberts, P.; Ellison, L.; Pickard, D.J.; Martin, M.J.; Connor, T.R.; Harris, S.R.; Fairley, D. Emergence and global spread of epidemic healthcare-associated *Clostridium difficile*. *Nat. Genet.* **2013**, *45*, 109–113. [CrossRef] [PubMed]
7. Czepiel, J.; Dróżdż, M.; Pituch, H.; Kuijper, E.J.; Perucki, W.; Mielimonka, A.; Goldman, S.; Wultańska, D.; Garlicki, A.; Biesiada, G. *Clostridium difficile* infection: Review. *Eur. J. Clin. Microbiol. Infect. Dis.* **2019**, *38*, 1211–1221. [CrossRef]
8. Leffler, D.A.; Lamont, J.T. *Clostridium difficile* infection. *N. Engl. J. Med.* **2015**, *373*, 287–288. [CrossRef]
9. Ofori, E.; Ramai, D.; Dhawan, M.; Mustafa, F.; Gasperino, J.; Reddy, M. Community-acquired *Clostridium difficile*: Epidemiology, ribotype, risk factors, hospital and intensive care unit outcomes, and current and emerging therapies. *J. Hosp. Infect.* **2018**, *99*, 436–442. [CrossRef] [PubMed]
10. McDonald, L.C.; Gerding, D.N.; Johnson, S.; Bakken, J.S.; Carroll, K.C.; Coffin, S.E.; Dubberke, E.R.; Garey, K.W.; Gould, C.V.; Kelly, C.; et al. Clinical practice guidelines for *Clostridium difficile* infection in adults and children: 2017 update by the Infectious Diseases Society of America (IDSA) and Society for Healthcare Epidemiology of America (SHEA). *Clin. Infect. Dis.* **2018**, *66*, e1–e48. [CrossRef]
11. Kwon, J.H.; Olsen, M.A.; Dubberke, E.R. The morbidity, mortality, and costs associated with *Clostridium difficile* infection. *Infect. Dis. Clin. N. Am.* **2015**, *29*, 123–134. [CrossRef]
12. Kyne, L.; Hamel, M.B.; Polavaram, R.; Kelly, C.P. Health care costs and mortality associated with nosocomial diarrhea due to *Clostridium difficile*. *Clin. Infect. Dis.* **2002**, *34*, 346–353. [CrossRef] [PubMed]
13. Miller, M.A.; Hyland, M.; Ofner-Agostini, M.; Gourdeau, M.; Ishak, M.; Canadian Hospital Epidemiology Committee. Canadian Nosocomial Infection Surveillance Program. Morbidity, mortality, and healthcare burden of nosocomial *Clostridium difficile*-associated diarrhea in Canadian hospitals. *Infect. Control. Hosp. Epidemiol.* **2002**, *23*, 137–140. [CrossRef]
14. Olson, M.M.; Shanholtzer, C.J.; Lee, J.T., Jr.; Gerding, D.N. Ten years of prospective *Clostridium difficile*-associated disease surveillance and treatment at the Minneapolis VA Medical Center, 1982–1991. *Infect. Control. Hosp. Epidemiol.* **1994**, *15*, 371–381. [CrossRef]
15. Dallal, R.M.; Harbrecht, B.G.; Boujoukas, A.J.; Sirio, C.A.; Farkas, L.M.; Lee, K.K.; Simmons, R.L. Fulminant *Clostridium difficile*: An underappreciated and increasing cause of death and complications. *Ann. Surg.* **2002**, *235*, 363–372. [CrossRef]
16. Vincent, J.L.; Rello, J.; Marshall, J.; Silva, E.; Anzueto, A.; Martin, C.D.; Moreno, R.; Lipman, J.; Gomersall, C.; Sakr, Y.; et al. International study of the prevalence and outcomes of infection in intensive care units. *JAMA* **2009**, *302*, 2323–2329. [CrossRef]
17. Sidler, J.A.; Battegay, M.; Tschudin-Sutter, S.; Widmer, A.F.; Weisser, M. *Enterococci*, *Clostridium difficile* and ESBL producing bacteria: Epidemiology, clinical impact and prevention in ICU patients. *Swiss Med. Wkly.* **2014**, *144*, 14009. [CrossRef] [PubMed]
18. Debast, S.B.; Bauer, M.P.; Kuijper, E.J.; ESCMID. European Society of Clinical Microbiology and Infectious Diseases: Update of the treatment guidance document for *Clostridium difficile* infection. *Clin. Microbiol. Infect.* **2014**, *20*, 1–26. [CrossRef]
19. Krutova, M.; Kinross, P.; Barbut, F.; Hajdu, A.; Wilcox, M.H.; Kuijper, E.J.; Allerberger, F.; Delmée, M.; Van Broeck, J.; Vatcheva-Dobrevska, R.; et al. How to: Surveillance of *Clostridium difficile* infections. *Microbiol. Infect.* **2018**, *24*, 469–475. [CrossRef] [PubMed]
20. Banks, A.; Moore, E.K.; Bishop, J.; Coia, J.E.; Brown, D.; Mather, H.; Wiuff, C. Trends in mortality following *Clostridium difficile* infection in Scotland, 2010–2016: A retrospective cohort and case control study. *J. Hosp. Infect.* **2018**, *100*, 133–141. [CrossRef] [PubMed]
21. Chintanaboina, J.; Navabi, S.; Suchniak-Mussari, K.; Stern, B.; Bedi, S.; Lehman, E.B.; Tinsley, A. Predictors of 30-day mortality in hospitalized patients with *Clostridium difficile* infection. *S. Med. J.* **2017**, *110*, 546–549. [CrossRef]
22. Abou Chakra, C.N.; Pepin, J.; Sirard, S.; Valiquette, L. Risk factors for recurrence, complications and mortality in *Clostridium difficile* infection: A systematic review. *PLoS ONE* **2014**, *9*, e98400. [CrossRef] [PubMed]
23. Johnson, S. Recurrent *Clostridium difficile* infection: A review of risk factors, treatments, and outcomes. *J. Infect.* **2009**, *58*, 403–410. [CrossRef]
24. Morrison, R.H.; Hall, N.S.; Said, M.; Rice, T.; Groff, H.; Brodine, S.K.; Slymen, D.; Lederman, E.R. Risk factors associated with complications and mortality in patients with *Clostridium difficile* infection. *Clin. Infect. Dis.* **2011**, *53*, 1173–1178. [CrossRef]
25. Takahashi, M.; Mori, N.; Bito, S. Multi-institution case–control and cohort study of risk factors for the development and mortality of *Clostridium difficile* infections in Japan. *BMJ Open* **2014**, *4*, e005665. [CrossRef]
26. Larentis, D.Z.; Rosa, R.G.; Dos Santos, R.P.; Goldani, L.Z. Outcomes and risk factors associated with *Clostridium difficile* diarrhea in hospitalized adult patients. *Gastroenterol. Res. Pract.* **2015**, *2015*, 346341. [CrossRef] [PubMed]

27. Appaneal, H.J.; Caffrey, A.R.; Beganovic, M.; Avramovic, S.; LaPlante, K.L. Predictors of mortality among a national cohort of veterans with recurrent *Clostridium difficile* infection. *Open Forum Infect. Dis.* **2018**, *5*, ofy175. [CrossRef] [PubMed]
28. Cozar-Llisto, A.; Ramos-Martinez, A.; Cobo, J. *Clostridium difficile* infection in special high-risk populations. *Infect. Dis. Ther.* **2016**, *5*, 253–269. [CrossRef] [PubMed]
29. Anand, A.; Glatt, A.E. *Clostridium difficile* infection associated with antineoplastic chemotherapy: A review. *Clin. Infect. Dis.* **1993**, *17*, 109–113. [CrossRef] [PubMed]
30. Loo, V.G.; Bourgault, A.M.; Poirier, L.; Lamothe, F.; Michaud, S.; Turgeon, N.; Toye, B.; Beaudoin, A.; Frost, E.H.; Gilca, R.; et al. Host and pathogen factors for *Clostridium difficile* infection and colonization. *N. Engl. J. Med.* **2011**, *365*, 1693–1703. [CrossRef] [PubMed]
31. Bishop, K.D.; Castillo, J.J. Risk factors associated with *Clostridium difficile* infection in adult oncology patients with a history of recent hospitalization for febrile neutropenia. *Leuk. Lymphoma* **2012**, *53*, 1617–1619. [CrossRef]
32. Delgado, A.; Reveles, I.A.; Cabello, F.T.; Reveles, K.R. Poorer outcomes among cancer patients diagnosed with *Clostridium difficile* infections in United States community hospitals. *BMC Infect. Dis.* **2017**, *17*, 448. [CrossRef]
33. Trifan, A.; Stanciu, C.; Stoica, O.; Girleanu, I.; Cojocariu, C. Impact of *Clostridium difficile* infection on inflammatory bowel disease outcome: A review. *World J. Gastroenterol.* **2014**, *20*, 11736–11742. [CrossRef] [PubMed]
34. Pant, C.; Deshpande, A.; Anderson, M.P.; Sferra, T.J. *Clostridium difficile* infection is associated with poor outcomes in end-stage renal disease. *J. Investig. Med.* **2012**, *60*, 529–532. [CrossRef]
35. Thongprayoon, C.; Cheungpasitporn, W.; Phatharacharukul, P.; Edmonds, P.J.; Kaewpoowat, Q.; Mahaparn, P.; Bruminhent, J.; Erickson, S.B. Chronic kidney disease and end-stage renal disease are risk factors for poor outcomes of *Clostridium difficile* infection: A systematic review and meta-analysis. *Int. J. Clin. Pract.* **2015**, *69*, 998–1006. [CrossRef] [PubMed]
36. López-de-Andrés, A.; Esteban-Vasallo, M.D.; de Miguel-Díez, J.; Hernández-Barrera, V.; de Miguel-Yanes, J.M.; Méndez-Bailón, M.; Jiménez-García, R. Incidence and in-hospital outcomes of *Clostridium difficile* infection among type 2 diabetes patients in Spain. *Int. J. Clin. Pract.* **2018**, *72*, e13251. [CrossRef]
37. Qu, H.Q.; Jiang, Z.D. *Clostridium difficile* infection in diabetes. *Diabetes Res. Clin. Pract.* **2014**, *105*, 285–294. [CrossRef]
38. Nathanson, B.H.; Higgins, T.L.; McGee, W.T. The dangers of extreme body mass index values in patients with *Clostridium difficile*. *Infection* **2017**, *45*, 787–793. [CrossRef] [PubMed]
39. Mansoor, M.S.; Feuerstadt, P. Underweight patients with *C. difficile* infection (CDI) are at higher risk of poor outcome than normal, overweight and obese patients. *Gastroenterology* **2015**, *148*, S484. [CrossRef]
40. Lawes, T.; Lopez-Lozano, J.M.; Nebot, C.A.; Macartney, G.; Subbarao-Sharma, R.; Wares, K.D.; Sinclair, C.; Gould, I.M. Effect of a national 4C antibiotic stewardship intervention on the clinical and molecular epidemiology of *Clostridium difficile* infections in a region of Scotland: A non-linear time-series analysis. *Lancet Infect. Dis.* **2017**, *17*, 194–206. [CrossRef]
41. Bhangu, S.; Bhangu, A.; Nightingale, P.; Michael, A. Mortality and risk stratification in patients with *Clostridium difficile*-associated diarrhoea. *Colorectal. Dis.* **2010**, *12*, 241–246. [CrossRef]
42. Pant, C.; Madonia, P.; Minocha, A.; Manas, K.; Jordan, P.; Bass, P. Laboratory markers as predictors of mortality in patients with *Clostridium difficile* infection. *J. Invest. Med.* **2010**, *58*, 43–45. [CrossRef]
43. Gujja, D.; Friedenberg, F.K. Predictors of serious complications due to *Clostridium difficile* infection. *Aliment. Pharmacol. Ther.* **2009**, *29*, 635–642. [CrossRef]
44. Czepiel, J.; Kędzierska, J.; Biesiada, G.; Birczyńska, M.; Perucki, W.; Nowak, P.; Garlicki, A. Epidemiology of *Clostridium difficile* infection: Results of a hospital-based study in Krakow, Poland. *Epidemiol. Infect.* **2015**, *143*, 3235–3243. [CrossRef]
45. Paláu-Dávila, L.; Lara-Medrano, R.; Negreros-Osuna, A.A.; Salinas-Chapa, M.; Garza-González, E.; Gutierrez-Delgado, E.M.; Camacho-Ortiz, A. Efficacy of computed tomography for the prediction of colectomy and mortality in patients with *Clostridium difficile* infection. *Ann. Med. Surg. (Lond.)* **2016**, *12*, 101–105. [CrossRef]
46. World Health Organization (WHO). *Ten Threats to Global Health in 2019*; WHO: Geneva, Switzerland, 2019. Available online: https://www.who.int/news-room/spotlight/ten-threats-to-global-health-in-2019 (accessed on 1 May 2019).
47. Di Gennaro, F.; Marotta, C.; Amicone, M.; Bavaro, D.F.; Bernaudo, F.; Frisicale, E.M.; Kurotschka, P.K.; Mazzari, A.; Veronese, N.; Murri, R.; et al. Italian young doctors' knowledge, attitudes and practices on antibiotic use and resistance: A national cross-sectional survey. *J. Glob. Antimicrob. Resist.* **2020**, *23*, 167–173. [CrossRef]
48. Gerding, D.N.; Cornely, O.A.; Grill, S.; Kracker, H.; Marrast, A.C.; Nord, C.E.; Talbot, G.H.; Buitrago, M.; Diaconescu, I.G.; de Oliveira, C.M.; et al. Cadazolid for the treatment of *Clostridium difficile* infection: Results of two double-blind, placebo-controlled, non-inferiority, randomised phase 3 trials. *Lancet Infect. Dis.* **2019**, *19*, 265–274. [CrossRef]
49. Abougergi, M.A.; Broor, A.; Cui, W.; Jaar, B.G. Intravenous immunoglobulin for the treatment of severe *Clostridium difficile* colitis: An observational study and review of the literature. *J. Hosp. Med.* **2010**, *5*, E1–E9. [CrossRef] [PubMed]
50. Shah, N.; Shaaban, H.; Spira, R.; Slim, J.; Boghossian, J. Intravenous immunoglobulin in the treatment of severe *Clostridium difficile* colitis. *J. Glob. Infect. Dis.* **2014**, *6*, 82–85. [PubMed]
51. Wilcox, M.H.; Gerding, D.N.; Poxton, I.R.; Kelly, C.; Nathan, R.; Birch, T.; Cornely, O.A.; Rahav, G.; Bouza, E.; Lee, C.; et al. Bezlotoxumab for prevention of recurrent *Clostridium difficile* infection. *N. Engl. J. Med.* **2017**, *376*, 305–317. [CrossRef] [PubMed]

antibiotics

Article

Clostridioides difficile Infection among Cirrhotic Patients with Variceal Bleeding

Mirela Nicoleta Voicu [1], Florica Popescu [1], Dan Nicolae Florescu [2], Ion Rogoveanu [2], Adina Turcu-Stiolica [3,*], Dan Ionut Gheonea [2], Vlad Florin Iovanescu [2], Sevastita Iordache [2], Sergiu Marian Cazacu [2] and Bogdan Silviu Ungureanu [2]

1 Department of Pharmacology, University of Medicine and Pharmacy of Craiova, 200349 Craiova, Romania; nicoletamirelavoicu@gmail.com (M.N.V.); prof_floricapopescu@hotmail.com (F.P.)
2 Department of Gastroenterology, University of Medicine and Pharmacy of Craiova, 200349 Craiova, Romania; dan.florescu@umfcv.ro (D.N.F.); ion.rogoveanu@umfcv.ro (I.R.); dan.gheonea@umfcv.ro (D.I.G.); vlad.iovanescu@umfcv.ro (V.F.I.); sevastita.iordache@umfcv.ro (S.I.); sergiu.cazacu@umfcv.ro (S.M.C.); bogdan.ungureanu@umfcv.ro (B.S.U.)
3 Department of Pharmacoeconomics, University of Medicine and Pharmacy of Craiova, 200349 Craiova, Romania
* Correspondence: adina.turcu@umfcv.ro

Abstract: *Clostridioides difficile* infection (CDI) stands as the leading cause of nosocomial infection with high morbidity and mortality rates, causing a major burden on the healthcare system. Driven by antibiotics, it usually affects older patients with chronic disease or immunosuppressed or oncologic management. Variceal bleeding secondary to cirrhosis requires antibiotics to prevent bacterial translocation, and thus patients become susceptible to CDI. We aimed to investigate the risk factors for CDI in cirrhotic patients with variceal bleeding following ceftriaxone and the mortality risk in this patient's population. We retrospectively screened 367 cirrhotic patients with variceal bleeding, from which 25 patients were confirmed with CDI, from 1 January 2017 to 31 December 2019. We found MELD to be the only multivariate predictor for mortality (odds ratio, OR = 1.281, 95% confidence interval, CI: 0.098–1.643, $p = 0.042$). A model of four predictors (age, days of admission, Charlson index, Child–Pugh score) was generated (area under the receiver operating characteristics curve, AUC = 0.840, 95% CI: 0.758–0.921, $p < 0.0001$) to assess the risk of CDI exposure. Determining the probability of getting CDI for cirrhotic patients with variceal bleeding could be a tool for doctors in taking decisions, which could be integrated in sustainable public health programs.

Keywords: *Clostridioides difficile*; risk factors; Charlson comorbidity index; Child–Pugh score

Citation: Voicu, M.N.; Popescu, F.; Florescu, D.N.; Rogoveanu, I.; Turcu-Stiolica, A.; Gheonea, D.I.; Iovanescu, V.F.; Iordache, S.; Cazacu, S.M.; Ungureanu, B.S. *Clostridioides difficile* Infection among Cirrhotic Patients with Variceal Bleeding. *Antibiotics* **2021**, *10*, 731. https://doi.org/10.3390/antibiotics10060731

Academic Editor: Guido Granata

Received: 1 May 2021
Accepted: 15 June 2021
Published: 17 June 2021

1. Introduction

Clostridioides difficile infection (CDI) represents the leading cause of nosocomial infection and is associated with high morbidity and mortality as well as increased healthcare costs [1]. A European multicentre study involving 482 hospitals showed a rate of seven cases per 10,000 patients and also revealed a suboptimal laboratory diagnosis in the eastern European countries [2]. While it seems that CDI is shifting towards community spreading, there are still many hospital-acquired cases, especially in patients with comorbidities and if antibiotics are used.

Chronic disease, older age, immunosuppressive and oncologic medication are considered risk factors for patients acquiring hospital CDI [3]. Additionally, the increased use of proton pump inhibitors (PPI) [4] and nonsteroidal anti-inflammatory drugs (NSAID) [5] has been associated with an increase in CDI. Even though any antibiotic may be incriminated for inducing hospital-based infection by disrupting the gut barrier, clindamycin, cephalosporins and fluoroquinolones have been frequently linked to CDI [6]. Liver cirrhosis is the 13th cause of death worldwide, even though the viral aetiology seems to be diminishing [7]. When portal hypertension is present, oesophageal varices will appear and approximately 20% will bleed in the first three years from diagnosis. Despite standard endoscopic therapy for oesophageal varices, some patients will rebleed and other complications may occur either due to portal hypertension or liver insufficiency [8].

Cirrhotic patients are vulnerable to developing CDI infection due to their frequent admission and infections, as well as dysbiosis and a low immune system [9]. Bacterial infection is frequently encountered in cirrhotic patients with variceal bleeding. Both the American Association for the Study of Liver Diseases (AASLD) and the European Association for the Study of the Liver (EASL) recommends the use of ceftriaxone as a prophylaxis for bacterial infection, rebleeding and reduced hospital stay [10,11]. Nonetheless, patients admitted with variceal bleeding have a higher mortality rate and are usually present in an advanced cirrhotic stage with additional possible complications. While the use of ceftriaxone is recommended for 5–7 days, this time, it might be enough for patients to acquire CDI depending on their status.

Additional methods might be required to prevent widespread CDI incidence in cirrhotic patients. Both local and global strategies should ensure new public health actions to consider sustainability in restraining the rate of CDI for vulnerable entities such as cirrhotic patients [12]. Despite the prevalence of CDI among hospitalized patients, few studies assessed the impact of CDI on patients with cirrhosis and variceal bleeding. The aim of our study is to provide an overview on patients with cirrhosis and variceal bleeding, which developed CDI after antibiotic prophylaxis.

2. Materials and Methods

2.1. Study Design

This was a retrospective, single-centre cohort study involving the assessment of information from cirrhotic patient records with or without CDI, who presented to the University County Hospital of Craiova, Romania, from 1 January 2017 to 31 December 2019. All patients signed an informed consent form at the hospital upon admission, conforming to the Declaration of Helsinki, 1967. The study was approved by the University of Medicine and Pharmacy of Craiova Ethics Commission no. 88/2020.

The patients-related variables included demographics, age, alcoholism, comorbidities, previous use of PPI, or antibiotics. Medical history was registered: cardiovascular and pulmonary diseases, diabetes mellitus, chronic renal failure, hepatocellular carcinoma (CHC). The variables related to admission were analysed: Child–Pugh score (total bilirubin, albumin, INR, ascites, encephalopathy), Atlas score (age, systemic antibiotics during CDI therapy, leukocyte count, albumin, creatinine), MELD (dialysis at least twice in the past week, creatinine, bilirubin, INR, sodium), Charlson comorbidity index (age, myocardial infarction, peripheral vascular disease, history of cerebrovascular accident, dementia, COPD, connective tissue disease, peptic ulcer disease, liver disease, diabetes mellitus, hemiplegia, chronic kidney disease, solid tumour, leukaemia, lymphoma, aids), albumin (g/dL), C-reactive protein (CRP, mg/dL), leukocytes (cells/µL), neutrophils (%), erythrocytes (cells/µL), haemoglobin (g/dL), haematocrit (%), platelet count (cells/µL), creatinine (mg/dL), urea (mg/mL), glomerular filtration rate (mL/min/1.73 m^2), Na (mEq/L), K (mEq/L). Costs were also considered in the outcomes' analysis.

2.2. Patient Admission Protocol

We only included patients $\geq$ 18 years old, admitted with variceal bleeding secondary to liver cirrhosis at their first episode. We followed the European Society of Gastrointestinal Endoscopy (ESGE) and American Gastroenterological Association (AGA) guidelines for variceal bleeding with immediate resuscitation, if necessary, terlipressin prescription as well as antibiotic use to prevent bacterial dissemination. Endoscopy was performed as soon as possible, pointing out either oesophageal or gastric varices. Endoscopic signs such as active bleeding, oozing and white nipple are red signs requiring immediate therapy. Band ligation was performed for oesophageal varices and sclerotherapy with n-butyl-2-

cyanoacrylate for gastric varices. According to their status, patients were followed up for the next few days in the intensive care unit (ICU) or in our clinic with medical management. If rebleeding reappeared, another upper endoscopy was performed. All patients received antibiotics (ceftriaxone) according to the European Association for the Study of the Liver (EASL) recommendations [11] before or after endoscopy. Patients were also given lactulose to prevent hepatic encephalopathy.

Patients were excluded if they previously received treatment with metronidazole or vancomycin, had a recent positive test for CDI and had CDI treatment before testing. Additionally, if other antibiotics were used during their hospitalization before CDI positive results, patients were not included. Patients redirected from other hospitals that did not respect our upper gastrointestinal bleeding (UGIB) protocol were not included.

2.3. CDI Diagnosis

Patients developing symptoms 48 h after admission with more than 3 watery stools/per day for two consecutive days associated with abdominal pain were tested for CDI by A/B stool assay. Results were further confirmed by an enzyme immunoassay (EIA) for detecting glutamate dehydrogenase according to the European Society of Clinical Microbiology and Infectious Disease (ESCMID) [13]. We also checked the prescription records for all patients, as well as if other antibiotics were prescribed in the previous months, recent admissions for other conditions. Only one test result was used in this study. Patients received vancomycin or vancomycin +/− metronidazole depending on disease severity and therapeutic response.

2.4. Statistical Analysis

Continuous variables for the study sample were described as using mean and standard deviation or median (interquartile range). Percentages were used to describe the categorical variables. Comparison among groups was conducted with the Mann–Whitney U test for continuous variables and with the chi-square test for categorical variables. We created violin plots to visually compare measured parameters between two groups. Violin plots are like box plots, but also show the probability density of the data at different values. Univariate and multivariate analyses were performed to find the significant independent predictors of mortality. Variables that had a univariate association with overall mortality in CDI patients at p-value < 0.5 were included in the multivariate analysis. The same method was used to identify the risk factors of CDI. Correlogram with hierarchical clustering of covariates was drawn to reveal the best models for predictors of CDI. The Hosmer and Lemeshow test was used to assess how well the model fit with the data (the null hypothesis is that the model is an adequate fit). The 95% confidence interval for the odds ratio was assessed for every predictor. The area under the receiver operating characteristic (AUC) and its 95% CI was used to assess prognostic accuracy for models. A model is considered outstanding if AUC is bigger than 0.9, excellent if AUC is between 0.80 and 0.89, and acceptable if its AUC is between 0.7 and 0.8, and its 95% CI of AUC exceeds 0.7. All results were considered significant at a significance probability below 5%. All data were analysed using the GraphPad Prism 9.1.0 software (GraphPad Software, San Diego, CA, USA) and R *corrplot* and *pROC* packages (version 4.0.3).

3. Results

3.1. Patient Characteristics

A total of 367 patients with cirrhosis were identified during the study period, meeting inclusion criteria. From these patients, 25 patients were confirmed with CDI. The clinical features, comorbidities, and characteristics of patients with CDI are summarized in Table 1. The mean age of cirrhotic patients with CDI was 65.8 years (SD: 8.06 years), and 76% of the patients were male.

Table 1. Demographics and clinical characteristics of the study population.

	Cirrhotic with CDI Patients Mean (±S.D.)/Number of Patients (%) Total *n* = 25
Age (years)	65.8 (±8.06)
Alcohol	20 (80%)
Death (yes)	11 (44%)
Time between admission and CDI diagnosis	4.16 (±1.4)
Viral	
HBV	3 (12%)
HCV	5 (20%)
No	17 (68%)
Hepatic cancer	7 (28%)
ICU	15 (60%)
Atlas score	4.32 (2.3)
PPI	23 (92%)
Rifaximin	5 (20%)
Encephalopathy	20 (80%)
Ascites	25 (100%)
SBP	5 (20%)
CRP (mg/mL)	50.4 (±23.82)
Leukocytes (cells/μL)	15,610.68 (±6900.72)
Neutrophils (%)	79.61 (±9.78)
Erythrocytes (cells/μL)	5305.44 (±6422.44)
Haematocrit (%)	27.61 (±7.67)
Glomerular filtration rate (mL/min/1.73 m^2)	73.42 (±45.55)
Na (mEq/L)	129.96 (±4.84)
K (mEq/L)	4.45 (±0.85)

PPI, proton pump inhibitor; ICU, intensive care unit; SBP, spontaneous bacterial peritonitis; CRP, C-reactive protein.

There were no significant differences in MELD value, the level of haemoglobin, platelets, and urea between patients with CDI and without CDI. The number of the days of admission was higher for patients with CDI (Table 2). The Child–Pugh score was significantly higher for the CDI group ($p < 0.0001$). Patients with cirrhosis and CDI had higher albumin and creatinine level than the patients with cirrhosis, but without CDI. The percentage of deaths was lower in the group of patients without CDI ($n = 87$, 25%) than in the group of patients with CDI ($n = 11$, 44%). Cirrhotic with CDI patients had a significantly higher costs (EUR 1502.45 vs. 998.31, p-value = 0.0006) compared with those without CDI (on an average were 1.5-fold greater). Cirrhotic patients with CDI had a higher Charlson index than cirrhotic patients without CDI (8.64 vs. 6.31, p-value = 0.001).

There was a modest trend for a higher rebleeding rate in patients without CDI at 7% compared with 4% for CDI patients; however, this did not reach the level of statistical significance (p-value = 0.53). There was a statistically significant trend for higher outpatients PPI usage in the patients with CDI at 92% compared with 48% without CDI.

The comparison of the violin plots demonstrated that patients with CDI tended to have a more skewed distribution of Charlson index, Child–Pugh score, costs, creatinine, urea or admission's days than patients without CDI, with their values toward higher values, as shown in Figure 1.

Table 2. Comparison of Cirr+CDI+ and Cirr+CDI−.

Characteristics	Cirr+CDI+ *n* = 25	Cirr+CDI− *n* = 342	*p*-Value
Death (yes)	11 (44%)	89 (25.6%)	0.0446 *
Rebleeding rate	1 (4%)	23 (6.73%)	0.5321
Proton pump inhibitor (yes)	23 (92%)	164 (47.95%)	<0.0001 *
Days admission	14.84 (8.87) 12 (9–19)	8.08 (5.22) 7 (5–10)	<0.0001 *
Child–Pugh score	11.20 (2.14) 12 (9–13)	7.9 (3.83) 9 (7–10)	<0.0001 *
MELD	10.9 (15.64) 8.32 (6.54–9.25)	14.79 (69.35) 8.3 (6.66–10.5)	0.98
Albumin (g/dL)	2.33 (0.52) 2.2 (2–2.65)	2.45 (0.88) 2.6 (2.1–3)	0.013 *
Haemoglobin (g/dL)	8.73 (2.55) 8.8 (7.03–10.15)	13.7 (69.37) 8.09 (6.48–10)	0.368
Platelet count (cells/μL)	136,661.6 (111,271.56) 114,000 (80,500–168,000)	110,425.07 (77,579.62) 93,000 (64,112.5–137,000)	0.095
Creatinine (mg/dL)	1.35 (0.81) 1.1 (0.73–1.88)	0.96 (0.75) 0.74 (0.63–0.92)	0.037 *
Urea (mg/dL)	101.68 (62.79) 110 (44.5–131.5)	64.03 (42.24) 55.5 (36–77)	0.368
Costs (EUR)	1502.45 (1125.94) 1448.47 (558.99–1898.34)	998.31 (1253.4) 618.41 (412.38–1142.08)	0.0006 *
Charlson index	8.64 (3.46) 8.0 (5.50–12.00)	6.31 (1.83) 6.0 (5.0–8.0)	0.001 *

Mean (S.D.) and median (interquartile range) for continuous variables; *n* (percentage) for categorical variables; MELD, Model for End-Stage Liver Disease; Cirr+CDI+, cirrhotic with CDI patients; Cirr+CDI−, cirrhotic without CDI patients; *, *p*-value < 0.05.

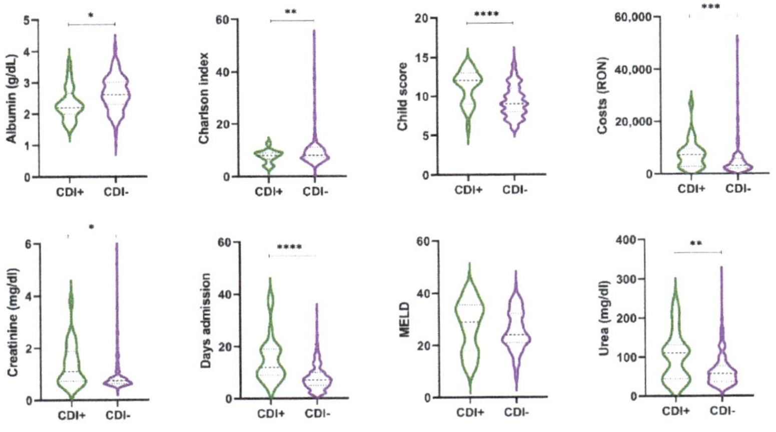

Figure 1. Violin plots showing the expression distribution of values of variables between Cirr+CDI+ and Cirr+CDI− patients. *, *p*-value < 0.05; **, *p*-value < 0.01; ***, *p*-value < 0.001; ****, *p*-value < 0.0001.

3.2. Factors Associated with Mortality in Cirrhotic Patients with CDI

As shown in Table 3, univariate predictors of mortality for the cirrhosis and CDI patients included Child–Pugh score (*p*-value = 0.026), leukocytes (*p*-value = 0.023), CRP (*p*-value = 0.012), Atlas score (*p*-value = 0.011) and MELD (*p*-value = 0.022).

Table 3. Univariate regression to explore factors associated with mortality.

Factors	COR	95%CI	*p*-Value
Age	1.03	0.929–1.142	0.57
Days admission	0.919	0.816–1.035	0.163
Child–Pugh score	3.787	1.174–12.208	0.026 *
Alcohol (yes)	2.25	0.304–16.632	0.427
Virala			
HBV	0.364	0.047–2.817	0.333
HCV	1.333	0.067–26.618	0.851
Diabetes (yes)	2.0	0.366–10.919	0.423
Hepatic cancer (yes)	5.0	0.74–33.777	0.099
Rifaximin (yes)	7.429	0.69–79.957	0.098
HDS (yes)	0.205	0.018–2.327	0.201
SBP (yes)	4.875	0.43–55.292	0.201
Proton pump inhibitor (yes)	0.00	-	0.99
Albumin (g/dL)	0.167	0.021–1.315	0.089
Platelet (cells/μL)	1	1–1	0.413
Leukocytes (cells/μL)	1	1–1.001	0.023 *
CRP	1.139	1.029–1.261	0.012 *
Atlas	4.22	1.387–12.837	0.011 *
MELD	1.48	1.058–2.07	0.022 *
Charlson index	63.32	0.0–96.1	0.996

COR, crude odds ratio; PPI, proton pump inhibitor; ICU, intensive care unit; SBP, spontaneous bacterial peritonitis; MELD, model for end-stage liver disease; *, $p < 0.05$, statistically significant.

According to the multivariate model, MELD is a predictor of mortality for patients with cirrhosis and CDI (Table 4). The logistic regression model was statistically significant, $\chi^2(6) = 7.21$, $p = 0.032$. The model explained 74.5% (Nagelkerke R^2) of the variance in mortality and correct classified 96% of cases. Increasing MELD was associated with an increase in the likelihood of mortality.

Table 4. Multivariate regression to explore factors associated with mortality.

Factors	AOR	95%CI	*p*-Value
Child–Pugh score	1.409	0.883–2.25	0.787
Liver cancer (yes)	14.082	0.245–89.231	0.201
Rifaximin (yes)	10.039	0.005–19.27	0.55
Leukocytes	1.0	1.0–1.001	0.147
CRP	1.016	0.032–31.933	0.993
Atlas	3.704	0.622–22.072	0.15
MELD	1.281	0.098–1.643	0.042 *

AOR, adjusted odds ratio; MELD, model for end-stage liver disease; *, $p < 0.05$, statistically significant.

3.3. Risk Factors Associated with CDI in Cirrhotic Patients with Variceal Bleeding

Table 5 summarize the results of the univariate analysis to describe the risk factors associated with CDI. Higher age (OR = 1.062; 95% CI: 1.017–1.109), higher length of hospital admission (OR = 1.115; 95% CI: 1.062–1.171), liver cancer (OR = 3.173; 95% CI: 1.245–8.087), the use of proton pump inhibitor (OR = 12.902; 95% CI: 2.995–55.566), higher level of urea (OR = 1.013; 95% CI: 1.006–1.020) and a higher Charlson index (OR = 1.609; 95% CI: 1.33–1.947) were the risk factors for CDI during the hospitalization.

Table 5. Univariate regression to explore factors associated with CDI.

Factors	COR	95%CI	*p*-Value
Age	1.062	1.017–1.109	0.006 *
Days admission	1.115	1.062–1.171	<0.0001 *
Child–Pugh score	1.543	1.262–1.887	<0.0001 *
Alcohol (yes)	1.5	0.52–4.3	0.451
Hepatic cancer (yes)	3.173	1.245–8.087	0.016 *
Creatinine	1.376	1.0–1.892	0.050
Urea	1.013	1.006–1.020	<0.0001 *
Proton pump inhibitor (yes)	12.902	2.996–55.566	0.001 *
Charlson index	1.609	1.330–1.947	<0.0001 *

COR, crude odds ratio; *, $p < 0.05$, statistically significant.

Multivariate analysis showed that a higher age (OR = 1.067; 95% CI: 1.004–1.134), longer hospital stay (OR = 1.159; 95% CI: 1.086–1.238), higher level of urea (OR = 1.013; 95% CI: 1.002–1.023), higher Charlson index (OR = 1.671; 95% CI: 1.326–2.106) and the use of proton pump inhibitor (OR = 23.015; 95% CI: 4.311–52.854) were risk factors for CDI in cirrhotic patients (Table 6).

Table 6. Multivariate regression to explore factors associated with CDI.

Factors	AOR	95%CI	*p*-Value
Age	1.067	1.004–1.134	0.037 *
Days admission	1.159	1.086–1.238	<0.0001 ****
Child–Pugh score	1.224	0.916–1.636	0.171
Liver cancer (yes)	2.829	0.81–9.879	0.103
Creatinine	0.784	0.305–2.016	0.614
Urea	1.013	1.002–1.023	0.020 *
Proton pump inhibitor (yes)	23.015	4.311–52.854	<0.0001 ****
Charlson index	1.671	1.326–2.106	<0.0001 ****

AOR, adjusted odds ratio; *, $p < 0.05$; ****, *p*-value < 0.0001, statistically significant.

The correlation values in the Spearman correlation matrix ordered by hierarchical clustering and visualized by correlogram (Figure 2) identified two clusters, which will be assessed as Model 1 (age, days of admission, Charlson index, Child–Pugh score) and Model 2 (HCC, PPI, creatinine, urea). The highest positively correlated parameters seen in the correlogram were Charlson with age (r = 0.47, *p*-value < 0.05), Child–Pugh score with PPI (r = 0.55, *p*-value < 0.05), and creatinine with urea (r = 0.64, *p*-value < 0.05).

The accuracy of the two models, evaluated by AUC, as in Figure 3, suggested Model 1 (covariates age, days of submission, Charlson index, Child–Pugh score) being the best to predict CDI in cirrhotic patients with variceal bleeding. According to our results, the probability p of developing CDI after antibiotic prophylaxis could be assessed with the formula as in Equation (1):

$$\log\left(\frac{p}{1-p}\right) = -14.884 + 0.067 \times \text{Age} + 0.122 \times \text{DaysAdm} + 0.281 \times \text{Charlson} + 0.463 \times \text{ChildScore} \quad (1)$$

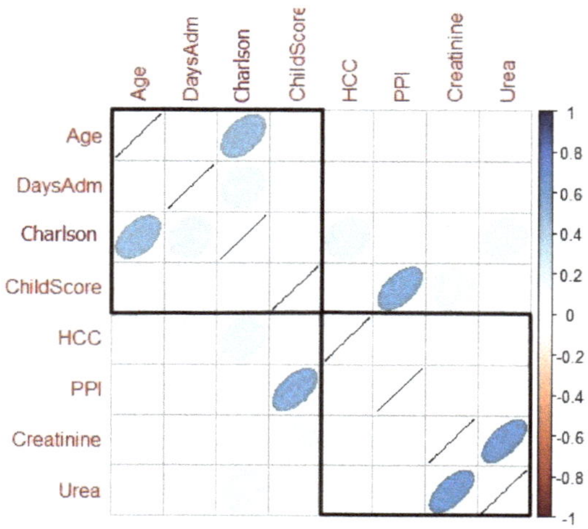

Figure 2. Correlogram with a hierarchical clustering of covariates included in the logistic regression analysis. Positive correlations are displayed in blue and negative correlations in red. Colour intensity and the size of the ellipse are proportional to the correlation coefficients.

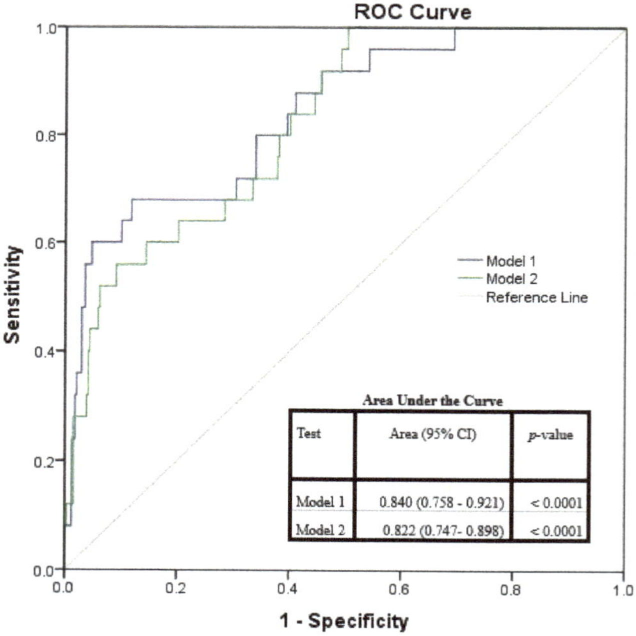

Figure 3. The ROC curves for Model 1 and Model 2. The ROC of a perfect predictive model has sensibility (true positive rate) equal to 1 and 1-specificity (false positive rate) equal to 0.

4. Discussion

As the most frequent hospital-associated infection, CDI will presumably first target chronic patients, which also tend to be more susceptible to bacterial infection. However, the healthcare systems are all aware of this potential threat, as CDI should have been discussed at a rather global scale since it has also shifted to community onset [14]. The environment stands as a high-ground factor in disease evolution, namely because of asymptomatic colonization as well as spore-resistant circumstances within medical care systems, which will eventually lead to new virulent strains [15]. Thus, first focusing on a targeted group of patients who require specific antibiotics might help restrain morbidity and health costs and enable new approaches to prevent widespread infection.

Antibiotic exposure represents the highest risk for CDI, with the most common agents represented by the second and third generation of cephalosporins [16]. Depending on the patient status, even a brief exposure may be incriminated for CDI appearance. Our study focused on a specific group of cirrhotic patients who presented with variceal bleeding, pointing out a 7.20% development of CDI after ceftriaxone administration in order to prevent bacterial translocation. In addition to antibiotic prophylaxis, patients suffering from advanced chronic liver disease are at risk of acquiring nosocomial infections due to their recurrent need for hospitalizations and the additional complications they develop over time [17]. Moreover, cirrhosis may lead to an impaired local gut immune response with a low motility level which may cause bacterial overgrowth, thus hampering the CDI exposure [18].

Variceal bleeding is a major complication of cirrhosis and portal hypertension with high mortality, ranging from 15 to 20% [19]. Available guidelines suggest the use of cephalosporines for antibiotic prophylaxis for patients admitted with variceal bleeding [10,11]. Cirrhotic patients have an increased risk for bacterial infection due to increased intestinal permeability, immune dysfunction and bacterial translocation [20]. The recommendation is to use antibiotics as soon as possible, since the bacterial infection may lead to a high mortality rate. The main choice remains ceftriaxone 1 g/24 h for up to seven days followed by norfloxacin 400 mg if patients do not have advanced liver disease [11]. Antibiotic use was proved to be efficient and to decrease early bacterial infection in cirrhotic patients [21]. However, the use of antibiotics on cirrhotic patients and the potential hospital-acquired infection is not extensively discussed. Only one study analysed the CDI relevance after antibiotic administration [22]. However, the results are rather doubtable since they used metronidazole, which is not actually indicated for variceal bleeding infection risk, but also included in the CDI management.

While all antibiotics may be incriminated for hospital-related CDI, some antimicrobial agents are known to associate a higher risk than others such as fluorochinolones, cephalosporins, carbapenems and clindamycin [23]. Ceftriaxone, a third generation cephalosporine, is commonly used for bacterial prevention in patients with variceal bleeding. However, since its elimination occurs through the biliary system, the bile concentration of antibiotic will be higher within the gut, which may cause a dysbiosis in the microbiota [24].

PPIs are frequently prescribed in patients with cirrhosis, even though their indication is limited to gastroduodenal ulcers or after band ligation. Their benefit outside these causes is controversial, and their long-term use has been linked to cirrhosis complications such as spontaneous bacterial peritonitis and hepatic encephalopathy [25]. PPI influence on CDI development has been well documented. Several meta-analyses concluded that their use may foster CDI appearance, thus promoting them as an independent risk factor [26–29]. Several theories were suggested, mainly based on the PPI's effect with acid suppression [30] and gene expression decrease, which maintain the colonocyte integrity [31] or by decreasing microbial diversity [32]. While histamine-2-receptor antagonists may be less harmful, the use of PPI along with antibiotics may enhance the risk of CDI [33]. Our study confirms that PPI might influence CDI development since patients were on a long-term therapy.

Our first objective was to highlight possible risk factors that may lead to CDI. We identified that older patients, longer admission, urea, higher Charlson index, liver cancer and PPI may influence CDI appearance. Thus, our results are similar with other studies which assessed CDI and cirrhosis. Furthermore, we tried to develop a patient profile to statistically identify a model that might help differentiate high risk patients. By hierarchical clustering, we identified two models that suggested what patients might be more predisposed to develop CDI. While Model 2 consisted of HCC, PPI, creatinine and urea, the best prediction model seemed to correspond to Model 1 which followed age, days of admission, Charlson index and the Child–Pugh score. Nevertheless, this might enhance awareness when antibiotics are used for cirrhotic patients with variceal bleeding and also help identify early additional complications. Hence, the medical system will also benefit, since this tool will help in early decision making and integrate it in sustainable public health programs through economic and environmental domains. The CDI risk tool will be helpful and might be embedded in the local protocols and decision-making process.

CDI is known to prolong admission, and consecutively raises the health costs [9]. This was also observed in our study, with patients with CDI having significantly higher costs than the ones without CDI. This provides an additional burden to the healthcare system increasing hospital charges. Bajaj et al. [34] reported that patients with cirrhosis and CDI have a 2.2-fold greater costs than those without CDI. A strategy was proposed by Saab et al. [35] who tried to implement a screening strategy to reduce healthcare costs. They concluded that patients with cirrhosis might require screening regarding their symptoms, and consecutively, the cost will be reduced at least four times compared with patients without CDI.

Mortality in CDI patients might be related to age, albumin levels, leukocytes count and renal failure [36]. Several studies identified risk factors associated with mortality in cirrhotic patients, which acquired CDI [37–39]. While ICU admission and albumin were recognized as predictors of short-term mortality, we identified some risk factors related to CDI severity, such as leukocytes, CRP and Atlas score, and to the liver disease—mainly Child–Pugh score and MELD. Malignancy has also been reported to increase death rate; however, our patients with HCC with associated CDI did not have a worse prognosis than other CDI patients. Hong et al. [40] obtained a hazard ratio of 1.06 ± 0.02 for the MELD score, suggesting a 21.5% increase in mortality in CDI patients and concluding that this is the only reliable short-term mortality predictor. Our analysis also recognized the MELD score as the most reliable predictor of mortality and its increase was associated with the likelihood of mortality.

A major concern for CDI exposure should now be acknowledged along with the COVID-19 pandemic. Its impact on the healthcare system should not be considered only in the short term by affecting patient's status, medical workers [41] and the fact that some diseases might be neglected but also in the long-run by the use of specific medication and their effect on patients [42]. However, at first, the CDI rate might be on a lower trend, due to increase hand hygiene and contact precautions, but most of all due to extensive cleaning and general disinfection, along with more patients which develop severe disease, as antibiotics will be used more frequently to prevent additional bacterial pulmonary infection [43,44].

Extensive measures should be considered for dedicated patients with known risk factors when antibiotics are used. Preventing a possible CDI infection might be challenging in cirrhotic patients which require antibiotics, however, if a better knowledge of hand hygiene for both patients and medical staff is instated within hospital policies, it might prevent disease spread [45,46]. Nevertheless, isolating patients, chemical disinfection agents as well as glove use on CDI patients should be considered as infection control measures to limit other cases appearance [47].

Thus, new CDI policies on awareness should be developed and identifying a patient profile might ease day-to-day practice and decrease morbidity and healthcare costs, at least in our group of patients.

Several limitations should be considered in our study. First of all, this was a single-centre retrospective study, using a small number of CDI patients, thus, when compared to other dedicated institutions, results may differ. However, we tried to minimize potential errors by limiting to a specific set of patients and a specific antibiotic. Therapy consisted in vancomycin and vancomycin +/− metronidazole, but with no follow up in all patients for 14 days and also with no data included regarding recurrence rate. We also did not include data about CDI strains and long-term mortality. Moreover, the recurrence rate of CDI was not taken into account since we focused on the first diagnosis, risk factors and early mortality.

5. Conclusions

CDI infection should be considered whenever ceftriaxone is used to prevent bacterial infection after variceal bleeding and identifying the patients with a higher risk will have an impact on morbidity and on the healthcare system. Our model consisting of age, days of admission, Child–Pugh score and Charlson index could predict CDI development in cirrhotic patients with variceal bleeding following ceftriaxone. Furthermore, multicentre studies should be implemented to validate our results.

Author Contributions: Conceptualization, M.N.V., I.R. and B.S.U.; methodology, I.R., D.I.G. and B.S.U.; software, A.T.-S.; validation, F.P., D.N.F., V.F.I., S.I. and S.M.C.; formal analysis, A.T.-S., D.I.G. and B.S.U.; data curation, D.N.F., V.F.I. and S.M.C.; writing—original draft preparation, M.N.V., A.T.-S. and B.S.U.; writing—review and editing, I.R.; supervision, B.S.U. All authors have read and agreed to the published version of the manuscript.

Funding: This research received no external funding.

Institutional Review Board Statement: The study was conducted according to the guidelines of the Declaration of Helsinki and approved by the University of Medicine and Pharmacy of Craiova Ethics Commission no. 88/2020.

Informed Consent Statement: Informed consent was obtained from all subjects involved in the study.

Data Availability Statement: Data supporting the results of this study are available from the corresponding author on request.

Conflicts of Interest: The authors declare no conflict of interest.

References

1. Eberly, M.D.; Susi, A.; Adams, D.J.; Love, C.S.; Nylund, C.M. Epidemiology and outcomes of patients with healthcare facility-onset clostridioides difficile infection. *Mil. Med.* **2021**, usab116. [CrossRef]
2. Davies, K.A.; Longshaw, C.M.; Davis, G.L.; Bouza, E.; Barbut, F.; Barna, Z.; Delmee, M.; Fitzpatrick, F.; Ivanova, K.; Kuijper, E.; et al. Underdiagnosis of Clostridium difficile across Europe: The European, multicentre, prospective, biannual, point-prevalence study of Clostridium difficile infection in hospitalized patients with diarrhoea (EUCLID). *Lancet Infect. Dis.* **2014**, *14*, 1208–1219. [CrossRef]
3. Bowman, A.J.; Utter, H.G. Evolving strategies to manage clostridium difficile colitis. *J. Gastrointest. Surg.* **2020**, *24*, 484–491. [CrossRef] [PubMed]
4. Cao, F.; Chen, C.X.; Wang, M.; Liao, H.R.; Wang, M.X.; Hua, S.Z.; Huang, B.; Xiong, Y.; Zhang, J.Y.; Xu, Y.L. Updated meta-analysis of controlled observational studies: Proton-pump inhibitors and risk of Clostridium difficile infection. *J. Hosp. Infect.* **2018**, *98*, 4–13. [CrossRef] [PubMed]
5. Maseda, D.; Zackular, J.P.; Trindade, B.; Kirk, L.; Roxas, J.L.; Rogers, L.M.; Washington, M.K.; Du, L.; Koyama, T.; Viswanathan, V.K.; et al. Nonsteroidal anti-inflammatory drugs alter the microbiota and exacerbate Clostridium difficile colitis while dysregulating the inflammatory response. *mBio* **2019**, *10*, e02282-18. [CrossRef] [PubMed]
6. Mendo-Lopez, R.; Villafuerte-Gálvez, J.; White, N.; Mahoney, M.V.; Kelly, C.P.; Alonso, C.D. Recent developments in the management of recurrent Clostridioides difficile infection. *Anaerobe* **2020**, *62*, 102108. [CrossRef] [PubMed]
7. Lesmana, C.R.A.; Raharjo, M.; Gani, R.A. Managing liver cirrhotic complications: Overview of esophageal and gastric varices. *Clin. Mol. Hepatol.* **2020**, *26*, 444–460. [CrossRef]
8. Plaz Torres, M.C.; Best, L.M.; Freeman, S.C.; Roberts, D.; Cooper, N.J.; Sutton, A.J.; Roccarina, D.; Benmassaoud, A.; Iogna Prat, L.; Williams, N.R.; et al. Secondary prevention of variceal bleeding in adults with previous oesophageal variceal bleeding due to decompensated liver cirrhosis: A network meta-analysis. *Cochrane Database Syst. Rev.* **2021**, *3*, CD013122.
9. Trifan, A.; Stoica, O.; Stanciu, C.; Cojocariu, C.; Singeap, A.M.; Girleanu, I.; Miftode, E. Clostridium difficile infection in patients with liver disease: A review. *Eur. J. Clin. Microbiol. Infect. Dis.* **2015**, *34*, 2313–2324. [CrossRef]
10. Garcia-Tsao, G.; Abraldes, J.G.; Berzigotti, A.; Bosch, J. Portal hypertensive bleeding in cirrhosis: Risk stratification, diagnosis, and management: 2016 practice guidance by the American Association for the study of liver diseases. *Hepatology* **2017**, *65*, 310–335. [CrossRef]

11. European Association for the Study of the Liver. EASL Clinical Practice Guidelines for the management of patients with decompensated cirrhosis. *J. Hepatol.* **2018**, *69*, 406–460. [CrossRef] [PubMed]
12. Negrut, N.; Nistor-Cseppento, D.C.; Khan, S.A.; Pantis, C.; Maghiar, T.A.; Maghiar, O.; Aleya, S.; Rus, M.; Tit, D.M.; Aleya, L.; et al. Clostridium difficile Infection Epidemiology over a Period of 8 Years—A Single Centre Study. *Sustainability* **2020**, *12*, 4439. [CrossRef]
13. Tschudin-Sutter, S.; Kuijper, E.J.; Durovic, A.; Vehreschild, M.J.G.T.; Barbut, F.; Eckert, C.; Fitzpatrick, F.; Hell, M.; Norèn, T.; O'Driscoll, J.; et al. Guidance document for prevention of Clostridium difficile infection in acute healthcare settings. *Clin. Microbiol. Infect.* **2018**, *24*, 1051–1054. [CrossRef] [PubMed]
14. Adelman, M.W.; Goodenough, D.; Sefton, S.; Mackey, C.; Thomas, S.; Fridkin, S.K.; Woodworth, M.H. Changes in treatment of community-onset Clostridioides difficile infection after release of updated guidelines, Atlanta, Georgia, 2018. *Anaerobe* **2021**, *13*, 102364.
15. Skinner, A.M.; Phillips, S.T.; Merrigan, M.M.; O'Leary, K.J.; Sambol, S.P.; Siddiqui, F.; Peterson, L.R.; Gerding, D.N.; Johnson, S. The Relative Role of Toxins A and B in the Virulence of Clotridioides difficile. *J. Clin. Med.* **2020**, *10*, 96. [CrossRef]
16. Wilcox, M.H.; Chalmers, J.D.; Nord, C.E.; Freeman, J.; Bouza, E. Role of cephalosporins in the era of Clostridium difficile infection. *J. Antimicrob. Chemother.* **2017**, *72*, 1–18. [CrossRef]
17. Abdalla, A.O.; Pisipati, S.; Elnaggar, M.; Rishi, M.; Doshi, R.; Gullapalli, N. Outcomes of Clostridioides difficile Infection in Patients with Liver Cirrhosis: A Nationwide Study. *Gastroenterol. Res.* **2020**, *13*, 53–57. [CrossRef]
18. Rosenblatt, R.; Mehta, A.; Cohen-Mekelburg, S.; Shen, N.; Snell, D.; Lucero, C.; Jesudian, A.; Fortune, B.; Crawford, C.V.; Kumar, S. The rise of Clostridioides difficile infections and fall of associated mortality in hospitalized advanced cirrhotics. *Liver Int.* **2019**, *39*, 1263–1270. [CrossRef]
19. Roberts, D.; Best, L.M.; Freeman, S.C.; Sutton, A.J.; Cooper, N.J.; Arunan, S.; Begum, T.; Williams, N.R.; Walshaw, D.; Milne, E.J.; et al. Treatment for bleeding oesophageal varices in people with decompensated liver cirrhosis: A network meta-analysis. *Cochrane Database Syst. Rev.* **2021**, *1*, CD013155. [CrossRef]
20. Tandon, P.; Garcia-Tsao, G. Bacterial infections, sepsis, and multiorgan failure in cirrhosis. *Semin. Liver Dis.* **2008**, *28*, 26–42. [CrossRef]
21. Soares-Weiser, K.; Brezis, M.; Tur-Kaspa, R.; Leibovici, L. Antibiotic prophylaxis for cirrhotic patients with gastrointestinal bleeding. *Cochrane Database Syst. Rev.* **2002**, *2*, CD002907.
22. Brown, M.R.; Jones, G.; Nash, K.L.; Wright, M.; Guha, I.N. Antibiotic prophylaxis in variceal hemorrhage: Timing, effectiveness and Clostridium difficile rates. *World J. Gastroenterol.* **2010**, *16*, 5317–5323. [CrossRef]
23. Slimings, C.; Riley, T.V. Antibiotics and hospital-acquired Clostridium difficile infection: Update of systematic review and meta-analysis. *J. Antimicrob. Chemother.* **2014**, *69*, 881–891. [CrossRef]
24. Brogard, J.M.; Blickle, J.F.; Jehl, F.; Arnaud, J.P.; Paris-Bockel, D.; Monteil, H. High biliary elimination of ceftriaxone in man. *Int. J. Clin. Pharmacol. Ther. Toxicol.* **1988**, *26*, 167–172.
25. Chavez-Tapia, N.C.; Tellez-Avila, F.I.; Garcia-Leiva, J.; Valdovinos, M.A. Use and overuse of proton pump inhibitors in cirrhotic patients. *Med. Sci. Monit.* **2008**, *14*, CR468–CR472.
26. Khan, M.A.; Kamal, S.; Khan, S.; Lee, W.M.; Howden, C.W. Systematic review and meta-analysis of the possible association between pharmacological gastric acid suppression and spontaneous bacterial peritonitis. *Eur. J. Gastroenterol. Hepatol.* **2015**, *27*, 1327–1336. [CrossRef]
27. Trifan, A.; Stanciu, C.; Girleanu, I.; Stoica, O.C.; Singeap, A.M.; Maxim, R.; Chiruac, S.A.; Ciobica, A.; Boiculese, L. Proton pump inhibitors therapy and risk of Clostridium difficile infection: Systematic review and meta-analysis. *World J. Gastroenterol.* **2017**, *23*, 6500–6515. [CrossRef]
28. Wu, X.; Zhang, D.; Yu, Y.; Lou, L.; Li, X. Proton pump inhibitor use and mortality in patients with cirrhosis: A meta-analysis of cohort studies. *Biosci. Rep.* **2020**, *40*, BSR20193890. [CrossRef]
29. Wang, J.; Wu, Y.; Bi, Q.; Zheng, X.; Zhang, J.; Huang, W. Adverse outcomes of proton pump inhibitors in chronic liver disease: A systematic review and meta-analysis. *Hepatol. Int.* **2020**, *14*, 385–398. [CrossRef]
30. Howell, M.D.; Novack, V.; Grgurich, P.; Soulliard, D.; Novack, L.; Pencina, M.; Talmor, D. Iatrogenic gastric acid suppression and the risk of nosocomial Clostridium difficile infection. *Arch. Intern. Med.* **2010**, *170*, 784–790. [CrossRef]
31. Hegarty, J.P.; Sangster, W.; Harris, L.R., 3rd; Stewart, D.B. Proton pump inhibitors induce changes in colonocyte gene expression that may affect Clostridium difficile infection. *Surgery* **2014**, *156*, 972–978. [CrossRef] [PubMed]
32. Seto, C.T.; Jeraldo, P.; Orenstein, R.; Chia, N.; DiBaise, J.K. Prolonged use of a proton pump inhibitor reduces microbial diversity: Implications for Clostridium difficile susceptibility. *Microbiome* **2014**, *2*, 42. [CrossRef] [PubMed]
33. Kwok, C.S.; Arthur, A.K.; Anibueze, C.I.; Singh, S.; Cavallazzi, R.; Loke, Y.K. Risk of Clostridium difficile infection with acid suppressing drugs and antibiotics: Meta-analysis. *Am. J. Gastroenterol.* **2012**, *107*, 1011–1019. [CrossRef] [PubMed]
34. Bajaj, J.S.; Ananthakrishnan, A.N.; Hafeezullah, M.; Zadvornova, Y.; Dye, A.; McGinley, E.L.; Saeian, K.; Heuman, D.; Sanyal, A.J.; Hoffmann, R.G. Clostridium difficile is associated with poor outcomes in patients with cirrhosis: A national and tertiary center perspective. *Am. J. Gastroenterol.* **2010**, *105*, 106–113. [CrossRef]
35. Saab, S.; Alper, T.; Sernas, E.; Pruthi, P.; Alper, M.A.; Sundaram, V. Hospitalized Patients with Cirrhosis Should Be Screened for Clostridium difficile Colitis. *Dig. Dis. Sci.* **2015**, *60*, 3124–3129. [CrossRef]

36. Sbeit, W.; Kadah, A.; Shahin, A.; Abed, N.; Haddad, H.; Jabbour, A.; Said Ahmad, H.; Pellicano, R.; Khoury, T.; Mari, A. Predictors of in-hospital mortality among patients with clostridium difficile infection: A multicenter study. *Minerva Med.* **2021**, *112*, 124–129. [CrossRef]
37. Bednarska, A.; Bursa, D.; Podlasin, R.; Paciorek, M.; Skrzat-Klapaczyńska, A.; Porowski, D.; Raczyńska, J.; Puła, J.; Krogulec, D.; Makowiecki, M.; et al. Advanced age and increased CRP concentration are independent risk factors associated with Clostridioides difficile infection mortality. *Sci. Rep.* **2020**, *10*, 14681. [CrossRef]
38. Kruger, A.J.; Durkin, C.; Mumtaz, K.; Hinton, A.; Krishna, S.G. Early Readmission Predicts Increased Mortality in Cirrhosis Patients after Clostridium difficile Infection. *J. Clin. Gastroenterol.* **2019**, *53*, e322–e327. [CrossRef]
39. Czepiel, J.; Krutova, M.; Mizrahi, A.; Khanafer, N.; Enoch, D.A.; Patyi, M.; Deptuła, A.; Agodi, A.; Nuvials, X.; Pituch, H.; et al. Mortality Following Clostridioides difficile Infection in Europe: A Retrospective Multicenter Case-Control Study. *Antibiotics* **2021**, *10*, 299. [CrossRef]
40. Hong, S.J.; Feuerstadt, P.; Brandt, L.J. MELD is the only predictor of short-term mortality in cirrhotic patients with C. difficile infection. *Dig. Liver Dis.* **2019**, *51*, 275–280. [CrossRef]
41. Ungureanu, B.S.; Vladut, C.; Bende, F.; Sandru, V.; Tocia, C.; Turcu-Stiolica, R.A.; Groza, A.; Balan, G.G.; Turcu-Stiolica, A. Impact of the COVID-19 Pandemic on Health-Related Quality of Life, Anxiety, and Training among Young Gastroenterologists in Romania. *Front. Psychol.* **2020**, *11*, 579177. [CrossRef]
42. Spigaglia, P. Clostridioides difficile infection in the COVID-19 era: Old and new problems. *Pol. Arch. Intern. Med.* **2021**, *131*, 118–120. [CrossRef]
43. Hazel, K.; Skally, M.; Glynn, E.; Foley, M.; Burns, K.; O'Toole, A.; Boland, K.; Fitzpatrick, F. The other 'C': Hospital-acquired Clostridioides difficile infection during the coronavirus disease 2019 (COVID-19) pandemic. *Infect. Control Hosp. Epidemiol.* **2021**. [CrossRef]
44. Ochoa-Hein, E.; Rajme-López, S.; Rodríguez-Aldama, J.C.; Huertas-Jiménez, M.A.; Chávez-Ríos, A.R.; de Paz-García, R.; Haro-Osnaya, A.; González-Colín, K.K.; González-González, R.; González-Lara, M.F.; et al. Substantial reduction of healthcare facility-onset Clostridioides difficile infection (HO-CDI) rates after conversion of a hospital for exclusive treatment of COVID-19 patients. *Am. J. Infect. Control* **2020**. [CrossRef]
45. Kabała, M.; Aptekorz, M.; Martirosian, G. Rola środowiska szpitalnego i rąk personelu medycznego w szerzeniu się zakażeń Clostridioides (Clostridium) difficile [The role of hospital environment and the hands of medical staff in the transmission of the Clostridioides (Clostridium) difficile infection]. *Med. Pract.* **2019**, *70*, 739–745. (In Polish)
46. Ragusa, R.; Giorgianni, G.; Lupo, L.; Sciacca, A.; Rametta, S.; La Verde, M.; Mulè, S.; Marranzano, M. Healthcare-associated Clostridium difficile infection: Role of correct hand hygiene in cross-infection control. *J. Prev. Med. Hyg.* **2018**, *59*, E145–E152.
47. Marra, A.R.; Perencevich, E.N.; Nelson, R.E.; Samore, M.; Khader, K.; Chiang, H.Y.; Chorazy, M.L.; Herwaldt, L.A.; Diekema, D.J.; Kuxhausen, M.F.; et al. Incidence and Outcomes Associated With Clostridium difficile Infections: A Systematic Review and Meta-analysis. *JAMA Netw. Open* **2020**, *3*, e1917597. [CrossRef]

antibiotics

MDPI

Article

Nonalcoholic Fatty Liver Disease—A Novel Risk Factor for Recurrent *Clostridioides difficile* Infection

Lara Šamadan [1], Mia Jeličić [2], Adriana Vince [1,2] and Neven Papić [1,2,*]

1 School of Medicine, University of Zagreb, 10000 Zagreb, Croatia; lsamadan@mef.hr (L.Š.); avince@bfm.hr (A.V.)
2 University Hospital for Infectious Diseases, 10000 Zagreb, Croatia; majdukovic@bfm.hr
* Correspondence: npapic@bfm.hr

Abstract: Recurrent *Clostridioides difficile* infections (rCDI) have a substantial impact on healthcare systems, with limited and often expensive therapeutic options. Nonalcoholic fatty liver disease (NAFLD) affects about 25% of the adult population and is associated with metabolic syndrome, changes in gut microbiome and bile acids biosynthesis, all possibly related with rCDI. The aim of this study was to determine whether NAFLD is a risk factor associated with rCDI. A retrospective cohort study included patients ≥ 60 years hospitalized with CDI. The cohort was divided into two groups: those who were and were not readmitted with CDI within 3 months of discharge. Of the 329 patients included, 107 patients (32.5%) experienced rCDI. Patients with rCDI were older, had higher Charlson Age–Comorbidity Index (CACI) and were more frequently hospitalized within 3 months. Except for chronic kidney disease and NAFLD, which were more frequent in the rCDI group, there were no differences in other comorbidities, antibiotic classes used and duration of antimicrobial therapy. Multivariable Cox regression analysis showed that age >75 years, NAFLD, CACI >6, chronic kidney disease, statins and immobility were associated with rCDI. In conclusion, our study identified NAFLD as a possible new host-related risk factor associated with rCDI.

Keywords: *Clostridioides difficile* associated disease; CDI; nonalcoholic fatty liver disease; NAFLD; NASH; recurrent disease

Citation: Šamadan, L.; Jeličić, M.; Vince, A.; Papić, N. Nonalcoholic Fatty Liver Disease—A Novel Risk Factor for Recurrent *Clostridioides difficile* Infection. *Antibiotics* **2021**, *10*, 780. https://doi.org/10.3390/antibiotics10070780

Academic Editor: Guido Granata

Received: 14 May 2021
Accepted: 25 June 2021
Published: 27 June 2021

1. Introduction

Clostridioides difficile infection (CDI), with increasing prevalence and mortality rates, is the leading cause of healthcare-associated diarrhea [1]. On hospital admission, 7% of patients are already colonized with *C. difficile* and another 21% become infected during hospitalization [2]. Furthermore, 20 to 30% of patients will develop symptomatic CDI recurrence within 2 weeks of completion of accurate therapy, and each episode increases the risk of future episodes by about 20% [3,4]. Therefore, recurrent *C. difficile* infections (rCDI) cause substantial impact on healthcare systems with limited and often expensive therapeutic options [5]. This requires identification of patients at high risk of rCDI. So far, major risk factors suggested to be associated with rCDI were age, use of antibiotics for non-*C. difficile* infection, gastric acid suppression and infection with a hypervirulent strain (NAP1/BI/027) [5]. Age is the most frequently reported risk factor for rCDI; the probability of rCDI is 27% in the age group between 18 and 64 and 58.4% in patients older than 65 years [4,6]. However, the literature data on other host risk factors are inconsistent and often contradictory. Severe underlying comorbidities, chronic renal disease, CDI severity, prolonged hospital stay, and nursing home residency were inconsistently reported as additional risk factors [5–8]. Recently, it was suggested that metabolic syndrome and its components, primarily obesity and diabetes mellitus (DM), might be associated with rCDI [8,9]. Metabolic syndrome is linked with changes in gut microbiome that might serve as protective intestinal flora for *C. difficile* germination and disease development [10].

Nonalcoholic fatty liver disease (NAFLD) is the most common chronic liver disease, affecting about 25% of the adult Western population [11,12]. NAFLD represents a spectrum of chronic liver pathologies, from simple steatosis to nonalcoholic steatohepatitis, cirrhosis, and hepatocellular carcinoma [11,12]. There is a close relationship between NAFLD and metabolic syndrome, clustering visceral overweight, dyslipidemia, insulin resistance and arterial hypertension [11–13]. Some consider NAFLD as the hepatic manifestation of metabolic syndrome. Importantly, it is well described that changes in the gut microbiome promote the development of NAFLD through inflammatory processes, insulin resistance and bile acids metabolism, all possibly related with increased susceptibility to CDI [14,15]. We have recently shown that NAFLD is an independent risk factor for in-hospital CDI in elderly patients treated with systemic antimicrobial therapy [16]. Similarly, a case–control study showed that hospitalized patients with CDI more frequently have NAFLD and metabolic syndrome, as compared to age- and gender-matched controls hospitalized for non-CDI diarrhea [17]. However, the question remains if NAFLD is a risk factor for CDI recurrence. Due to the high and increasing burden of NAFLD in the Western population, identification of NAFLD as a novel and common risk factor could improve current CDI management strategies.

Therefore, the aim of this retrospective cohort study was to determine whether NAFLD is an independent risk factor associated with CDI recurrence in elderly patients who are at the highest risk for increased mortality, hospitalization, complications and healthcare costs.

2. Results

A total of 329 patients were included in the study (196, 59.6% females with the median age of 77, interquartile range (IQR) 71–83 years). Among the entire cohort, 107 (32.5%) patients developed recurrent CDI within 90 days of index hospitalization discharge or by the end of index CDI therapy (total of 171 episodes). Of those, 67 patients developed rCDI by 28 days (a cumulative probability of recurrence of 20.7%, 95% CI = 13.5–28.9%) and 40 patients by 90 days (33.3%, 26.5–40.4%). Three, four and five or more documented episodes were registered in the studied period in 38, 11 and 5 patients, respectively.

Patients with rCDI were older (78 years, IQR 74–84 vs. 77 years, 71–81), had higher Charlson Age–Comorbidity Index (CACI) (6, IQR 5–7 vs. 5, IQR 4–6) and were more frequently hospitalized within 3 months (81.3% vs. 68.9%). Except for chronic kidney disease (CKD) (26.2% vs. 6.8%) and NAFLD (34.6% vs. 18.5%), which were more frequent in the rCDI group, there were no differences in other comorbidities, as presented in Table 1. Notably, the majority of patients with CKD in our cohort did not undergo chronic dialysis; two patients in CDI and four in rCDI group were in a dialysis program.

High proportions of patients in both groups were nursing home residents (37.4% vs. 33.3%). Regarding chronic medications, patients without recurrence were more frequently receiving statins (23.4% vs. 13.1%), while there were no differences in prescription of perioral anti-diabetic, metformin or insulin. The majority of patients in both groups were receiving histamine-2 receptor antagonist and/or proton pump inhibitors (47.7% vs. 43.7%).

Use of specific of antibiotic classes per patient and duration of therapy prior the first episode of CDI were similar; fluoroquinolones were most frequently prescribed (29.9% vs. 27.0%), followed by 3rd generation cephalosporins (20.5% vs. 13.5%) and amoxicillin/clavulanate (19.6% vs. 22.1%). The reasons for antibiotic prescription prior the first episode of CDI were similar in both groups—most commonly for urinary tract infections (28.9% vs. 30.2%), respiratory infections (26.2% vs. 23.4%) and skin/soft tissue infections (11.2% vs. 5.9%). However, there were 9 patients with rCDI (8.4%) and 42 (18.9%) with CDI, for whom the reason for antibiotic prescription was not clear.

On index hospitalization, the majority of patients presented with severe CDI, median ATLAS score of 5 (IQR 4–7) in both groups, and elevated inflammatory markers (C-reactive protein and white blood cells count), as presented in Table 2. There were no differences in APRI or FIB4 scores between groups; APRI score >1.5 had 4.0% of patients in CDI and 2.8% in rCDI group. FIB4 score >3.25 had 10.8% in CDI and 10.3% of patients in rCDI group.

Table 1. Baseline patients' characteristics.

Characteristics	*Clostridioides difficile* Infection (*n* = 222)	Recurrent *Clostridioides difficile* Infection (*n* = 107)	*p*-Value [a]
Age, median (IQR [b])	77 (71–81)	78 (74–84)	0.011
Female, No. (%)	135 (60.8%)	61 (57.0%)	0.549
Nursing Home Resident	74 (33.3%)	40 (37.4%)	0.536
Charlson Age–Comorbidity Index	5 (4–6)	6 (5–7)	<0.001
Hospital Admission within 3 months	153 (68.9%)	87 (81.3%)	0.018
Comorbidities			
Diabetes Mellitus	54 (24.3%)	34 (31.8%)	0.183
Arterial Hypertension	108 (48.6%)	59 (55.1%)	0.291
Cardiovascular Disease	57 (25.7%)	18 (16.8%)	0.092
Peripheral Vascular Disease	20 (9.0%)	9 (8.4%)	>0.999
Hyperlipidemia	54 (24.3%)	25 (23.4%)	0.891
Solid Tumor	22 (9.9%)	14 (13.1%)	0.451
Chronic Kidney Disease	15 (6.8%)	28 (26.2%)	<0.001
Chronic Obstructive Pulmonary Disease	51 (22.9%)	19 (17.8%)	0.316
Neurological Diseases	51 (22.9%)	27 (25.2%)	0.679
Obesity (BMI > 30 kg/m^2)	23 (10.4%)	18 (16.8%)	0.109
Body Mass Index (BMI) [c]	25 (23–28)	27 (24–30)	0.010
Nonalcoholic Fatty Liver Disease	41 (18.5%)	37 (34.6%)	0.002
Use of Chronic Medications			
Statins	52 (23.4%)	14 (13.1%)	0.028
Metformin	15 (6.8%)	13 (12.1%)	0.138
Other Perioral Anti-diabetic	13 (5.9%)	10 (9.3%)	0.255
Insulin	22 (9.9%)	15 (14.0%)	0.269
Histamine-2 Receptor Antagonist and/or Proton Pump Inhibitor	97 (43.7%)	51 (47.7%)	0.554
Immunosuppressive Agents	20 (9.0%)	7 (6.5%)	0.525
Antibiotic Therapy before the 1st Episode of CDI			
Fluoroquinolones	60 (27.0%)	32 (29.9%)	0.510
1st Generation Cephalosporins	1 (0.4%)	1 (0.9%)	0.545
2nd Generation Cephalosporins	18 (8.1%)	7 (6.5%)	0.824
3rd Generation Cephalosporins	30 (13.5%)	22 (20.5%)	0.108
4th Generation Cephalosporins	3 (1.3%)	1 (0.9%)	>0.999
Amoxicillin/Clavulanate	49 (22.1%)	21 (19.6%)	0.668
Piperacillin/Tazobactam	18 (8.1%)	9 (8.4%)	>0.999
Carbapenems	7 (3.1%)	5 (4.7%)	0.536
Macrolides	22 (9.9%)	8 (7.5%)	0.544
Clindamycin	12 (5.4%)	10 (9.3%)	0.237
Others	6 (2.7%)	6 (5.6%)	0.214

[a] Fisher exact or Mann–Whitney U test, as appropriate; [b] IQR, interquartile range; [c] data available for 299 patients.

There was no difference in the choice of CDI treatment between groups; 118 patients were treated with metronidazole, 182 with vancomycin and 29 received combined therapy. There were 39 patients considered metronidazole unresponsive who were switched to vancomycin. Importantly, the majority of our cohort received non-CDI antibiotics during hospitalization (62.6% in rCDI and 67.6% in CDI group). As shown in Table 2, the most commonly used antibiotics were piperacillin/tazobactam (23.4% vs. 18.5%), 3rd generation cephalosporins (23.4% vs. 21.6%) and carbapenems (10.3% vs. 14.9%). The reasons for non-CDI therapy were respiratory tract infection (15.5%), urinary tract infection (30.7%), sepsis (7.9%) and suspected bacteriaemia of gastrointestinal origin (6.1%). There were no differences between groups in the choice of antibiotic therapy, number of antibiotic classes prescribed or duration of antimicrobial therapy.

Table 2. Clinical, laboratory and treatment characteristics during the first episode of CDI.

Characteristics	*Clostridioides difficile* Infection (n = 222)	Recurrent *Clostridioides difficile* Infection (n = 107)	p-Value [a]
CDI Severity			
Nonsevere	95 (42.8%)	45 (42.0%)	
Severe	100 (45.0%)	54 (50.5%)	0.377
Fulminant	27 (12.2%)	8 (7.5%)	
ATLAS Score	5 (4–7)	5 (4–7)	0.503
Laboratory Findings on Admission			
C-reactive Protein, mg/L	107.5 (54–172)	94.1 (54.6–147.0)	0.294
White Blood Cells Count, $\times 10^9$/L	14.5 (10.0–20.0)	13.2 (10.1–19.6)	0.487
Hemoglobin, g/L	120 (107–129)	120 (108–130)	0.851
Platelets, $\times 10^9$	251 (198–327)	256 (190–327)	0.859
Urea, mmol/L	8.1 (5.3–13.0)	7.1 (4.97–11.63)	0.256
Creatinine, µmol/L	103 (77.0–153.0)	109 (75–145)	0.890
Aspartate Aminotransferase, IU/L	19 (14–28)	19 (13–24)	0.146
Alanine Aminotransferase, IU/L	15 (10–23)	14 (10–22)	0.581
Serum Albumins, g/L	27.8 (23.9–32.4)	28.8 (24.8–33.9)	0.194
CDI Treatment Regiment			
Metronidazole	77 (34.7%)	41 (38.3%)	0.541
Vancomycin	122 (54.9%)	60 (56.1%)	0.906
Metronidazole + vancomycin	23 (10.4%)	6 (5.6%)	0.212
Other Antimicrobials (not for *C. difficile*)			
Any Systemic Antibiotic	150 (67.6%)	67 (62.6%)	0.387
Fluoroquinolones	9 (4.0%)	8 (7.5%)	0.194
1st Generation Cephalosporins	2 (0.9%)	0	>0.999
2nd Generation Cephalosporins	2 (0.9%)	1 (0.9%)	>0.999
3rd Generation Cephalosporins	48 (21.6%)	25 (23.4%)	0.777
4th Generation Cephalosporins	2 (0.9%)	2 (1.9%)	0.598
Amoxicillin Clavulanate	18 (8.1%)	8 (7.5%)	>0.999
Piperacillin/Tazobactam	41 (18.5%)	25 (23.4%)	0.307
Carbapenems	33 (14.9%)	11 (10.3%)	0.301
Macrolides	5 (2.2%)	5 (4.7%)	0.304
Clindamycin	1 (0.4%)	1 (0.9%)	0.545
Others	8 (3.6%)	5 (4.7%)	0.763
No. of Antibiotic Classes Used per Patient	1 (0–3)	1 (0–3)	0.889

[a] Fisher exact or Mann–Whitney U test, as appropriate.

In order to identify potential risk factors for CDI recurrence, we performed a multivariable Cox regression analysis. After adjustment for potential cofounders, Charlson Age–Comorbidity Index >6 (Hazard ratio (HR) 1.97, 95% CI 1.32–2.92), age > 75 years (HR 1.88, 95% CI 1.20–2.97), NAFLD (HR 1.81, 95% CI 1.19–2.74, Figure 1), chronic kidney disease (HR 1.86, 95% CI 1.19–2.88) and immobility (HR 1.73, 95% CI 1.16–2.56) were associated with rCDI, as presented in Table 3. Chronic therapy with statins was associated with a decreased risk of rCDI (HR 0.24, 95% CI 0.11–0.52). Interestingly, some of the expected risk factors such as diabetes mellitus or obesity, nasogastric tube feeding and nursing home residency, as well as previous hospital admissions, choice of previous antibiotic therapy or concomitantly used antibiotics were not associated with rCDI in our model.

In addition, when NAFLD was combined with age > 75 years, chronic kidney disease and immobility, the risk of rCDI was even higher, as shown in Figure 2. Statin use was associated with lower rCDI in both patients with and without NAFLD (Figure 2, Panel d).

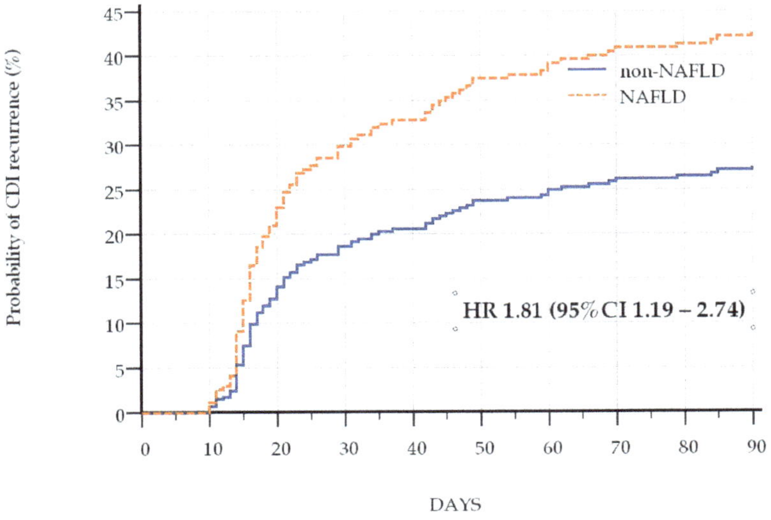

Figure 1. Kaplan–Meier curves and Cox proportional hazard ratios (HR) for recurrence of *Clostridioides difficile* infection in patients with and without nonalcoholic fatty liver disease.

Table 3. Multivariable Cox regression analysis of risk factors for the development recurrent *Clostridioides difficile* infection.

Variable	Hazard Ratio	95% CI	*p*-Value
Age > 75 Years	1.88	1.20 to 2.97	0.006
Charlson Age-Comorbidity Index (CACI) > 6	1.97	1.32 to 2.92	<0.001
Immobility	1.73	1.16 to 2.56	0.006
Nonalcoholic Fatty Liver Disease	1.81	1.19 to 2.74	0.005
Chronic Kidney Disease	1.86	1.19 to 2.88	0.006
Statins	0.24	0.11 to 0.52	<0.001

The strength of association was expressed as hazard ratio (HR) and its corresponding 95% confidence interval (CI). The area under the ROC curve in the fully adjusted model was AUC 0.72 (95% CI 0.66 to 0.77).

Finally, we report the demographic and clinical characteristics of patients with NAFLD. As previously shown, they had significantly higher incidence of rCDI (47.4% vs. 27.9%). They were younger than patients without NAFLD (median of 76, IQR 71–81 vs. 78, IQR 72–83 years), more commonly had BMI > 30 (38.5% vs. 9.6%), diabetes mellitus (41.0% vs. 22.3%) and hyperlipidemia (33.3% vs. 21.1%) (data not shown). Consequently, they were more frequently prescribed statins (26.9% vs. 17.9%), metformin (11.5% vs. 7.9%) and insulin (17.9% vs. 9.2%) (data not shown). There was no difference in other comorbidities, chronic medications or antibiotics used. The 1st episode disease severity was similar to patients without NAFLD (ATLAS score of 5, IQR 4–6 vs. 6, IQR 4–7, $p = 0.103$) (data not shown).

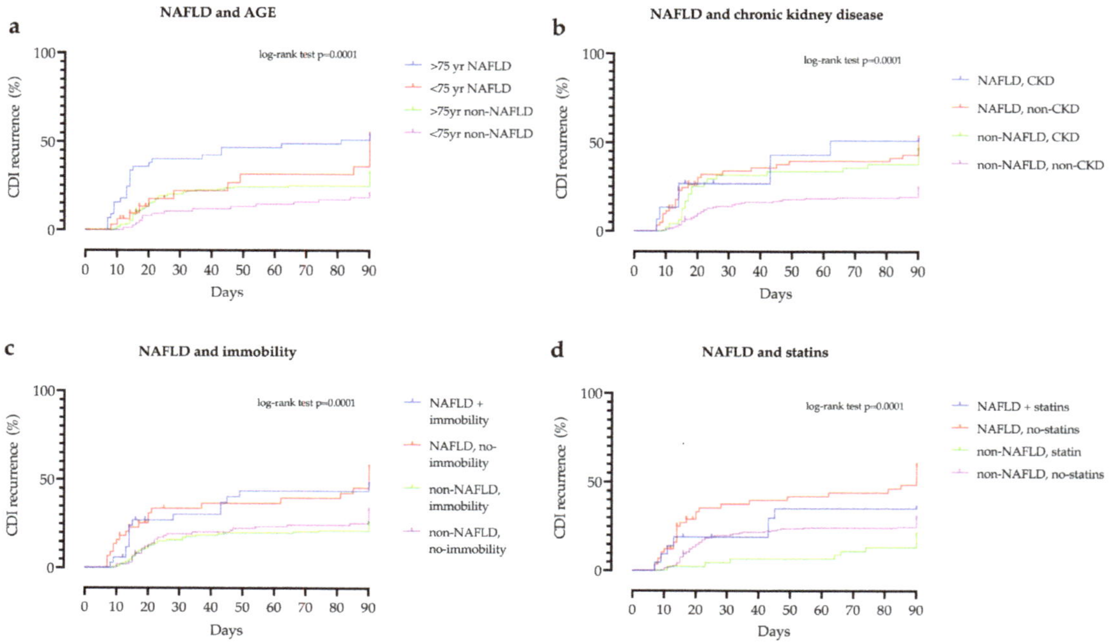

Figure 2. Kaplan–Meier curves for recurrence of *Clostridioides difficile* infection (CDI). Using the Kaplan–Meier method, a proportion of patients with CDI recurrence stratified by the concomitant presence of NAFLD and (**a**) age, (**b**) chronic kidney disease, (**c**) immobility and (**d**) statins during the follow-up period.

3. Discussion

Over the last decade, there has been a marked increase in the incidence and severity of CDI, with relapsing episodes now occurring at a higher frequency, especially in the elderly. Notably, recurrent CDI is associated with a significantly higher risk of death within six months after initial CDI treatment completion, compared with CDI patients who do not develop a recurrence [18,19].

In this retrospective cohort study, we found a significant association between recurrent CDI and NAFLD in elderly patients. Moreover, this appears to be independent of a number of potential confounders, specifically other components of metabolic syndrome.

While there are several well-established risk factors for primary infection with *C. difficile*, the studies examining risk factors for CDI recurrence had variable results depending on the population studied. To the best of our knowledge, none of them have analyzed the impact of NAFLD on CDI recurrence.

Surprisingly, the investigation of the role of NAFLD in bacterial infections has only recently been initiated. Although patients with NAFLD might have a higher risk for infections due to the concomitant presence of obesity or diabetes mellitus, few studies that included NAFLD in the analysis consistently showed its outcome impact independently of the metabolic syndrome components [20]. So far, this was suggested for community-acquired pneumonia, bacteriaemia of gastrointestinal origin, sepsis and urinary tract infections [21–25]. Recently, we have shown that NAFLD is a risk factor for in-hospital CDI development in elderly patients treated with systemic antimicrobial therapy [16].

The possible explanation of increased risk of CDI in NAFLD patients includes changes in intestinal microbiota linked to the development and progression of NAFLD [13]. While *Bacteroides* and *Bifidobacterium* play an important role in the mechanism, preventing colonization by *C. difficile*, patients with NAFLD were shown to have a relative decrease in the proportion of *Bacteroides* to *Firmicutes* [13,26,27]. Notably, NAFLD is now considered a multisystem disease due to the persistent low-level inflammation with impaired immune response that might predispose patients to a variety of infections [13,28].

In our cohort, DM and obesity were not associated with rCDI. The current medical literature is contradictory on the association between obesity and *C. difficile* infection. Two case–control studies that examined the association of CDI with BMI showed different results. While Bishara et al., based on data collected from 148 adult patients with CDI, showed an association of BMI with CDI (OR = 1.196 per 1-unit increase in BMI scale) [9], Punni et al. in their study on 189 patients did not [29]. There was no association of obesity with the risk of *C. difficile* infection among patients with ulcerative colitis and according to another study, obesity was even associated with decreased risk of CDI in hospitalized patients with pouchitis [30,31].

Meanwhile, several studies have shown that DM increases the risk of CDI recurrence, but none of them included NAFLD as a variable. A large Spanish cohort study showed a significantly higher incidence of CDI in DM patients, with an increasing trend between 2011 and 2015 [32]. In addition, patients with DM have significantly higher probability for hospital readmission due to CDI (adjusted OR of 3.79 to 5.46) and the development of severe CDI [8,33]. DM was also recognized as an independent risk factor in patients with toxigenic *C. difficile* colonization to develop *C. difficile*-associated diarrhea [7].

Interestingly, it was shown that metformin increases the *Bacteroidetes/Firmicutes* ratio; therefore, it may yield a protective effect against CDI in patients with DM [34]. A retrospective, case–control study compared CDI diabetic patients to diabetic patients without CDI and found metformin treatment to be associated with significant reduction in CDI (OR 0.58) [35]. This could be partially explained by the study that showed that metformin reduces vegetative cell growth of *C. difficile* in vitro, as well as ex vivo in human microbiome culture system [36]. Metformin modified human gut microbiome by decreasing *C. difficile* growth while increasing the growth of non-pathogenic Clostridium strains [36].

Other risk factors for rCDI in our study were age, significant comorbidities measured with Charlson Age–Comorbidity Index (CACI), chronic kidney disease and immobility.

Several studies examined the association of CKD with CDI. While the association of severe CKD requiring dialysis with CDI severity and mortality is clear, there are inconsistent data on if patients not undergoing dialysis are at higher risk for CDI [37–40]. We provide additional data that patients with CKD not requiring chronic dialysis are at increased risk for rCDI.

Meanwhile, antibiotics and proton pump inhibitors, which are well-known risk factors for initial CDI and rCDI, were not associated with rCDI in our study. This might be due to the characteristics of our cohort and widespread use of these medications, which might have predisposed the development of CDI in the first place.

Next, we found that statin use was associated with lower rCDI in patients both with and without NAFLD. Due to the global epidemic of cardiovascular diseases, obesity and metabolic syndrome, statins are considered as one of the most commonly used medications worldwide [41]. Other than their cholesterol-lowering effect, they also have an anti-inflammatory and immunomodulatory properties [42]. According to a recent meta-analysis of available data, the risk of developing CDI was approximately 25% lower in statin users compared with non-users [43]. However, this meta-analysis included eight observational studies with significant heterogeneity. There are no randomized control trials published so far. Although the exact mechanisms of risk decrease in CDI in statin users remains unknown, some studies demonstrated that statins have an influence on gut microbiota and could change its composition [44–46]. Vieira-Silva et al. recently identified statins as a key covariate of gut microbiome diversification [45]. In their study examining obesity-associated microbiota alterations, they showed that obesity is linked with intestinal microbiota configuration characterized by a high proportion of *Bacteroides*, a low proportion of *Faecalibacterium* and low microbial cell densities (the so called Bact2 enterotype) [45]. However, patients treated with statins had significantly lower Bact2 prevalence [45]. A systematic review of both human and animal data showed that statins modulate the gut microbiome, but the effect of change is unclear, probably due to the differences in populations studied [46]. It seems reasonable to speculate that modulation of the gut microbiome by statins might aid in the restoration of colonization resistance and lower recurrence of CDI. Alternatively, as statins have anti-inflammatory properties, their use may decrease the inflammatory response to *C. difficile* infection, which may lead to the decreased severity of CDI [47].

The major limitation of this study comes from its retrospective, monocentric design, and despite adjustment for a variety of demographics, comorbidities and medications, residual confounding may exist. The diagnosis of NAFLD was based on abdominal US, which is operator-dependent, and patients were not systematically screened for other causes of liver steatosis, but from data available in medical charts. Importantly, US has limited sensitivity and does not reliably detect steatosis when <20% or in individuals with high body mass index (BMI) (>40 kg/m^2) and is inferior to MRI or CT scan for detection and grading of steatosis [48,49]. Next, while any potential effects of NAFLD should be interpreted in connection with metabolic syndrome, due to the retrospective design, we could not include waist circumference, type of dyslipidemia, levels of triglycerides or HDL cholesterol. However, we included diabetes mellitus and obesity (defined by BMI > 30 kg/m^2), which might have the highest confounding impact, and have both been previously shown to be associated with rCDI. Since only a minority of patients had a significant risk of advanced fibrosis, as measured by APRI and FIB4 score, we were not able to determine the effect of advanced NAFLD on rCDI. Another limitation was the lack of data on *C. difficile* strain, which might be important since 027/BI/NAP1 strain has been associated with increased risk of CDI recurrence [50]. The study was designed to investigate the effect of NAFLD in elderly who are at the highest risk for rCDI and included only patients who were rehospitalized during a 3-month period. Therefore, patients diagnosed and treated for rCDI entirely as outpatients would not have been identified as having a recurrence. However, this would underestimate, rather than overestimate, the impact of NAFLD on patient outcomes.

Nevertheless, we report the first data examining the association of NAFLD with rCDI.

4. Materials and Methods

4.1. Study Design and Patients

This was a retrospective cohort study conducted at the University Hospital for Infectious Diseases Zagreb (UHID), Croatia, which is a national referral center for infectious diseases. We reviewed the hospital records of all adult patients hospitalized at UHID with a diagnosis of *Clostridium difficile* infection over a 5-year period (2016–2019). We included patients > 60 years diagnosed with the first episode of CDI. Patients who had a previous episode of CDI within three months before index hospitalization were excluded, as well as patients with known alcohol abuse and/or those diagnosed with chronic viral hepatitis or with a history of other known liver diseases. Next, only patients with performed ultrasonography examination to assess liver steatosis were included in study. During the period studied, a total of 841 patients were hospitalized with diagnosis of CDI. Of those, 730 were >60 years (total of 999 episodes of CDI). A total of 401 patients were excluded: 31 had CDI within 3 months, significant alcohol intake in 38, chronic viral hepatitis in 21, cirrhosis in 11 and hepatotoxic medications in 14 patients. There were 267 patients who did not have abdominal imaging, and 19 patients died during initial hospitalization. In the end, 329 patients were included in the study. The cohort was divided into two groups, those who were and were not readmitted with CDI within 3 months of discharge, as described in a flowchart (Figure 3).

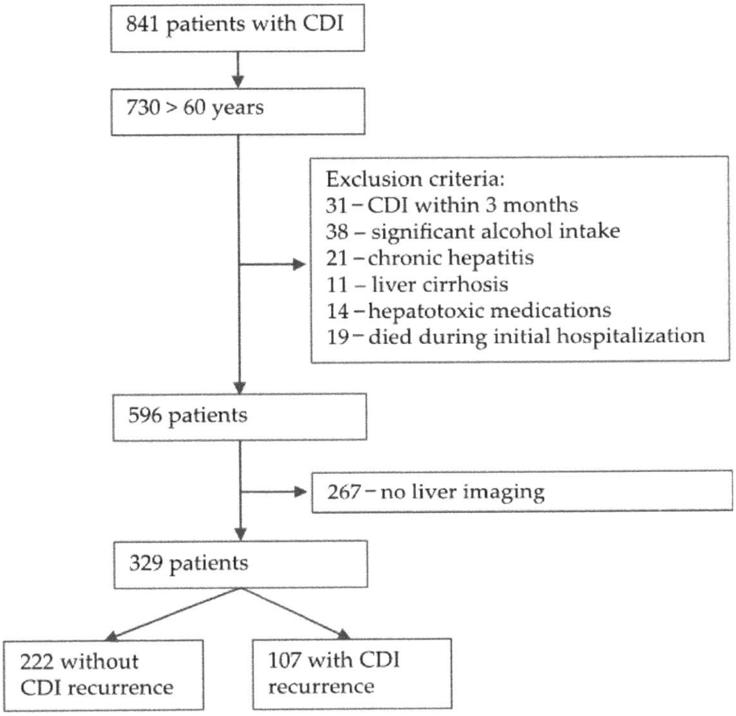

Figure 3. Study design flow chart.

4.2. Data Collection, Outcomes, and Definitions

We collected multiple variables that could be associated with patient outcomes. These variables included demographic data (age, sex and residence in nursing homes) and medical history (comorbidities (measured by Charlson Age–Comorbidity Index, CACI [51]), chronic medications, hospital admission within 3 months, administration of antibiotics within 90 days). CDI was defined as the presence of 3 or more unformed stools in 24 or fewer consecutive hours, confirmed with positive two-stage *C. difficile* stool tests (screening GDH test confirmed with toxin A/B PCR), according to current guidelines [52–54]. CDI severity was determined by ATLAS score calculation [55]. CDI treatment regimen, its duration and the use of other non-CDI antimicrobials were collected. Selected blood laboratory data at the admission were analyzed: C-reactive protein level, white blood cell count, platelet count, hemoglobin, blood urea nitrogen, serum creatinine, aspartate aminotransferase, alanine aminotransferase, gamma-glutamyl transferase, alkaline phosphatase, bilirubin and serum albumin concentration. In addition, as a surrogate marker of liver injury, APRI and FIB-4 score were calculated for all patients [56]. Using the CKD-EPI equation, we calculated estimated glomerular filtration rate (eGFR) [57]. The diagnosis of NAFLD was made based on the results of abdominal ultrasound and by the absence of a secondary cause of NAFLD, according to current guidelines [11,12]. The liver steatosis was assessed by ultrasound in all patients by an experienced radiologist, and defined as finding liver parenchyma with increased echogenicity and sound attenuation [49].

The primary study outcome was rCDI, defined as CDI occurring within 14–90 days of the initial CDI diagnosis date. Same as CDI, rCDI was defined based on compatible symptoms accompanied by a positive laboratory test.

4.3. Statistical Analysis

The clinical characteristics, laboratory and demographic data were evaluated and descriptively presented. We used Fisher's exact test and the Mann–Whitney U test to compare the groups. All tests were two-tailed; a p value < 0.05 was considered statistically significant. Time to CDI recurrence was evaluated using the Kaplan–Meier method, and the comparison of CDI recurrence risk between patients with and without NAFLD was made using the log-rank test. Risk factors for the development of the rCDI were investigated using a univariate, and subsequently, a multivariable Cox regression model by estimating the hazard ratio (HR) and its 95% CI for the time from cure date of the primary CDI to the first episode of rCDI. Variables with $p < 0.2$ on univariate analysis or with clinical/biological plausibility were included in initial multivariable models. Multivariable Cox proportional hazards models were developed using backward elimination with $p < 0.1$ to retain variables in the model. Statistical analyses were performed using the GraphPad Prism Software version 9.1.1. (San Diego, CA, USA) and MedCalc version 20.008 (MedCalc Software, Ostend, Belgium).

5. Conclusions

In conclusion, we have shown that NAFLD is a novel host-related risk factor for recurrent CDI in elderly patients. This might be relevant for several reasons. Firstly, this highlights the need to include NAFLD as a variable in future studies, examining both CDI and rCDI. Secondly, patients with NAFLD might benefit from screening strategies, preemptive treatment or prophylactic measures, such as antibiotic prophylaxis that has recently been investigated [58,59]. The finding that statins reduce the risk of rCDI in both patients with and without NAFLD might be a novel treatment option that warrants further examination. Finally, there is growing evidence that immunological changes in patients with NAFLD might have a profound impact in the course of bacterial infections, the place where we have not been looking so far.

Author Contributions: Conceptualization, N.P. and A.V.; methodology, N.P.; validation, A.V.; resources, N.P.; data curation, L.Š., M.J.; writing—original draft preparation, L.Š., M.J.; writing—review and editing, N.P., A.V.; supervision, A.V.; funding acquisition, N.P. All authors have read and agreed to the published version of the manuscript.

Funding: This research was funded by the Croatian Science Foundation, for the project entitled "The role of immune semaphorins in NAFLD and sepsis" (principal investigator Neven Papić, project number UIP-2019–04–7194).

Institutional Review Board Statement: The study was conducted according to the guidelines of the Declaration of Helsinki and approved by the Institutional Review Board (or Ethics Committee) of the University Hospital for Infectious Diseases Zagreb (protocol code 01–1247–2–2019, date of approval 30 August 2019).

Informed Consent Statement: Patient consent was waived due to retrospective design of the study.

Data Availability Statement: The datasets generated and/or analyzed during the current study are available from the corresponding author on reasonable request.

Conflicts of Interest: The authors declare no conflict of interest. The funders had no role in the design of the study; in the collection, analyses, or interpretation of data; in the writing of the manuscript, or in the decision to publish the results.

References

1. Magill, S.S.; Edwards, J.R.; Bamberg, W.; Beldavs, Z.G.; Dumyati, G.; Kainer, M.A.; Lynfield, R.; Maloney, M.; McAllister-Hollod, L.; Nadle, J.; et al. Multistate point-prevalence survey of health care-associated infections. *N. Engl. J. Med.* **2014**, *370*, 1198–1208. [CrossRef]
2. Crobach, M.J.T.; Vernon, J.J.; Loo, V.G.; Kong, L.Y.; Pechine, S.; Wilcox, M.H.; Kuijper, E.J. Understanding Clostridium difficile Colonization. *Clin. Microbiol. Rev.* **2018**, *31*. [CrossRef] [PubMed]
3. Louie, T.J.; Miller, M.A.; Mullane, K.M.; Weiss, K.; Lentnek, A.; Golan, Y.; Gorbach, S.; Sears, P.; Shue, Y.K.; Group, O.P.T.C.S. Fidaxomicin versus vancomycin for Clostridium difficile infection. *N. Engl. J. Med.* **2011**, *364*, 422–431. [CrossRef] [PubMed]

4. Pepin, J.; Alary, M.E.; Valiquette, L.; Raiche, E.; Ruel, J.; Fulop, K.; Godin, D.; Bourassa, C. Increasing risk of relapse after treatment of Clostridium difficile colitis in Quebec, Canada. *Clin. Infect. Dis.* **2005**, *40*, 1591–1597. [CrossRef]
5. Song, J.H.; Kim, Y.S. Recurrent Clostridium difficile Infection: Risk Factors, Treatment, and Prevention. *Gut Liver* **2019**, *13*, 16–24. [CrossRef] [PubMed]
6. Deshpande, A.; Pasupuleti, V.; Thota, P.; Pant, C.; Rolston, D.D.; Hernandez, A.V.; Donskey, C.J.; Fraser, T.G. Risk factors for recurrent Clostridium difficile infection: A systematic review and meta-analysis. *Infect. Control Hosp. Epidemiol.* **2015**, *36*, 452–460. [CrossRef]
7. Lin, H.J.; Hung, Y.P.; Liu, H.C.; Lee, J.C.; Lee, C.I.; Wu, Y.H.; Tsai, P.J.; Ko, W.C. Risk factors for Clostridium difficile-associated diarrhea among hospitalized adults with fecal toxigenic C. difficile colonization. *J. Microbiol. Immunol. Infect.* **2015**, *48*, 183–189. [CrossRef]
8. Shakov, R.; Salazar, R.S.; Kagunye, S.K.; Baddoura, W.J.; DeBari, V.A. Diabetes mellitus as a risk factor for recurrence of Clostridium difficile infection in the acute care hospital setting. *Am. J. Infect. Control* **2011**, *39*, 194–198. [CrossRef]
9. Bishara, J.; Farah, R.; Mograbi, J.; Khalaila, W.; Abu-Elheja, O.; Mahamid, M.; Nseir, W. Obesity as a risk factor for Clostridium difficile infection. *Clin. Infect. Dis.* **2013**, *57*, 489–493. [CrossRef]
10. Czepiel, J.; Drozdz, M.; Pituch, H.; Kuijper, E.J.; Perucki, W.; Mielimonka, A.; Goldman, S.; Wultanska, D.; Garlicki, A.; Biesiada, G. Clostridium difficile infection: Review. *Eur. J. Clin. Microbiol. Infect. Dis.* **2019**, *38*, 1211–1221. [CrossRef]
11. European Association for the Study of The Liver; European Association for the Study of Diabetes; European Association for the Study of Obesity (EASO). EASL-EASD-EASO Clinical Practice Guidelines for the management of non-alcoholic fatty liver disease. *J. Hepatol.* **2016**, *64*, 1388–1402. [CrossRef] [PubMed]
12. Chalasani, N.; Younossi, Z.; Lavine, J.E.; Charlton, M.; Cusi, K.; Rinella, M.; Harrison, S.A.; Brunt, E.M.; Sanyal, A.J. The diagnosis and management of nonalcoholic fatty liver disease: Practice guidance from the American Association for the Study of Liver Diseases. *Hepatology* **2018**, *67*, 328–357. [CrossRef]
13. Haas, J.T.; Francque, S.; Staels, B. Pathophysiology and Mechanisms of Nonalcoholic Fatty Liver Disease. *Annu. Rev. Physiol.* **2016**, *78*, 181–205. [CrossRef]
14. Jayakumar, S.; Loomba, R. Review article: Emerging role of the gut microbiome in the progression of nonalcoholic fatty liver disease and potential therapeutic implications. *Aliment. Pharmacol. Ther.* **2019**, *50*, 144–158. [CrossRef] [PubMed]
15. Hopkins, M.J.; Macfarlane, G.T. Changes in predominant bacterial populations in human faeces with age and with Clostridium difficile infection. *J. Med. Microbiol.* **2002**, *51*, 448–454. [CrossRef]
16. Papic, N.; Jelovcic, F.; Karlovic, M.; Maric, L.S.; Vince, A. Nonalcoholic fatty liver disease as a risk factor for Clostridioides difficile infection. *Eur. J. Clin. Microbiol. Infect. Dis.* **2020**, *39*, 569–574. [CrossRef]
17. Nseir, W.B.; Hussein, S.H.H.; Farah, R.; Mahamid, M.N.; Khatib, H.H.; Mograbi, J.M.; Peretz, A.; Amara, A.E. Nonalcoholic fatty liver disease as a risk factor for Clostridium difficile-associated diarrhea. *QJM* **2020**, *113*, 320–323. [CrossRef]
18. Olsen, M.A.; Yan, Y.; Reske, K.A.; Zilberberg, M.D.; Dubberke, E.R. Recurrent Clostridium difficile infection is associated with increased mortality. *Clin. Microbiol. Infect.* **2015**, *21*, 164–170. [CrossRef]
19. Cozar, A.; Ramos-Martinez, A.; Merino, E.; Martinez-Garcia, C.; Shaw, E.; Marrodan, T.; Calbo, E.; Bereciartua, E.; Sanchez-Munoz, L.A.; Salavert, M.; et al. High delayed mortality after the first episode of Clostridium difficile infection. *Anaerobe* **2019**, *57*, 93–98. [CrossRef]
20. Adenote, A.; Dumic, I.; Madrid, C.; Barusya, C.; Nordstrom, C.W.; Rueda Prada, L. NAFLD and Infection, a Nuanced Relationship. *Can. J. Gastroenterol. Hepatol.* **2021**, *2021*, 5556354. [CrossRef] [PubMed]
21. Mari, A.; Abu Baker, F. Recurrent Urinary Tract Infection: Time to Recommend Weight Loss? *Isr. Med. Assoc. J.* **2019**, *21*, 412–413. [PubMed]
22. Nseir, W.; Artul, S.; Nasrallah, N.; Mahamid, M. The association between primary bacteremia of presumed gastrointestinal origin and nonalcoholic fatty liver disease. *Dig. Liver Dis.* **2016**, *48*, 343–344. [CrossRef] [PubMed]
23. Nseir, W.; Taha, H.; Khateeb, J.; Grosovski, M.; Assy, N. Fatty liver is associated with recurrent bacterial infections independent of metabolic syndrome. *Dig. Dis. Sci.* **2011**, *56*, 3328–3334. [CrossRef] [PubMed]
24. Nseir, W.B.; Mograbi, J.M.; Amara, A.E.; Abu Elheja, O.H.; Mahamid, M.N. Non-alcoholic fatty liver disease and 30-day all-cause mortality in adult patients with community-acquired pneumonia. *QJM* **2019**, *112*, 95–99. [CrossRef]
25. Gjurasin, B.; Butic, I.; Vince, A.; Papić, N. Non-Alcoholic Fatty Liver Disease is Associated with an Increased Mortality in Adult Patients with Group B Streptococcus Invasive Disease. *Croat. J. Infect.* **2020**, *40*, 124–128. [CrossRef]
26. Damms-Machado, A.; Mitra, S.; Schollenberger, A.E.; Kramer, K.M.; Meile, T.; Konigsrainer, A.; Huson, D.H.; Bischoff, S.C. Effects of surgical and dietary weight loss therapy for obesity on gut microbiota composition and nutrient absorption. *Biomed. Res. Int.* **2015**, *2015*, 806248. [CrossRef]
27. Loomba, R.; Seguritan, V.; Li, W.; Long, T.; Klitgord, N.; Bhatt, A.; Dulai, P.S.; Caussy, C.; Bettencourt, R.; Highlander, S.K.; et al. Gut Microbiome-Based Metagenomic Signature for Non-invasive Detection of Advanced Fibrosis in Human Nonalcoholic Fatty Liver Disease. *Cell Metab.* **2019**, *30*, 607. [CrossRef] [PubMed]
28. Van Herck, M.A.; Weyler, J.; Kwanten, W.J.; Dirinck, E.L.; De Winter, B.Y.; Francque, S.M.; Vonghia, L. The Differential Roles of T Cells in Non-alcoholic Fatty Liver Disease and Obesity. *Front. Immunol.* **2019**, *10*, 82. [CrossRef]
29. Punni, E.; Pula, J.L.; Asslo, F.; Baddoura, W.; DeBari, V.A. Is obesity a risk factor for Clostridium difficile infection? *Obes. Res. Clin. Pract.* **2015**, *9*, 50–54. [CrossRef]

30. Chandradas, S.; Khalili, H.; Ananthakrishnan, A.; Wayman, C.; Reidel, W.; Waalen, J.; Konijeti, G.G. Does Obesity Influence the Risk of Clostridium difficile Infection Among Patients with Ulcerative Colitis? *Dig. Dis. Sci.* **2018**, *63*, 2445–2450. [CrossRef]
31. Gosai, F.; Covut, F.; Alomari, M.; Hitawala, A.; Singh, A.; Kisangani, G.; Lopez, R.; Shen, B. Obesity Is Associated with Decreased Risk of Clostridium difficile Infection in Hospitalized Patients with Pouchitis. *Dig. Dis. Sci.* **2020**, *65*, 1423–1428. [CrossRef]
32. Lopez-de-Andres, A.; Esteban-Vasallo, M.D.; de Miguel-Diez, J.; Hernandez-Barrera, V.; de Miguel-Yanes, J.M.; Mendez-Bailon, M.; Jimenez-Garcia, R. Incidence and in-hospital outcomes of Clostridium difficile infection among type 2 diabetes patients in Spain. *Int. J. Clin. Pract.* **2018**, *72*, e13251. [CrossRef] [PubMed]
33. Wenisch, J.M.; Schmid, D.; Kuo, H.W.; Simons, E.; Allerberger, F.; Michl, V.; Tesik, P.; Tucek, G.; Wenisch, C. Hospital-acquired Clostridium difficile infection: Determinants for severe disease. *Eur. J. Clin. Microbiol. Infect. Dis.* **2012**, *31*, 1923–1930. [CrossRef]
34. Karlsson, F.H.; Tremaroli, V.; Nookaew, I.; Bergstrom, G.; Behre, C.J.; Fagerberg, B.; Nielsen, J.; Backhed, F. Gut metagenome in European women with normal, impaired and diabetic glucose control. *Nature* **2013**, *498*, 99–103. [CrossRef] [PubMed]
35. Eliakim-Raz, N.; Fishman, G.; Yahav, D.; Goldberg, E.; Stein, G.Y.; Zvi, H.B.; Barsheshet, A.; Bishara, J. Predicting Clostridium difficile infection in diabetic patients and the effect of metformin therapy: A retrospective, case-control study. *Eur. J. Clin. Microbiol. Infect. Dis.* **2015**, *34*, 1201–1205. [CrossRef] [PubMed]
36. Wang, S.; Yadav, H. Metformin reduces Clostridium difficile infection. *FASEB J.* **2021**, *35*. [CrossRef]
37. Eddi, R.; Malik, M.N.; Shakov, R.; Baddoura, W.J.; Chandran, C.; Debari, V.A. Chronic kidney disease as a risk factor for Clostridium difficile infection. *Nephrology* **2010**, *15*, 471–475. [CrossRef]
38. Yousuf, K.; Saklayen, M.G.; Markert, R.J.; Barde, C.J.; Gopalswamy, N. Clostridium difficile-associated diarrhea and chronic renal insufficiency. *South. Med. J.* **2002**, *95*, 681–683. [PubMed]
39. Kim, S.C.; Seo, M.Y.; Lee, J.Y.; Kim, K.T.; Cho, E.; Kim, M.G.; Jo, S.K.; Cho, W.Y.; Kim, H.K. Advanced chronic kidney disease: A strong risk factor for Clostridium difficile infection. *Korean J. Intern. Med.* **2016**, *31*, 125–133. [CrossRef]
40. Keddis, M.T.; Khanna, S.; Noheria, A.; Baddour, L.M.; Pardi, D.S.; Qian, Q. Clostridium difficile infection in patients with chronic kidney disease. *Mayo Clin. Proc.* **2012**, *87*, 1046–1053. [CrossRef]
41. Adedinsewo, D.; Taka, N.; Agasthi, P.; Sachdeva, R.; Rust, G.; Onwuanyi, A. Prevalence and Factors Associated With Statin Use Among a Nationally Representative Sample of US Adults: National Health and Nutrition Examination Survey, 2011–2012. *Clin. Cardiol.* **2016**, *39*, 491–496. [CrossRef] [PubMed]
42. Ferri, N.; Corsini, A.; Bellosta, S. Pharmacology of the new P2Y12 receptor inhibitors: Insights on pharmacokinetic and pharmacodynamic properties. *Drugs* **2013**, *73*, 1681–1709. [CrossRef] [PubMed]
43. Wijarnpreecha, K.; Panjawatanan, P.; Thongprayoon, C.; Ungprasert, P. Statins & risk of Clostridium difficile infection: A meta-analysis. *Indian J. Med. Res.* **2019**, *150*, 359–364. [CrossRef] [PubMed]
44. Nolan, J.A.; Skuse, P.; Govindarajan, K.; Patterson, E.; Konstantinidou, N.; Casey, P.G.; MacSharry, J.; Shanahan, F.; Stanton, C.; Hill, C.; et al. The influence of rosuvastatin on the gastrointestinal microbiota and host gene expression profiles. *Am. J. Physiol. Gastrointest. Liver Physiol.* **2017**, *312*, G488–G497. [CrossRef]
45. Vieira-Silva, S.; Falony, G.; Belda, E.; Nielsen, T.; Aron-Wisnewsky, J.; Chakaroun, R.; Forslund, S.K.; Assmann, K.; Valles-Colomer, M.; Nguyen, T.T.D.; et al. Statin therapy is associated with lower prevalence of gut microbiota dysbiosis. *Nature* **2020**, *581*, 310–315. [CrossRef]
46. Dias, A.M.; Cordeiro, G.; Estevinho, M.M.; Veiga, R.; Figueira, L.; Reina-Couto, M.; Magro, F.; the Clinical Pharmacology Unit, São João Hospital University Centre. Gut bacterial microbiome composition and statin intake-A systematic review. *Pharmacol. Res. Perspect.* **2020**, *8*, e00601. [CrossRef]
47. Al-Ani, B. Simvastatin inhibits neutrophil degranulation induced by anti-neutrophil cytoplasm auto-antibodies and N-formyl-methionine-leucine-phenylalanine (fMLP) peptide. *Saudi Med. J.* **2013**, *34*, 477–483.
48. Fishbein, M.; Castro, F.; Cheruku, S.; Jain, S.; Webb, B.; Gleason, T.; Stevens, W.R. Hepatic MRI for fat quantitation: Its relationship to fat morphology, diagnosis, and ultrasound. *J. Clin. Gastroenterol.* **2005**, *39*, 619–625. [CrossRef] [PubMed]
49. Siegelman, E.S.; Rosen, M.A. Imaging of hepatic steatosis. *Semin. Liver Dis.* **2001**, *21*, 71–80. [CrossRef] [PubMed]
50. Petrella, L.A.; Sambol, S.P.; Cheknis, A.; Nagaro, K.; Kean, Y.; Sears, P.S.; Babakhani, F.; Johnson, S.; Gerding, D.N. Decreased cure and increased recurrence rates for Clostridium difficile infection caused by the epidemic C. difficile BI strain. *Clin. Infect. Dis.* **2012**, *55*, 351–357. [CrossRef]
51. Charlson, M.E.; Pompei, P.; Ales, K.L.; MacKenzie, C.R. A new method of classifying prognostic comorbidity in longitudinal studies: Development and validation. *J. Chronic Dis.* **1987**, *40*, 373–383. [CrossRef]
52. McDonald, L.C.; Gerding, D.N.; Johnson, S.; Bakken, J.S.; Carroll, K.C.; Coffin, S.E.; Dubberke, E.R.; Garey, K.W.; Gould, C.V.; Kelly, C.; et al. Clinical Practice Guidelines for Clostridium difficile Infection in Adults and Children: 2017 Update by the Infectious Diseases Society of America (IDSA) and Society for Healthcare Epidemiology of America (SHEA). *Clin. Infect. Dis.* **2018**, *66*, e1–e48. [CrossRef] [PubMed]
53. Debast, S.B.; Bauer, M.P.; Kuijper, E.J.; European Society of Clinical, M.; Infectious, D. European Society of Clinical Microbiology and Infectious Diseases: Update of the treatment guidance document for Clostridium difficile infection. *Clin. Microbiol. Infect.* **2014**, *20* (Suppl. 2), 1–26. [CrossRef]
54. Ooijevaar, R.E.; van Beurden, Y.H.; Terveer, E.M.; Goorhuis, A.; Bauer, M.P.; Keller, J.J.; Mulder, C.J.J.; Kuijper, E.J. Update of treatment algorithms for Clostridium difficile infection. *Clin. Microbiol. Infect.* **2018**, *24*, 452–462. [CrossRef] [PubMed]

55. Miller, M.A.; Louie, T.; Mullane, K.; Weiss, K.; Lentnek, A.; Golan, Y.; Kean, Y.; Sears, P. Derivation and validation of a simple clinical bedside score (ATLAS) for Clostridium difficile infection which predicts response to therapy. *BMC Infect. Dis.* **2013**, *13*, 148. [CrossRef]
56. Sterling, R.K.; Lissen, E.; Clumeck, N.; Sola, R.; Correa, M.C.; Montaner, J.; Sulkowski, M.S.; Torriani, F.J.; Dieterich, D.T.; Thomas, D.L.; et al. Development of a simple noninvasive index to predict significant fibrosis in patients with HIV/HCV coinfection. *Hepatology* **2006**, *43*, 1317–1325. [CrossRef]
57. Levey, A.S.; Stevens, L.A.; Schmid, C.H.; Zhang, Y.L.; Castro, A.F., 3rd; Feldman, H.I.; Kusek, J.W.; Eggers, P.; Van Lente, F.; Greene, T.; et al. A new equation to estimate glomerular filtration rate. *Ann. Intern. Med.* **2009**, *150*, 604–612. [CrossRef]
58. Papic, N.; Maric, L.S.; Vince, A. Efficacy of oral vancomycin in primary prevention of Clostridium Difficile infection in elderly patients treated with systemic antibiotic therapy. *Infect. Dis.* **2018**, *50*, 483–486. [CrossRef] [PubMed]
59. Van Hise, N.W.; Bryant, A.M.; Hennessey, E.K.; Crannage, A.J.; Khoury, J.A.; Manian, F.A. Efficacy of Oral Vancomycin in Preventing Recurrent Clostridium difficile Infection in Patients Treated With Systemic Antimicrobial Agents. *Clin. Infect. Dis* **2016**, *63*, 651–653. [CrossRef]

antibiotics

MDPI

Article

Teicoplanin Suppresses Vegetative *Clostridioides difficile* and Spore Outgrowth

Suvash Chandra Ojha [1,2], Matthew Phanchana [3], Phurt Harnvoravongchai [4], Surang Chankhamhaengdecha [4], Sombat Singhakaew [4], Puey Ounjai [4] and Tavan Janvilisri [5,*]

1 Graduate Program in Molecular Medicine, Faculty of Science, Mahidol University, Bangkok 10400, Thailand; suvash_ojha@swmu.edu.cn
2 Department of Infectious Diseases, The Affiliated Hospital of Southwest Medical University, Luzhou 646000, China
3 Department of Molecular Tropical Medicine and Genetics, Faculty of Tropical Medicine, Mahidol University, Bangkok 10400, Thailand; matthew.pha@mahidol.edu
4 Department of Biology, Faculty of Science, Mahidol University, Bangkok 10400, Thailand; phurt.har@mahidol.edu (P.H.); surang.cha@mahidol.ac.th (S.C.); sombat.sin@mahidol.ac.th (S.S.); puey.oun@mahidol.edu (P.O.)
5 Department of Biochemistry, Faculty of Science, Mahidol University, Bangkok 10400, Thailand
* Correspondence: tavan.jan@mahidol.ac.th

Abstract: In recent decades, the incidence of *Clostridioides difficile* infection (CDI) has remained high in both community and health-care settings. With the increasing rate of treatment failures and its ability to form spores, an alternative treatment for CDI has become a global priority. We used the microdilution assay to determine minimal inhibitory concentrations (MICs) of vancomycin and teicoplanin against 30 distinct *C. difficile* strains isolated from various host origins. We also examined the effect of drugs on spore germination and outgrowth by following the development of OD_{600}. Finally, we confirmed the spore germination and cell stages by microscopy. We showed that teicoplanin exhibited lower MICs compared to vancomycin in all tested isolates. MICs of teicoplanin ranged from 0.03–0.25 μg/mL, while vancomycin ranged from 0.5–4 μg/mL. Exposure of *C. difficile* spores to broth supplemented with various concentrations of antimicrobial agents did not affect the initiation of germination, but the outgrowth to vegetative cells was inhibited by all test compounds. This finding was concordant with aberrant vegetative cells after antibiotic treatment observed by light microscopy. This work highlights the efficiency of teicoplanin for treatment of *C. difficile* through prevention of vegetative cell outgrowth.

Keywords: teicoplanin; *Clostridioides difficile*; spore; antibiotics

Citation: Ojha, S.C.; Phanchana, M.; Harnvoravongchai, P.; Chankhamhaengdecha, S.; Singhakaew, S.; Ounjai, P.; Janvilisri, T. Teicoplanin Suppresses Vegetative *Clostridioides difficile* and Spore Outgrowth. *Antibiotics* **2021**, *10*, 984. https://doi.org/10.3390/antibiotics10080984

Academic Editor: Guido Granata

Received: 13 July 2021
Accepted: 10 August 2021
Published: 15 August 2021

1. Introduction

Clostridioides difficile, previously known as *Clostridium difficile*, is a gram-positive anaerobic spore-forming bacterium. It accounts for about 20–25% of antibiotic associated diarrhea [1,2] and almost all cases of pseudomembranous colitis [3]. *C. difficile* infection (CDI) normally occurs after antibiotic administration, especially ampicillin and amoxicillin, cephalosporins, clindamycin, fluoroquinolones, and meropenem [3,4]. Studies have suggested that gut microbiota dysbiosis after antibiotic treatment allows colonization and growth of *C. difficile* [5]. CDI can cause clinical manifestations ranging from asymptomatic to severe diarrhea, pseudomembranous colitis, bowel perforation, and multi-organ dysfunction [6]. Ultimately, CDI can be fatal, mostly in older patients [7]. The total CDI incidence has decreased in the US according to the Center for Disease Control and Prevention (CDC) [8]. Although the number of cases is not on the rise, *C. difficile* is classified as a pathogen posing an urgent threat due to antibiotic resistance [9].

Treatment for CDI is now limited to a few antibiotics including fidaxomicin and vancomycin according to the new guideline by the Infectious Diseases Society of America

(IDSA) and the Society for Healthcare Epidemiology of America (SHEA) [10]. Metronidazole, which was suggested as a first line, is now recommended only when fidaxomicin or vancomycin is not available or is limited, owing to its inferiority to vancomycin and fidaxomicin, higher recurrence rate, and neurotoxicity in prolonged or repeated use [10,11]. Additionally, treatment failures have been reported for most regimens, mostly due to the recurrence of *C. difficile*, hence new antibiotics for CDI are of utmost importance [12].

Developing new drugs is a costly and time-consuming process. Therefore, drug repurposing or repositioning has come under the limelight in pharmaceutical research in recent years as it can cut down the development process to minimal [13,14]. Teicoplanin, a mixture of glycopeptide antibiotics, belongs to the same class as vancomycin, distinguished by glucosamine as the basic sugar and the presence of aliphatic acid residues. It binds to the terminal D-Ala-D-Ala sequence of peptides forming the bacterial cell wall and, by sterically hindering the transglycosylation reaction, inhibits the formation of peptidoglycan by an intracellular accumulation of UDP-*n*-acetylmuramyl-pentapeptide [15]. Teicoplanin exhibits great activity against multiple gram-positive bacteria, which fail for other regimens [16], including *C. difficile* [17]. Even though the activity of teicoplanin against vegetative cell *C. difficile* is well documented [17–19], no experimental evidence has been presented so far for spore and outgrowth of *C. difficile*. We investigated the effect of teicoplanin on spore germination and outgrowth in *C. difficile* isolates from different host origins and compared it to its vancomycin counterpart. In addition, we also examined the cell stage alterations marked by staining the affinity of germinating cells following antibiotic treatment. The data presented here provide experimental evidence for the inhibitory effect of teicoplanin on germinating *C. difficile* cells.

2. Results

2.1. MICs of Teicoplanin on C. difficile

Minimum inhibitory concentrations (MICs) of teicoplanin and vancomycin against 30 *C. difficile* isolates obtained from various sources were determined by the broth microdilution method as described earlier [20]. All strains tested were sensitive to both antibiotics with MIC ranges for teicoplanin and vancomycin of 0.03–0.25 μg/mL and 0.5–4.0 μg/mL, respectively. Teicoplanin showed lower MICs among all strains tested (Table 1). We also compared the effect of teicoplanin at sub-MICs to vancomycin on selected strains. At sub-MICs, both antibiotics were at least 1-log less potent than at their respective MICs. However, teicoplanin at sub-MIC concentrations reduced the number of colonies more than that of vancomycin (Figure 1). The MICs of antimicrobial agents for each respective vegetative strain were used as a platform to evaluate the effect of these drugs on *C. difficile* spore germination and outgrowth. We also evaluated minimum bactericidal concentrations (MBC) of both teicoplanin, and vancomycin and the results revealed that the MBC of both antibiotics were at the concentration of 2× MIC.

Table 1. Minimal inhibitory concentrations for teicoplanin and vancomycin for 30 *C. difficile* strains.

Strains	Origin	MIC (µg/mL)	
		Teicoplanin	Vancomycin
F101	Food	0.06	2
F102	Food	0.06	2
F103	Food	0.125	2
F104	Food	0.125	2
A121	Animal	0.25	4
A122	Animal	0.125	2
A123	Animal	0.25	4
A124	Animal	0.25	4
A125	Animal	0.25	4
A126	Animal	0.125	2
R20291	Human	0.03	0.5
H201	Human	0.06	1
H203	Human	0.125	2
H204	Human	0.06	1
H205	Human	0.25	4
H206	Human	0.25	4
H207	Human	0.25	4
H208	Human	0.25	4
H209	Human	0.125	2
H210	Human	0.125	2
H211	Human	0.25	4
H212	Human	0.125	2
H213	Human	0.25	2
H214	Human	0.25	4
H215	Human	0.25	4
H216	Human	0.125	2
H217	Human	0.125	2
H218	Human	0.25	4
32g57	Human	0.125	2

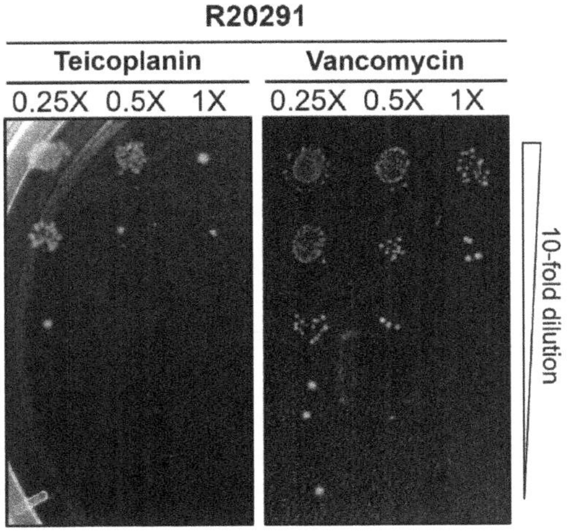

Figure 1. Antibacterial activity at sub-MICs of antibiotics using spot assay. A representative strain of *C. difficile* R20291 was attained to 0.1 OD_{600} in BHIS (brain heart infusion supplemented with 0.1% sodium taurocholate) medium supplemented with 0.25×, 0.5×, 1× MICs of teicoplanin or vancomycin. After 24-h incubation, cultures were 10-fold serially diluted and spotted onto BHIS agar plates, and plates were photographed following 24 h anaerobic incubation at 37 °C.

2.2. *Teicoplanin Does Not Inhibit C. difficile Spore Germination*

To determine the role of teicoplanin and vancomycin in its ability to block *C. difficile* spore germination, purified spores of 6 *C. difficile* strains were incubated for 1 h in the presence of BHIS supplemented with 0.5×, 1×, or 32× MIC of teicoplanin, and germination kinetics were monitored by observing the changes in OD_{600} of *C. difficile* cultures over a 1 h period. A drug-free control and 1× MIC of vancomycin were included as a comparator. As expected, *C. difficile* isolates germinated poorly in BHI broth without supplementation of 0.1% taurocholate. Nevertheless, teicoplanin and vancomycin did not inhibit spore germination at all concentrations tested ($p > 0.05$) (Figure 2), resulting in a significant drop of OD_{600}. The initiation of spore germination under treatment conditions was comparable to the drug-free control over time based on ANOVA at each time point.

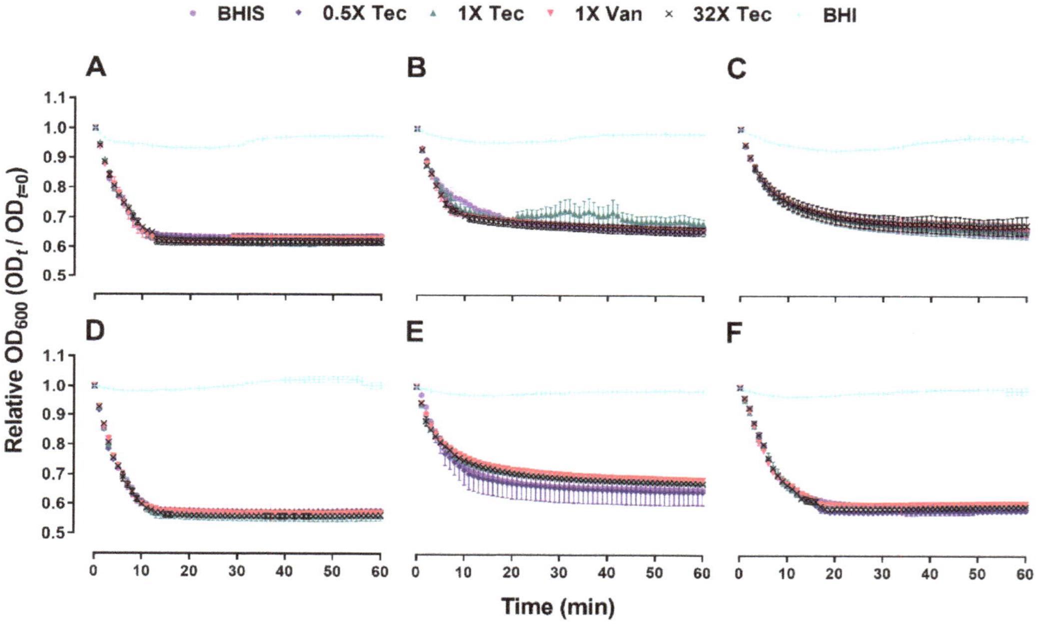

Figure 2. Teicoplanin and vancomycin do not inhibit spore germination. *C. difficile* spores were exposed to different concentration of antibiotics in relation to their respective MICs, and germination was followed by measuring loss of OD_{600} for 1 h at 1 min time interval. The growth control contained no antibiotic, and as a comparator, vancomycin was included. Data points represent the mean of the relative OD_{600} at the indicated time points normalized to $t = 0$ (control). All the experiments were performed in triplicates and error bars represent the standard errors. The results include the strains: (**A**) F101; (**B**) F102; (**C**) A125; (**D**) A126; (**E**) R20291; (**F**) H203. Circle (•), diamond (♦), triangle (▲), inverted tringle (▼), cross (×), and plus (+) denote the exposure to BHIS, 0.5× MIC teicoplanin, 1× MIC teicoplanin, 1× MIC vancomycin, 32× MIC teicoplanin, and BHI, respectively. Abbreviations: Tec = teicoplanin, Van = vancomycin, BHI = Brain heart infusion broth without 0.1% sodium taurocholate, BHIS = Brain heart infusion broth supplemented with 0.1% sodium taurocholate.

2.3. *Teicoplanin Inhibits C. difficile Spore Outgrowth*

Since both teicoplanin and vancomycin did not have either a positive or negative influence on the initiation of spore germination, we next evaluated the outgrowth to vegetative cells by monitoring the change in OD_{600}, to examine whether the later stage of germination would be affected. As expected, under the influence of 0.5× MIC of teicoplanin, growth differences were observed in contrast to the untreated control, although not significantly different (Figure 3). Sub-inhibitory concentrations of teicoplanin appeared to delay the onset of spore outgrowth and increased the time until the stationary phase was reached. However, they did not affect the outcome or the later stage of spore outgrowth. The outgrowth of spores in all tested strains exposed to a minimum of MIC of drugs was significantly inhibited compared to the drug-free control ($p < 0.0001$).

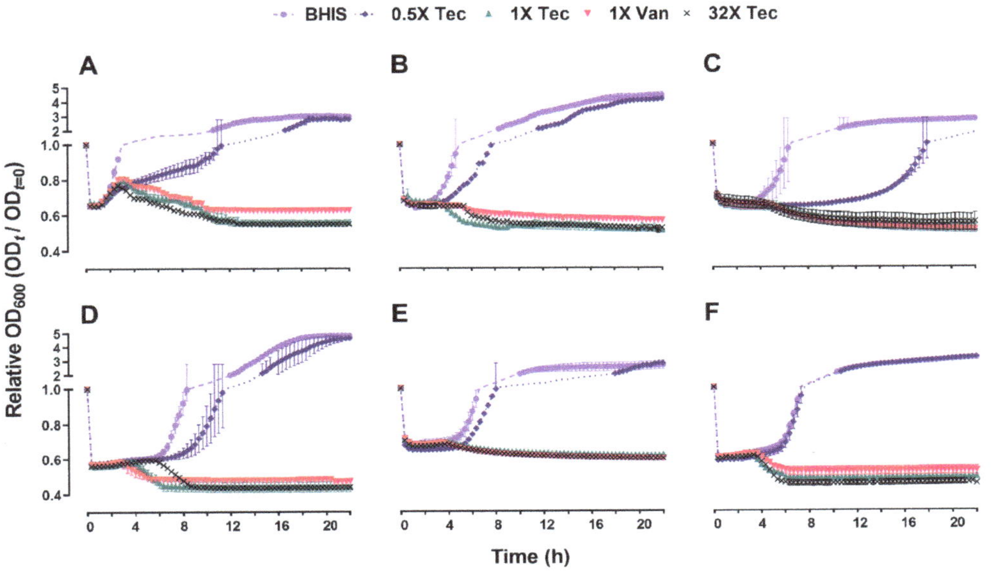

Figure 3. Teicoplanin and vancomycin at MIC inhibit spore outgrowth, while sub-MIC teicoplanin substantially delays outgrowth. Data points represent the mean of the relative OD_{600} at the indicated time points normalized to $t = 0$ (control). All the experiments were performed in triplicates and error bar represents the standard errors. The results include the strains: **(A)** F101; **(B)** F102; **(C)** A125; **(D)** A126; **(E)** R20291; **(F)** H203. Circle (•), diamond (♦), triangle (▲), inverted tringle (▼), and cross (×) denote the exposure to BHIS, 0.5× MIC teicoplanin, 1× MIC teicoplanin, 1× MIC vancomycin, and 32× MIC teicoplanin, respectively. Abbreviations: Tec = teicoplanin, Van = vancomycin, BHIS = Brain heart infusion broth supplemented with 0.1% sodium taurocholate. The dashed and dotted lines represent the data trend between the Y-axis break.

To further investigate the alteration under the influence of antibiotics on spore germination and outgrowth, we included strains that were the least and the most susceptible to teicoplanin, R20291 and A125, respectively. We next performed Wirtz–Conklin staining of untreated spores or spores treated with 1× MIC of teicoplanin or vancomycin following 3 h incubation in the growth medium. The number of spores estimated by visual inspection using light microscopic analysis revealed that >98% of spores germinated in both antibiotic treatment groups, which was not significantly different from the untreated control (Figure 4 and Figure 6). The control spores appeared as greenish-blue spheres, and the germinated cells appeared as pink spheres without shape alteration and no bacilli were detected. However, the inhibition of outgrowth by these antibiotics was more evident as determined by microscopic analysis (Figure 5), confirming that antibiotic exposure did inhibit outgrowth to vegetative cells. After 24 h incubation in a growth medium supplemented with 1× MIC of antibiotics, spores treated with both antibiotics appeared to lose their ability to change to bacillus vegetative cells. Spores were stained pink/purple or faintly stained with spherical or blunted rounded ends and showed structural degeneration and clear extrusion from the spore germinated structure (Figure 5). This suggested that the outgrowth was inhibited at the initial stage of germination. Both antibiotics at 1× MIC inhibited up to 80% of spore outgrowth to vegetative cells (Figures 5 and 6). Statistical analysis suggested that teicoplanin and vancomycin at their respective MICs inhibited spore outgrowth significantly ($p < 0.001$) when compared to untreated control. However, the effect of teicoplanin and vancomycin on spore outgrowth was not significantly different (Figure 6).

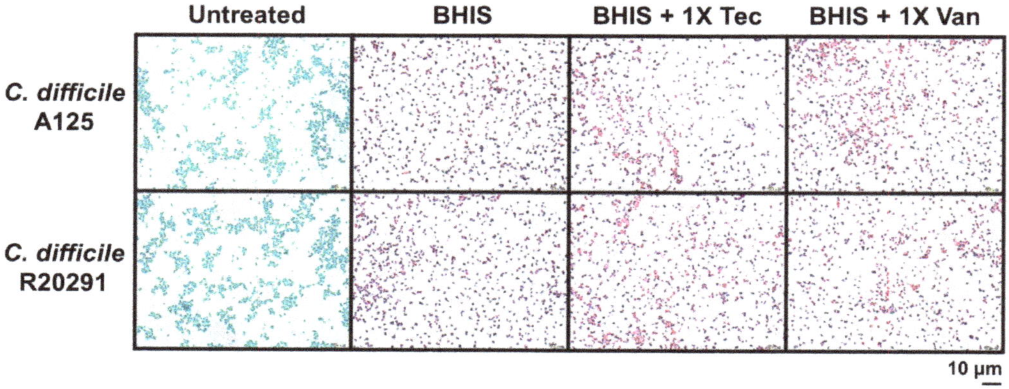

Figure 4. Teicoplanin and vancomycin at their respective MICs do not inhibit initiation of spore germination as revealed by differential staining. *C. difficile* spores were incubated with 1× MIC of either teicoplanin or vancomycin supplemented with BHIS medium for 3 h. Germinated cells were stained by Wirtz–Conklin staining (5% malachite green/0.5% safranin). Spores were greenish-blue spheres and germinated cells appeared to be pink/purple spheres. All the micrographs were taken at a magnification of 1000×. All the experiments were repeated in triplicates to ensure the reproducibility of the results. Abbreviations: Tec = teicoplanin, Van = vancomycin, BHIS = Brain heart infusion broth supplemented with 0.1% sodium taurocholate.

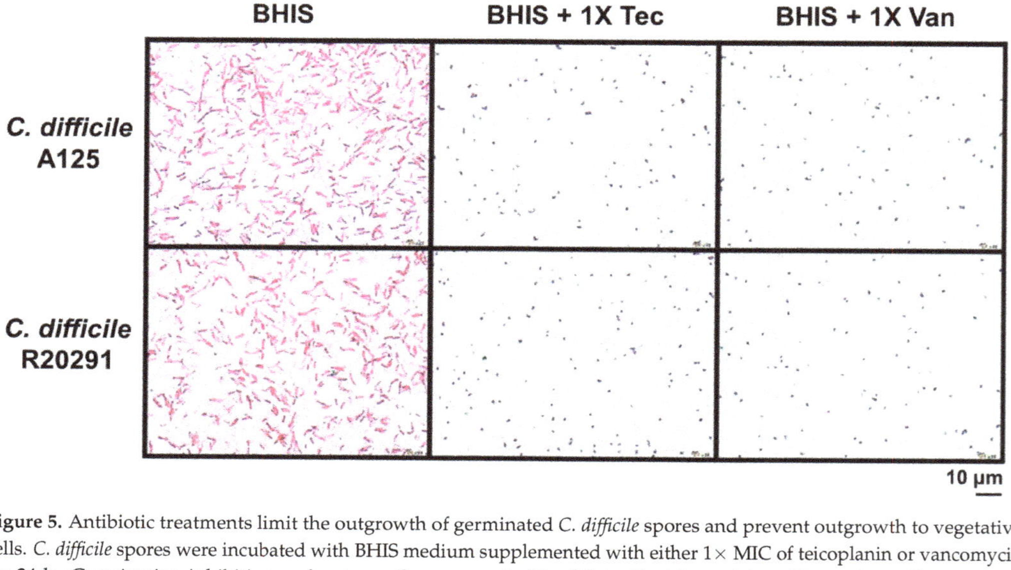

Figure 5. Antibiotic treatments limit the outgrowth of germinated *C. difficile* spores and prevent outgrowth to vegetative cells. *C. difficile* spores were incubated with BHIS medium supplemented with either 1× MIC of teicoplanin or vancomycin for 24 h. Germination inhibition and outgrowth were marked by Wirtz–Conklin staining. Vegetative cells were long filamentous and stained pink/purple, germinated cells were pink/purple spheres, outgrowths were pink/purple/faintly stained, blunted ends or extrusion from germinated cell. All the micrographs were taken at a magnification of 1000×, 5 fields counted, and repeated in triplicates to ensure the reproducibility of the results. Abbreviations: Tec = teicoplanin, Van = vancomycin, BHIS = Brain heart infusion broth supplemented with 0.1% sodium taurocholate (as negative control).

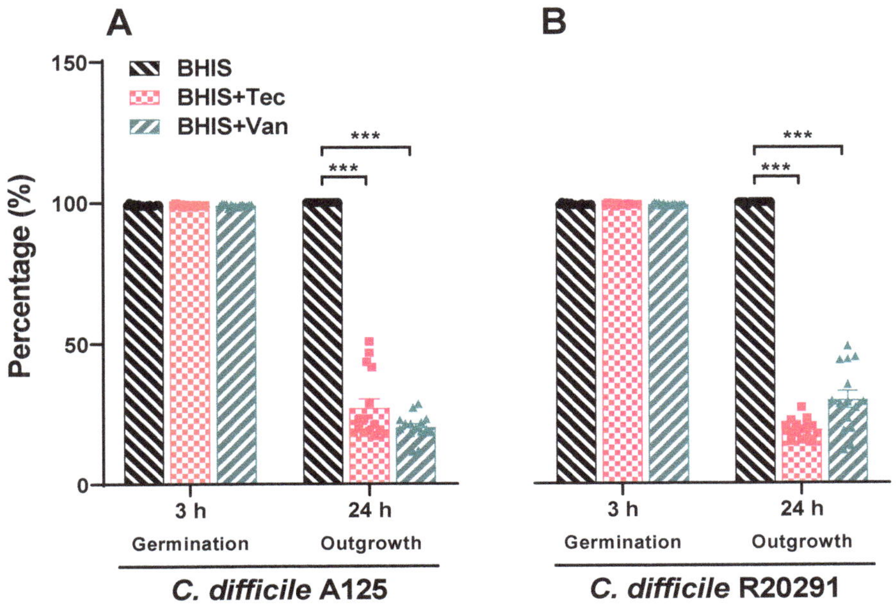

Figure 6. Teicoplanin and vancomycin significantly reduce outgrowth in *C. difficile* (**A**) A125 and (**B**) R20291 as determined by differential staining assay. *C. difficile* spores were incubated with BHIS medium alone or medium supplemented with 1× MIC of either teicoplanin or vancomycin for 24 h, then thoroughly washed and stained with a Wirtz–Conklin stain. All the micrographs were taken at a magnification of 1000×. Relative percentage of germinated spore and vegetative cells were calculated based on the count of five different fields by CellSens Dimension software. Bar graphs represent geometric means of three independent experiments and error bars represent the standard errors. Abbreviations: Tec = teicoplanin, Van = vancomycin and *** denotes p-value < 0.0001.

3. Discussion

CDI continues to be a major nosocomial pathogen and a particular source of morbidity and mortality among elderly and immune suppressed individuals [21]. Treatment failures have been more evident recently, which has raised a serious concern for clinicians across multiple specialties. Hence, there is a medical need to explore potential therapeutic drugs with improved properties. Previous studies have encouraged the use of teicoplanin over commonly used antibiotics in CDI treatment due to its longer half-life, lower relapse rate, relatively uncommon nephrotoxicity or cytotoxicity, and lack of requirement for routine serum monitoring [18,19,22,23] A study by Wenisch et al. (1996) also claimed to have 100% cure rate with the use of teicoplanin in patients endoscopically confirmed with pseudomembrane colitis [19]; however, direct comparisons with vancomycin are difficult because of inherent differences between studies.

As teicoplanin is fast acting at low concentrations and has poor absorption in the gut [24], it is incontestably an effective antimicrobial agent for the control of pathogens in the gut, including *C. difficile,* without permitting spore formation [25,26]. The activity of teicoplanin was at least 8–16 fold more potent than that of vancomycin, which was consistent with the studies done by Kunishima [27]. A set of 6 distinct target isolates obtained from humans, animals and food were used to account for the variation in the *C. difficile* spore germination and outgrowth under the influence of these antimicrobial agents. Examining the 0.5×, 1× or 32× of teicoplanin or 1× MIC of vancomycin on *C. difficile* spore germination revealed that none of the antimicrobial agents affected the initiation of germination compared to the drug-free control. At MIC or above, we observed that the outgrowth was inhibited by these antimicrobial agents. This is predictable as spores lose their dormancy upon germination, resume metabolism at the core region and subsequently an outgrowth begins by synthesizing new cell wall peptidoglycan [28,29]. The germinated spores are vulnerable to these glycopeptide antibiotics, which inhibit spore outgrowth. Although teicoplanin is functionally similar to vancomycin, its potent activity at relatively low concentration on vegetative cells and spore outgrowth may contribute to the lower recurrence rate in clinical trials [19,30–33]. Furthermore, transition from spores to vegetative cells is important and involves various metabolic changes. There are reports showing that some antibiotics can inhibit vegetative cells but not outgrowth [34]. Certain antibiotics inhibit both spore outgrowth and vegetative cells but at different concentrations, implying that there are underlying differences between these stages [35].

At sub-inhibitory concentration of teicoplanin, late growth had begun for most strains, which took an extended duration to reach their stationary phase; this could be due to the stress generated by the antibiotic at an early stage of spore germination.

To investigate further spore germination and outgrowth by light microscopy, we included 2 strains that were the least and the most susceptible to teicoplanin. Wirtz–Conklin staining displayed a clear distinction between different stages of spore germination following antibiotic treatment or untreated spores, which agreed with the studies done by Hamouda [36]. Untreated spores were dormant in structure and acquired greenish blue color following Wirtz–Conklin staining instead of pink/purple color spheres or rods [21,36,37]. Incubating spores with growth medium for 3 h displayed initiation of germination without complete transition to bacilli, where they appeared as pink spheres. This change in their staining affinity is associated with the initiation of germination in the presence of growth medium without complete outgrowth to the filamentous vegetative bacilli. The variability in spore germination appeared due to the asynchrony in spore population germination following exposure to spore germinants, which followed studies done by Moir [38]. Following complete germination, spores were transformed into filamentous vegetative cells that were stained purple rods. However, spores following treatment with antibiotics did not develop into bacilli for up to 24 h. The inhibitory action of those antibiotics affected their outgrowth to vegetative cells, which appeared as spheres or short rods with blunted ends, supporting the notion of being sporostatic agents.

4. Materials & Methods

4.1. *C. difficile* Strains and Growth Conditions

A total of 30 *C. difficile* isolates obtained from various sources, including food, animal, and human were used in this study (Table 1) [39]. *C. difficile* strain R20291 was kindly provided by Prof Nigel Minton, University of Nottingham. As described previously [40,41], all *C. difficile* strains were grown at 37 °C in an anaerobic workstation (85% N_2, 10% H_2, and 5% CO_2; Don Whitley Scientific, UK) in the brain heart infusion supplemented with 0.1% (*w*/*v*) sodium taurocholate, 0.1% L-cysteine, and 5 mg/mL yeast extract broth or agar (BHIS).

4.2. Spore Preparation

A total of 6 strains of *C. difficile* obtained from various sources were included for spore purification. Briefly, a single colony was inoculated into BHIS broth and incubated overnight at 37 °C. A 100-µL aliquot of overnight culture was spread onto BHIS agar, supplemented with 250 µg/mL cycloserine and 8 µg/mL cefoxitin, and incubated anaerobically at 37 °C for 10 days to allow efficient sporulation. Sporulation-induced lawns were harvested in 1 mL sterile distilled water (dH_2O) using cell scrapers. The suspension was then centrifuged at 5000× *g* for 15 min and washed 5 times with sterile dH_2O. To inactivate viable vegetative cells, spore suspensions were then treated with 0.3 mg/mL proteinase K at 37 °C for 2 h with gentle shaking, followed by incubation at 65 °C for 1 h. Subsequently, spore suspensions were washed 5 additional times to remove any residuals from proteinase K. Purified spores were examined by phase-contrast microscopy to ensure that they were free of vegetative cells and debris, and subsequently stored at 4 °C.

4.3. Antimicrobial Assay

To determine minimal inhibitory concentrations (MICs), a single colony from overnight culture was resuspended in 5 mL BHIS broth and incubated anaerobically for 12 h. Next day, 100 µL of aliquots were transferred to a new BHIS broth and incubated for another 6 h to minimize spore carryover and dilute the pre-formed toxin effect. The diluted vegetative cell suspension (100 µL) was aliquoted to the wells of flat-bottomed 96-well plates containing equal volumes of BHIS medium supplemented with defined concentrations of antibiotics, with the initial inoculum concentration maintained at OD_{600} of 0.6. An antibiotic-free control was included in each experiment. After 24 h incubation, the plates were measured for OD_{600} as an indicator of bacterial growth using a microplate reader (Tecan, Switzerland). MIC is defined by the concentration that has no visible growth. These assays were repeated at least 3 times to ensure reproducibility of the results. To compare the effect of sub-inhibitory concentrations of teicoplanin and vancomycin, *C. difficile* was exposed to 0.25×, 0.5×, and 1× MIC values, and was serially diluted before stamping on to BHIS plate, then incubated anaerobically for 24 h.

Minimal bactericidal concentration (MBC) was performed as previously described [42]. Briefly, the assay plate containing various concentrations of antibiotics was inoculated with bacterial suspension as per MIC and incubated for 24 h, then the bacterial suspensions around MIC value were transferred to the BHIS plate by the stamping technique and incubated for 24 h. MBC is defined by the concentration where no bacterial colony was observed on the BHIS plate.

4.4. Spore Germination and Outgrowth

Spore suspensions were heat activated at 65 °C for 30 min, vortexed to obtain a homogenous suspension and checked for clumping by microscopy. The time-kill kinetics of teicoplanin against 6 *C. difficile* strains were performed at the 0.5×, 1×, 2×, and 32× MIC of antibiotics supplemented in BHIS medium, with the final inoculum concentration maintained at OD_{600} of 0.6. Spore germination was followed anaerobically at 37 °C by measuring the loss of OD_{600} at 1 min time intervals for 1 h using a microplate reader. Reduction of OD_{600} reflects spore germination as it changes with the refractility of the spore coat [43]. Following germination, the differences in spore outgrowth efficiency were recorded by measuring OD_{600} at 20 min time intervals for 22 h using the same protocol. The ratio of the OD_{600} at time t and the control (t = 0) was then plotted against time. A drug-free control, and as a comparator, the spore suspensions treated with 1× MIC of vancomycin were included for every strain tested.

4.5. Wirtz–Conklin Staining

The staining protocol for differentiation of spores from germinating and vegetative cells was adapted from Hamouda [36]. The spore suspension was anaerobically incubated at 37 °C for 3 h or for 24 h with BHIS medium alone or medium supplemented with MIC concentrations of antibiotics. Following incubation, the spore suspension was washed thoroughly 5 times with sterile distilled water and resuspended with 15 µL dH_2O (OD_{600}~0.1). Five microliters of spore suspension were transferred to a clean glass slide and smeared uniformly. Henceforth, slides were air dried, and heat fixed and stained with Wirtz–Conklin stain. The specimen was visualized under oil immersion objective of a light microscope (Olympus BX53, Tokyo, Japan). Five fields of each slide were imaged from 3 independent biological replicates, counted by using software CellSens Dimension software version 1.11 (Olympus Software, Imaging System, Hamburg, Germany). Based on their color differences, relative percentages of germinated spores and vegetative cells were calculated. The percentage of spores in each image was also calculated as [Number of spores/Total number of cells (spores + vegetative cells)] × 100.

4.6. Statistical Analysis

All data presented were of at least 3 independent experiments. Statistical analyses were performed by the nonparametric one-way analysis of variance (ANOVA), using GraphPad Prism software (GraphPad Software Inc., La Jolla, CA, USA) to compare each condition with the corresponding controls. *p*-values less than 0.05 indicated statistically significant difference.

5. Conclusions

In conclusion, our results indicated that teicoplanin could be a potential therapeutic drug for *C. difficile* due to its potent activity at low concentrations, as well as having predetermined broad-spectrum activity against gram-positive anaerobes. Teicoplanin did not interrupt spore germination, but instead inhibited the outgrowth to vegetative cells from the germinated spore. Our data bridge the experimental gap on the effect of teicoplanin on spores as its effects on spore germination and outgrowth in *C. difficile* have not yet been reported. As most *C. difficile*-associated diseases are multifactorial, further in-depth studies, including many hypervirulent strains, animal models and human trials must be warranted to elucidate the therapeutic role of teicoplanin.

Author Contributions: Conceptualization, T.J.; formal analysis, S.C.O. and M.P.; methodology, S.C.O., M.P., P.H., S.C., S.S., and P.O.; investigation, S.C.O.; validation, T.J.; writing-original draft preparation, S.C.O.; writing-review and editing, M.P. and T.J.; project administration, T.J. All authors have read and agreed to the published version of the manuscript.

Funding: This research project is supported by Research Cluster: Multi-generation Researchers Grant from Mahidol University to S.C., T.J. and P.H. M.P. received the ICTM grant from the Faculty of Tropical Medicine, Mahidol University.

Institutional Review Board Statement: Not applicable.

Informed Consent Statement: Not applicable.

Data Availability Statement: Data are contained within the article.

Conflicts of Interest: The authors declare no conflict of interest.

References

1. Ayyagari, A.; Agarwal, J.; Garg, A. Antibiotic-associated diarrhea: Infectious causes. *Indian J. Med Microbiol.* **2003**, *21*, 6–11.
2. Bartlett, J.G. Antibiotic-Associated Diarrhea. *N. Engl. J. Med.* **2002**, *346*, 334–339. [CrossRef] [PubMed]
3. Kelly, C.P.; Pothoulakis, C.; Lamont, J.T. *Clostridium difficile* Colitis. *N. Engl. J. Med.* **1994**, *330*, 257–262. [CrossRef] [PubMed]
4. King, R.N.; Lager, S.L. Incidence of *Clostridium difficile* Infections in Patients Receiving Antimicrobial and Acid-Suppression Therapy. *Pharmacother. J. Hum. Pharmacol. Drug Ther.* **2011**, *31*, 642–648. [CrossRef]
5. Seekatz, A.M.; Young, V.B. *Clostridium difficile* and the microbiota. *J. Clin. Investig.* **2014**, *124*, 4182–4189. [CrossRef] [PubMed]
6. Smits, W.K.; Lyras, D.; Lacy, B.; Wilcox, M.H.; Kuijper, E.J. *Clostridium difficile* infection. *Nat. Rev. Dis. Primers* **2016**, *2*, 1–20. [CrossRef]
7. Czepiel, J.; Dróżdż, M.; Pituch, H.; Kuijper, E.J.; Perucki, W.; Mielimonka, A.; Goldman, S.; Wultańska, D.; Garlicki, A.; Biesiada, G. *Clostridium difficile* infection: Review. *Eur. J. Clin. Microbiol. Infect. Dis.* **2019**, *38*, 1211–1221. [CrossRef]
8. Guh, A.Y.; Mu, Y.; Winston, L.G.; Johnston, H.; Olson, D.; Farley, M.M.; Wilson, L.E.; Holzbauer, S.M.; Phipps, E.C.; Dumyati, G.K.; et al. Trends in U.S. Burden of *Clostridioides difficile* Infection and Outcomes. *N. Engl. J. Med.* **2020**, *382*, 1320–1330. [CrossRef]
9. CDC. *Antibiotic Resistance Threats in the United States*; CDC: Atlanta, GA, USA, 2019.
10. McDonald, L.C.; Gerding, D.N.; Johnson, S.; Bakken, J.S.; Carroll, K.C.; Coffin, S.E.; Dubberke, E.R.; Garey, K.W.; Gould, C.V.; Kelly, C.; et al. Clinical Practice Guidelines for *Clostridium difficile* Infection in Adults and Children: 2017 Update by the Infectious Diseases Society of America (IDSA) and Society for Healthcare Epidemiology of America (SHEA). *Clin. Infect. Dis.* **2018**, *66*, e1–e48. [CrossRef]
11. Musher, D.M.; Aslam, S.; Logan, N.; Nallacheru, S.; Bhaila, I.; Borchert, F.; Hamill, R.J. Relatively Poor Outcome after Treatment of *Clostridium difficile* Colitis with Metronidazole. *Clin. Infect. Dis.* **2005**, *40*, 1586–1590. [CrossRef] [PubMed]
12. Harnvoravongchai, P.; Pipatthana, M.; Chankhamhaengdecha, S.; Janvilisri, T. Insights into drug resistance mechanisms in *Clostridium difficile*. *Essays Biochem.* **2017**, *61*, 81–88. [CrossRef]
13. Pushpakom, S.; Iorio, F.; Eyers, P.A.; Escott, K.J.; Hopper, S.; Wells, A.; Doig, A.; Guilliams, T.; Latimer, J.; McNamee, C.; et al. Drug repurposing: Progress, challenges and recommendations. *Nat. Rev. Drug Discov.* **2019**, *18*, 41–58. [CrossRef]
14. Yssel, A.; Vanderleyden, J.; Steenackers, H.P. Repurposing of nucleoside- and nucleobase-derivative drugs as antibiotics and biofilm inhibitors. *J. Antimicrob. Chemother.* **2017**, *72*, 2156–2170. [CrossRef] [PubMed]

15. Reynolds, P.E. Structure, biochemistry and mechanism of action of glycopeptide antibiotics. *Eur. J. Clin. Microbiol. Infect. Dis.* **1989**, *8*, 943–950. [CrossRef]
16. Schaison, G.; Graninger, W.; Bouza, E. Teicoplanin in the Treatment of Serious Infection. *J. Chemother.* **2000**, *12*, 26–33. [CrossRef]
17. de Lalla, F.; Privitera, G.; Rinaldi, E.; Ortisi, G.; Santoro, D.; Rizzardini, G. Treatment of *Clostridium difficile*-associated disease with teicoplanin. *Antimicrob. Agents Chemother.* **1989**, *33*, 1125–1127. [CrossRef] [PubMed]
18. Pantosti, A.; Luzzi, I.; Cardines, R.; Gianfrilli, P. Comparison of the in vitro activities of teicoplanin and vancomycin against *Clostridium difficile* and their interactions with cholestyramine. *Antimicrob. Agents Chemother.* **1985**, *28*, 847–848. [CrossRef]
19. Wenisch, C.; Parschalk, B.; Hasenhundl, M.; Hirschl, A.M.; Graninger, W. Comparison of Vancomycin, Teicoplanin, Metronidazole, and Fusidic Acid for the Treatment of *Clostridium difficile*—Associated Diarrhea. *Clin. Infect. Dis.* **1996**, *22*, 813–818. [CrossRef] [PubMed]
20. Peterson, L.R.; Shanholtzer, C.J. Tests for bactericidal effects of antimicrobial agents: Technical performance and clinical relevance. *Clin. Microbiol. Rev.* **1992**, *5*, 420–432. [CrossRef] [PubMed]
21. Ochsner, U.A.; Bell, S.J.; O'Leary, A.L.; Hoang, T.; Stone, K.C.; Young, C.L.; Critchley, I.A.; Janjic, N. Inhibitory effect of REP3123 on toxin and spore formation in *Clostridium difficile*, and in vivo efficacy in a hamster gastrointestinal infection model. *J. Antimicrob. Chemother.* **2009**, *63*, 964–971. [CrossRef] [PubMed]
22. Kureishi, A.; Jewesson, P.J.; Rubinger, M.; Cole, C.D.; E Reece, D.; Phillips, G.L.; A Smith, J.; Chow, A.W. Double-blind comparison of teicoplanin versus vancomycin in febrile neutropenic patients receiving concomitant tobramycin and piperacillin: Effect on cyclosporin A-associated nephrotoxicity. *Antimicrob. Agents Chemother.* **1991**, *35*, 2246–2252. [CrossRef] [PubMed]
23. Wood, M.J. The comparative efficacy and safety of teicoplanin and vancomycin. *J. Antimicrob. Chemother.* **1996**, *37*, 209–222. [CrossRef]
24. Wilson, A.P.R. Clinical Pharmacokinetics of Teicoplanin. *Clin. Pharmacokinet.* **2000**, *39*, 167–183. [CrossRef]
25. Amidon, S.; Brown, J.E.; Dave, V.S. Colon-Targeted Oral Drug Delivery Systems: Design Trends and Approaches. *AAPS PharmSciTech* **2015**, *16*, 731–741. [CrossRef]
26. Davido, B.; Leplay, C.; Bouchand, F.; Dinh, A.; Villart, M.; Le Quintrec, J.-L.; Teillet, L.; Salomon, J.; Michelon, H. Oral Teicoplanin as an Alternative First-Line Regimen in *Clostridium difficile* Infection in Elderly Patients: A Case Series. *Clin. Drug Investig.* **2017**, *37*, 699–703. [CrossRef] [PubMed]
27. Kunishima, H.; Saito, M.; Kaku, M.; Chiba, J.; Honda, Y. Antimicrobial susceptibilities of *Clostridium difficile* isolated in Japan. *J. Infect. Chemother.* **2013**, *19*, 360–362. [CrossRef]
28. Lawler, A.J.; Lambert, P.; Worthington, T. A Revised Understanding of *Clostridioides difficile* Spore Germination. *Trends Microbiol.* **2020**, *28*, 744–752. [CrossRef]
29. Tocheva, E.I.; López-Garrido, J.; Hughes, H.V.; Fredlund, J.; Kuru, E.; VanNieuwenhze, M.S.; Brun, Y.V.; Pogliano, K.; Jensen, G.J. Peptidoglycan transformations during *Bacillus subtilis* sporulation. *Mol. Microbiol.* **2013**, *88*, 673–686. [CrossRef]
30. Allen, C.A.; Babakhani, F.; Sears, P.; Nguyen, L.; Sorg, J.A. Both Fidaxomicin and Vancomycin Inhibit Outgrowth of *Clostridium difficile* Spores. *Antimicrob. Agents Chemother.* **2013**, *57*, 664–667. [CrossRef] [PubMed]
31. de Lalla, F.; Nicolin, R.; Rinaldi, E.; Scarpellini, P.; Rigoli, R.; Manfrin, V.; Tramarin, A. Prospective study of oral teicoplanin versus oral vancomycin for therapy of pseudomembranous colitis and *Clostridium difficile*-associated diarrhea. *Antimicrob. Agents Chemother.* **1992**, *36*, 2192–2196. [CrossRef]
32. Popovic, N.; Korac, M.; Nesic, Z.; Milosevic, B.; Urosevic, A.; Jevtović, Đ.; Mitrovic, N.; Markovic, A.; Jordovic, J.; Katanic, N.; et al. Oral teicoplanin versus oral vancomycin for the treatment of severe *Clostridium difficile* infection: A prospective observational study. *Eur. J. Clin. Microbiol. Infect. Dis.* **2018**, *37*, 745–754. [CrossRef] [PubMed]
33. Wu, K.-S.; Syue, L.-S.; Cheng, A.; Yen, T.-Y.; Chen, H.-M.; Chiu, Y.-H.; Hsu, Y.-L.; Chiu, C.-H.; Su, T.-Y.; Tsai, W.-L.; et al. Recommendations and guidelines for the treatment of *Clostridioides difficile* infection in Taiwan. *J. Microbiol. Immunol. Infect.* **2020**, *53*, 191–208. [CrossRef] [PubMed]
34. Gut, I.M.; Blanke, S.R.; Van Der Donk, W.A. Mechanism of Inhibition of *Bacillus anthracis* Spore Outgrowth by the Lantibiotic Nisin. *ACS Chem. Biol.* **2011**, *6*, 744–752. [CrossRef]
35. Sun, L.; Atkinson, K.; Zhu, M.; D'Amico, D.J. Antimicrobial effects of a bioactive glycolipid on spore-forming spoilage bacteria in milk. *J. Dairy Sci.* **2021**, *104*, 4002–4011. [CrossRef]
36. Hamouda, T.; Shih, A.Y.; Baker, J.R., Jr. A rapid staining technique for the detection of the initiation of germination of bacterial spores. *Lett. Appl. Microbiol.* **2002**, *34*, 5. [CrossRef]
37. Hamouda, T.; Hayes, M.M.; Cao, Z.; Tonda, R.; Johnson, K.; Wright, D.C.; Brisker, J.; Baker, J.J.R. A Novel Surfactant Nanoemulsion with Broad-Spectrum Sporicidal Activity against *Bacillus* Species. *J. Infect. Dis.* **1999**, *180*, 1939–1949. [CrossRef] [PubMed]
38. Moir, A.; Lafferty, E.; Smith, D.A. Genetic Analysis of Spore Germination Mutants of *Bacillus subtilis* 168: The Correlation of Phenotype with Map Location. *J. Gen. Microbiol.* **1979**, *111*, 165–180. [CrossRef] [PubMed]
39. Ojha, S.C.; Chankhamhaengdecha, S.; Singhakaew, S.; Ounjai, P.; Janvilisri, T. Inactivation of *Clostridium difficile* spores by microwave irradiation. *Anaerobe* **2016**, *38*, 14–20. [CrossRef]
40. Harnvoravongchai, P.; Chankhamhaengdecha, S.; Ounjai, P.; Singhakaew, S.; Boonthaworn, K.; Janvilisri, T. Antimicrobial Effect of Asiatic Acid Against *Clostridium difficile* Is Associated With Disruption of Membrane Permeability. *Front. Microbiol.* **2018**, *9*, 2125. [CrossRef]

41. Phanchana, M.; Phetruen, T.; Harnvoravongchai, P.; Raksat, P.; Ounjai, P.; Chankhamhaengdecha, S.; Janvilisri, T. Repurposing a platelet aggregation inhibitor ticagrelor as an antimicrobial against *Clostridioides difficile*. *Sci. Rep.* **2020**, *10*, 1–8. [CrossRef] [PubMed]
42. Koburger, T.; Hubner, N.-O.; Braun, M.; Siebert, J.; Kramer, A. Standardized comparison of antiseptic efficacy of triclosan, PVP-iodine, octenidine dihydrochloride, polyhexanide and chlorhexidine digluconate. *J. Antimicrob. Chemother.* **2010**, *65*, 1712–1719. [CrossRef] [PubMed]
43. Trunet, C.; Carlin, F.; Coroller, L. Investigating germination and outgrowth of bacterial spores at several scales. *Trends Food Sci. Technol.* **2017**, *64*, 60–68. [CrossRef]

antibiotics

Article

Alteration of Intestinal Microbiome of *Clostridioides difficile*-Infected Hamsters during the Treatment with Specific Cow Antibodies

Hans-Jürgen Heidebrecht [1,*], Ilias Lagkouvardos [2], Sandra Reitmeier [2], Claudia Hengst [1], Ulrich Kulozik [1] and Michael W. Pfaffl [3]

1 Food- and Bioprocess Engineering, TUM School of Life Science, Technical University of Munich, Weihenstephaner Berg 1, 85354 Freising, Germany; claudia.hengst@tum.de (C.H.); ulrich.kulozik@tum.de (U.K.)
2 ZIEL—Institute for Food & HealthCore Facility Microbiome, Technical University of Munich, Weihenstephaner Berg 3, 85354 Freising, Germany; ilias.lagkouvardos@tum.de (I.L.); sandra.reitmeier@tum.de (S.R.)
3 Animal Physiology and Immunology, TUM School of Life Science, Technical University of Munich, Weihenstephaner Berg 3, 85354 Freising, Germany; michael.pfaffl@wzw.tum.de
* Correspondence: hans-juergen.heidebrecht@tum.de; Tel.: +49-8161713481

Abstract: *Clostridioides difficile* infection (CDI) often develops after pretreatment with antibiotics, which can lead to damage of the intestinal microbiome. The approach of this study was to use specific polyclonal antibodies isolated from the milk of immunized cows to treat CDI, in contrast to the standard application of nonspecific antibiotics. To gain a deeper understanding of the role of the microbiome in the treatment of CDI with bovine antibodies, stool and intestinal fluid samples of hamsters were collected in large quantities from various treatments (>400 samples). The results show that the regeneration of the microbiome instantly begins with the start of the antibody treatment, in contrast to the Vancomycin-treated group where the diversity decreased significantly during the treatment duration. All antibody-treated hamsters that survived the initial phase also survived the entire study period. The results also show that the regeneration of the microbiome was not an antibody-induced regeneration, but a natural regeneration that occurred because no microbiota-inactivating substances were administered. In conclusion, the treatment with bovine antibodies is a functional therapy for both the acute treatment and the prevention of recurrence in hamsters and could meet the urgent need for CDI treatment alternatives in humans.

Keywords: microbiome; *C. difficile*; hamsters; bovine immunoglobulins; 16S rRNA; next generation sequencing

Citation: Heidebrecht, H.-J.; Lagkouvardos, I.; Reitmeier, S.; Hengst, C.; Kulozik, U.; Pfaffl, M.W. Alteration of Intestinal Microbiome of *Clostridioides difficile*-Infected Hamsters during the Treatment with Specific Cow Antibodies. *Antibiotics* **2021**, *10*, 724. https://doi.org/10.3390/antibiotics10060724

Academic Editor: Guido Granata

Received: 6 May 2021
Accepted: 10 June 2021
Published: 16 June 2021

1. Introduction

Clostridioides difficile infection (CDI) is a leading healthcare-acquired infection characterized by severe diarrhea and high morbidity rates [1]. Risk factors for CDI are exposure to *C. difficile* spores through (a) community sources such as hospitals or long-term care facilities, (b) host factors such as immune status or comorbidities and (c) substances that interfere with the native commensal intestinal microbiome, such as antibiotics, surgery or other drugs [2]. The risk of CDI is six-fold higher within one month following antibiotic treatment [3]. Disruption of the indigenous microbiota creates conditions that allow the germination and further proliferation of *C. difficile* even though the mechanism is not yet fully understood. In its vegetative state, virulent strains of the obligate anaerobic bacteria *C. difficile* produce the toxins A (TcdA) and B (TcdB), that damage the intestinal epithelium, and which ultimately may cause the death of the patient. Paradoxically, CDI which is induced by antibiotic alteration of the native gut flora, is also treated with antibiotics by default (>95% of the cases). The standard antibiotics to fight and cure CDI are Metronidazole, Fidaxomicin and Vancomycin. These antibiotics suppress the growth of vegetative *C. difficile* and, thus, the initial response is typically good. However, the drawback is that these antibiotics are not specific for *C. difficile* but also cause a further destruction of the already damaged gastrointestinal microbiota. Thus, after discontinuation, patients are susceptible for recurrence of CDI due to the germination of resident and resistant spores, or due to reinfection with spores from an environmental source. In consequence 10–30% of the patient suffer from recurrent CDI after initial apparently successful therapy [2], which increases to 50–65% after the second recurrence [4].

The approach of this work is an alternative way to fight and cure CDI by using specific polyclonal antibodies obtained from bovine milk of immunized cows. Applying a cocktail of inactivated antigens in the vaccine (*C. difficile*, TcdA and TcdB), it is possible to simultaneously induce the formation of a mixture of polyclonal antibodies. The effectiveness of this approach for oral CDI treatment was demonstrated in our previous study [5], and before that in animal models such as hamsters [6,7], gnotobiotic piglets [8], mice [9] and human studies [6,10,11]. However, there is a lack of information about how the microbiota actually changes its composition, diversity and richness while treatment with bovine antibodies is ongoing. The only study touching this aspect was published by Sponseller et al. (2015) [8]. However, only stool samples from two hyper bovine colostrum treated pigs were compared with samples from two untreated pigs, so that no deeper or statistical analysis between the groups was made. To gain a deeper understanding of the role of the microbiome in the treatment of CDI with bovine polyclonal antibodies, in our study stool and intestinal fluid samples of the hamsters were collected on a large scale in various treatment groups (>400 samples). High-throughput deep sequencing was performed on an Illumina MiSeq targeting the V3–V4 hypervariable region of the 16S rRNA gene. The objective of this study was to show which treatment revealed a faster and better regeneration of the natural (pretreatment) gastrointestinal microbiome, either the specific antibodies against *C. difficile* or commonly used antibiotics. To extend the understanding of the role of the microbiome in CDI, independent of the applied treatments, different metabolites were quantified and correlated with *C. difficile* spore or vegetative cell numbers and the respective sequencing data.

2. Results

2.1. Comparison of Treatment Groups

Figure 1 shows the richness, i.e., the number of OTUs in a sample and the Simpson effective index, of the six different treatment groups on days three, six and 10. It is clear from the richness that around 200 different bacterial species were detected in each stool sample before therapy. The number of species in all groups decreased significantly compared to before the treatment to about 60–80 by treatment day three ($p < 0.001$). The individual significance levels are shown in the graphs. There were no significant differences within the groups, except for the group treated with Vancomycin, where the number was significantly ($p < 0.05$ for WPI 10,000, $p < 0.01$ for all other groups) lower, compared to all other groups. (Figure 1A). The decrease from day one to day three was due to the administration of the susceptibility antibiotic Clindamycin, according to the study design. Analogous to the pretreatment with antibiotics in humans, the antibiotic causes a reduction of intestinal microorganisms, which reduces the competition for *C. difficile* and thus enables the germination of its spores. The survival of the hamsters was WPI 10,000 = 100%; WPI 1000 = 50%; WPI 100 = 80%; Control-WPI = 10%; Vancomycin 10%; vehicle = 0% [5]. The significantly lower number in the treatment group can be explained by the antibiotic treatment, which is known to reduce the number of microbial species and diversity when applied. The increase in the significance level compared to the other treatment groups shows that the difference was even more pronounced after six days. While the number of OTUs in the group treated with antibiotics continued to decrease ($p < 0.01$) the number of species in all other groups increased again (Figure 1B).

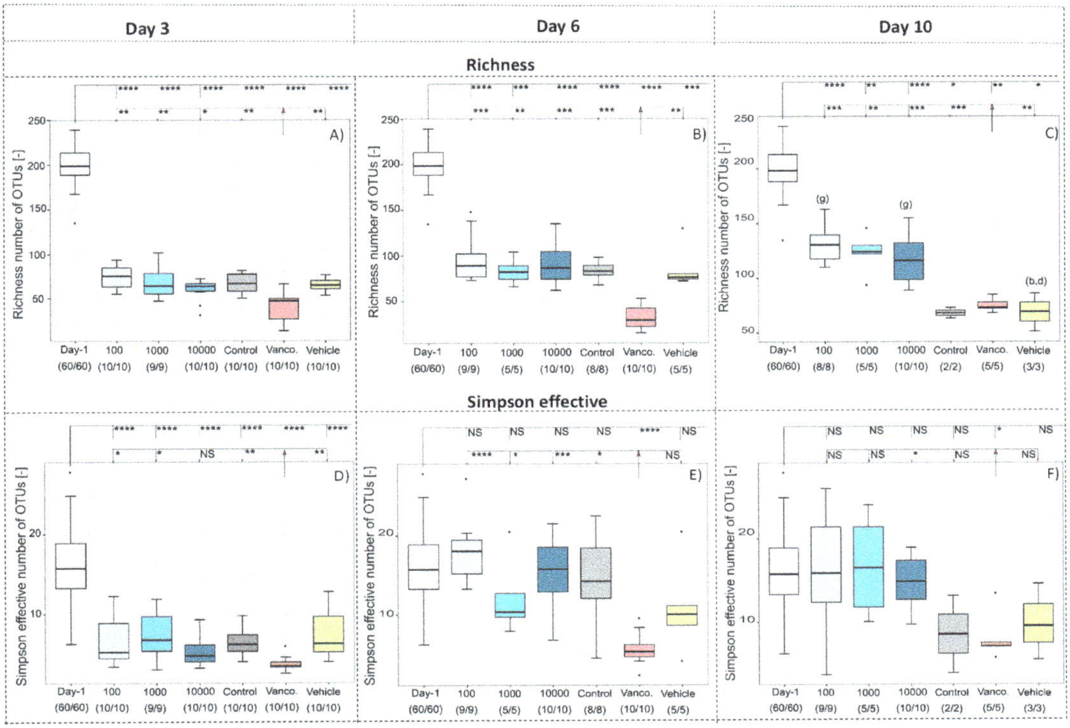

Figure 1. Richness (**A–C**) and Simpson effective index (**D–F**) during the six different treatments (WPI 10,000, WPI 1000, WPI 100, control WPI, Vancomycin, Vehicle) after 3 (**A**,**D**), 6 (**B**,**E**) and 10 (**C**,**F**) days compared to the 60 values of the hamsters before treatment (day -1). Significance values are $p < 0.05$ = *, $p < 0.01$ = **, $p < 0.001$ = ***, $p < 0.0001$ = ****, NS = not significant. Significant differences between the groups are marked by small letters. The number in parentheses indicates the number of samples and correlates with the number of hamsters surviving at that time.

By day 10, many hamsters in the control groups died from CDI; therefore, there is a clear difference from the antibody-treated groups (Figure 1C). Richness, however, does not provide any information about the relative diversity of the different OTUs. For a better representation of the community structures, therefore, the Simpson effective index was calculated (Figure 1D,E). The Simpson effective index is a measure of how equally diverse a community is, whereby high numbers stand for high diversity and low numbers for lower diversity. Analogous to the richness, intestinal microbial diversity decreased significantly ($p < 0.001$) in all groups by day three (Figure 1D). However, already from day six onwards (Figure 1E,F), there was no significant difference between the different treatment groups compared to the pretreatment group, except for the group treated with Vancomycin, which showed a significantly lower diversity ($p < 0.05$–0.0001). This means that the intestinal microbiome from day six onwards was equally diverse in all groups as before treatment, except the group treated with Vancomycin. Combining the results of richness and Simpson effective index, the number of bacterial species was not as high as before, probably because reduced occurrence of rare species, but the microbiome regenerated in terms of diversity from day six. There were only minor differences in the regeneration of diversity between the groups treated with polyclonal antibodies and the control groups. Based on the results it can be concluded that the regeneration of the microbiome was probably not an active antibody-induced regeneration. It was rather based on the fact that no microbiota-inactivating substances were administered, which led to natural microbiome regeneration, e.g., by ingestion of food. However, the comparison also revealed that the regeneration of the microorganisms alone was not sufficient for the survival of the hamsters, since almost all hamsters in the control groups died although the diversity of the microbiome increased, as the numbers in brackets show [5]. It should also be noted that the informative value of the microbiome within the control groups decreased over the course of the study due to the high mortality rate of hamsters. Nevertheless, this means that an active and antibody-induced mechanism must have taken place in addition to the regeneration of the microbiome, which caused survival and needs to be investigated further.

Looking at taxonomic differences, we focused on changes on phyla level (Figures 2 and 3). All levels of significance compared to pretreatment and compared to the Vancomycin treated group are marked on the graph. It shows that the relative abundance of Firmicutes ($p < 0.001$,Figure 2A) and Actinobacteria ($p < 0.05$, Figure 3D) was significantly lower in all groups by day 3 due to the susceptibility to the antibody Clindamycin, whereas the relative abundance of Proteobacteria ($p < 0.001$, Figure 2A) and Bacteroidetes ($p < 0.05$, Figure 3A) increased significantly), except for the Vancomycin-treated group where Firmicutes, Actinobacteria and Bacteroidetes were significantly eliminated, indicating susceptibility to the antibiotic. In contrast, the relative frequency of Proteobacteria in the Vancomycin-treated group increased from hardly detectable to over 85%, which is consistent with the result reported by [12]. In the three groups treated with different concentrations of antibodies after day 6 and 10, the frequency of Bacteroidetes was similar (Figure 3B,C). Firmicutes were less frequent (Figure 2B,C), while Proteobacteria (Figure 2E,F) and Actinobacteria (Figure 3E,F) were significantly more frequent compared to before treatment The change of the microbiota can also be seen in Figure 4, which shows a de novo clustering of all samples based on the distance of their microbial profile. Cluster 1 (red) shows the intestinal community of the hamsters before treatment. The application of Clindamycin changed the intestinal microbiome, and the microbiome of the hamsters of all treatment groups differed on day three resulting in a new cluster (green) ($p < 0.001$). However, the microbiome of all treatment groups changed again until day six (blue cluster) ($p = 0.001$). The only exception was the group treated with antibiotics, where the microbial distance of the bacteria changed so little that they were assigned to group two over the entire study period. This means that although the diversity was equally diverse from day six onwards compared to before treatment, the relative composition changed in relation to the abundance. In the future, it should be investigated whether there was no change in the microbiome without the susceptibility antibiotic or whether the administration of milk proteins led to a change due to the actual treatment.

2.2. Over-Time Comparison of Treatment Groups

Interindividual changes over time and between groups were analyzed as well. There was no significant difference in the number of surviving animals (23/30) within the three groups (WPI 100, 1000, 10,000) in terms of number of species present, overall diversity or relative composition. Therefore, they were combined and fused into one group (Figure 5). At the end of treatment, the relative abundance of Firmicutes, Bacteroidetes and Actinobacteria (Figure 5C–E) was again at the same level as before treatment, while the relative abundance of Proteobacteria (Figure 5F) was still significantly ($p < 0.001$) increased.

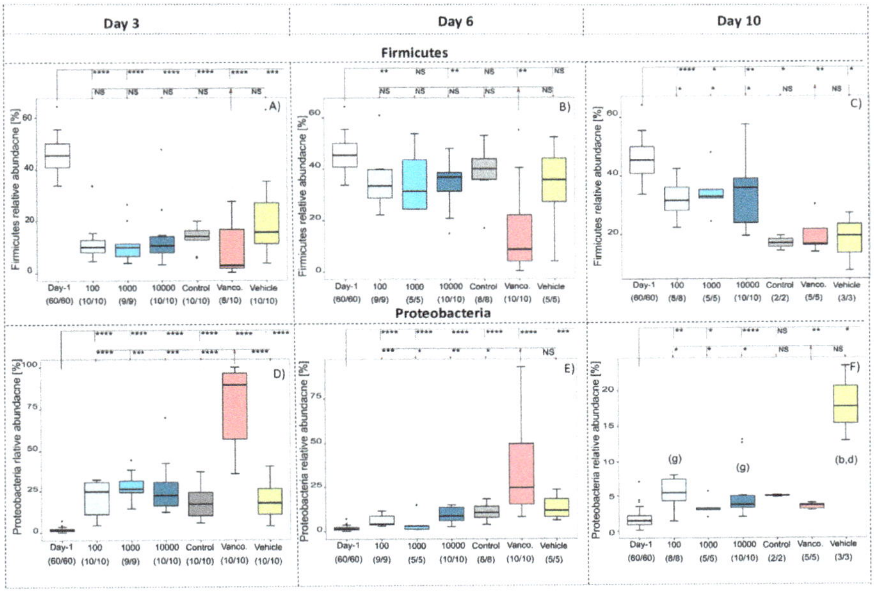

Figure 2. Relative abundance at phylum level of Firmicutes (**A–C**), Proteobacteria (**D–F**) after 3 (**A**,**D**), 6 (**B**,**E**) and 10 (**C**,**F**) days at indicated treatment compared to the relative abundance before treatment (day -1). Significance compared to before treatment and vancomycin values are $p < 0.05$ = *, $p < 0.01$ = **, $p < 0.001$ = ***, $p < 0.0001$ = ****, NS = not significant. Significant differences between the groups are marked by small letters.

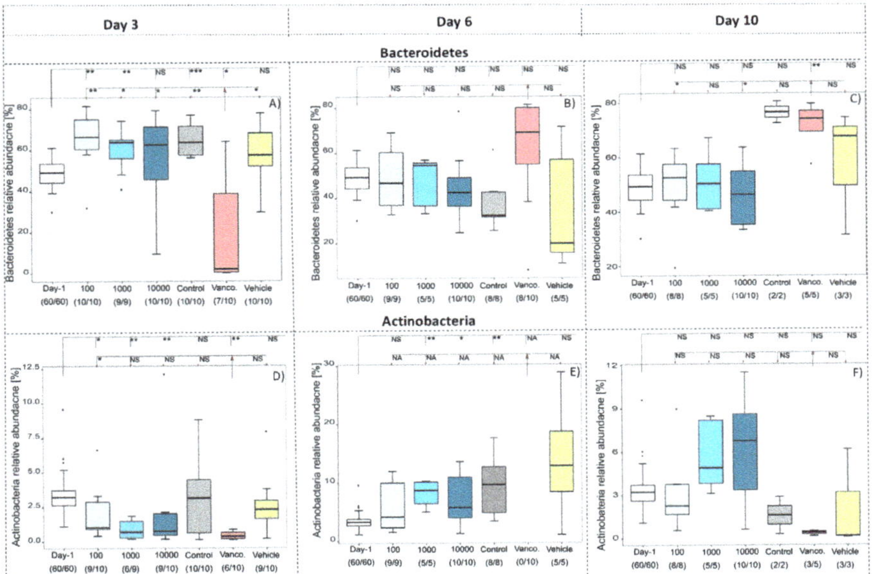

Figure 3. Relative abundance at phylum level of Bacteroidetes (**A–C**) and Actinobacteria (**A–E**) after 3 (**A**,**D**), 6 (**B**,**E**) and 10 (**C**,**F**) days at indicated treatment compared to the relative abundance before treatment (day -1). Significance compared to before treatment and Vancomycin values are $p < 0.05$ = *, $p < 0.01$ = **, $p < 0.001$ = ***, NS = not significant. Significant differences between the groups are marked by small letters.

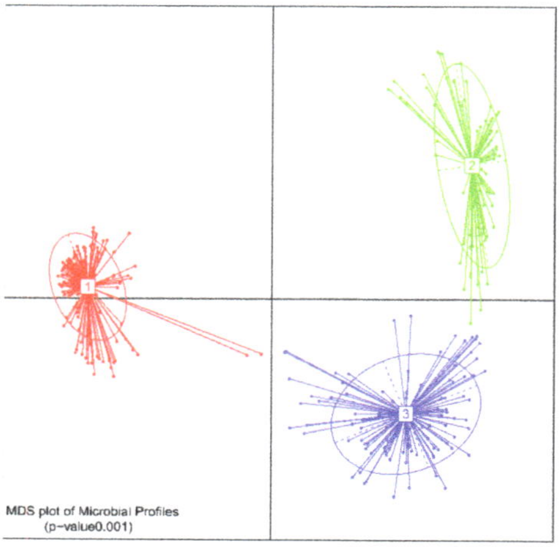

Figure 4. De novo clustering of all samples. Cluster 1 (red) shows the intestinal community of the hamsters before treatment, cluster 2 all treatment groups on day 3 as well as the Vancomycin-treated group throughout the study and cluster 3, all treatment groups from day 6 except the Vancomycin-treated group.

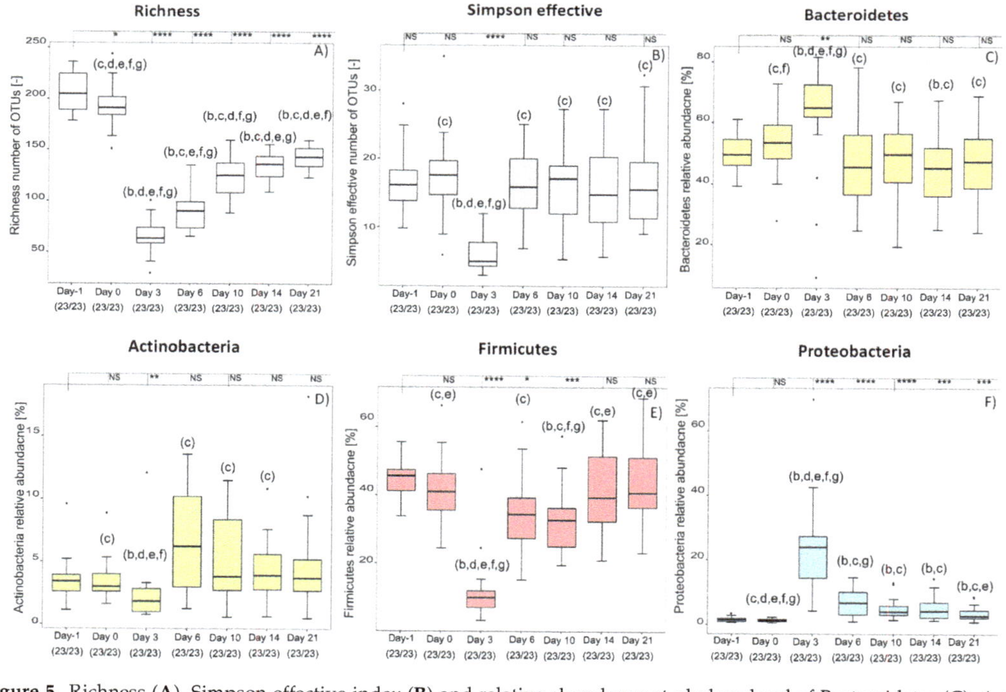

Figure 5. Richness (**A**), Simpson effective index (**B**) and relative abundance at phylum level of Bacteroidetes (**C**), Actinobacteria (**D**), Firmicutes (**E**), Proteobacteria (**F**) of the 23 hamster that survived due to the treatment with anti-CD-WPI (WPI 100, 1000, 10,000). Significance values are $p < 0.05$ = *, $p < 0.01$ = **, $p < 0.001$ = ***, $p < 0.001$ = ****, NS = not significant. Given significance values are in comparison to before treatment, significant differences between the groups are marked by small letters.

2.3. Expanding the Level of Understanding of the Role of the Microbiome in CDI

The commensal gut microbiota is a complex community of microorganisms that exist in the gastrointestinal tract, consisting of about 300 ± 150 different species in humans [13]. The balance of this microecosystem is essential for the homeostasis of the host. It protects the intestine by providing colonization stability and resistance against the infection by pathogens [14]. Mechanisms involved in this protection are direct inhibition of *C. difficile* through bacteriocins [15] or indirect by bacteria-derived metabolites, nutrient depletion [16] or stimulation of host immune defenses [17]. Even though several studies on the role of the microbiome in CDI have been carried out, there are still many gaps in knowledge regarding to the role of the microbiome in CDI [2,14]

Therefore, irrespective of the therapy used, the linearized cell and spore numbers of *C. difficile* [5] were correlated with the different metabolites measured by RP-HPLC (Table A1) in intestinal fluid (Figure 6) and with the relative abundance of different species (Figure 7). *C. difficile* was significantly positively (correlation coefficient >0.5) correlated with the metabolites ethanol, succinate and lactic acid, and significantly negatively (correlation coefficient <−0.5) correlated with the metabolites phosphate/citrate (no differentiation possible with the used RP-HPLC method), glucose, galactose, butyric acid and alpha diversity indicators, richness and Simpson effective. In addition to the Simpson effective index, the Shannon effective index was also considered in this evaluation. In analogy to the Simpson effective index, the Shannon effective index is a measure of the equality of microbiome diversity, with a slightly different weighting on the abundance of the species present. Since both parameters are used in the literature, both are shown here. The individual pairwise correlation coefficients and *p*-values are shown in Table A2 and for some selected values in the body text in brackets.

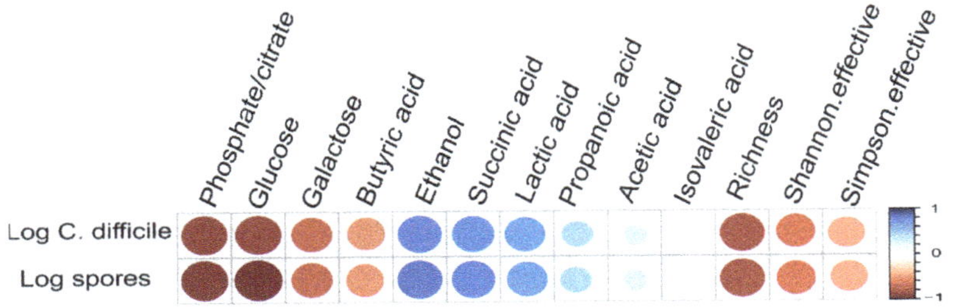

Figure 6. Heat map of pairwise correlation of *C. difficile* cell and spore counts (data from 5) with the metabolites phosphate/citrate, glucose, galactose, butyric acid, ethanol, succinate, lactic acid, propionic acid and isovaleric acid, and the alpha diversity indicators richness, Shannon effective index and Simpson effective index.

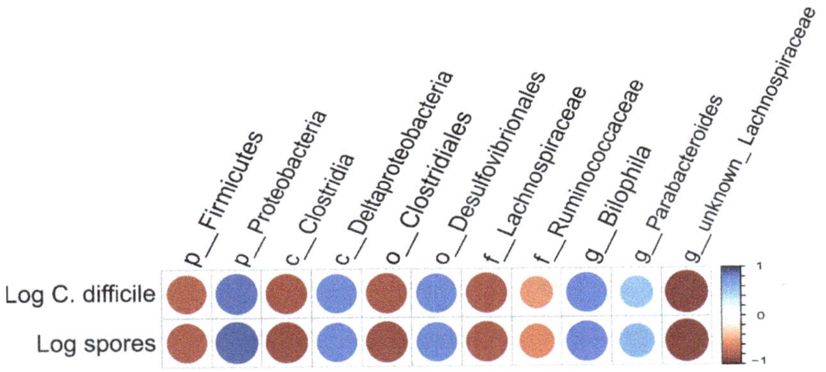

Figure 7. Simplified heatmap on different taxonomic levels where there is a significant correlation (>/< ±0.7) with *C. difficile*.

The role of the indigenous intestinal microbiota for the CDI, which has been extended by our findings, is shown in Figure 8, hence the individual steps or processes are numbered. Although the exact mechanism by which a healthy microbiota suppresses the growth of *C. difficile* is not known, it is known that bile acids play an important role. The intact microbiota converts the primary bile acids into secondary bile acids (step 1 & 6), thereby inhibiting vegetative *C. difficile* by detergent-induced toxicity (Ridlon and Hylemon 2012). Correlation values of *C. difficile* spores/cells are given in brackets and the significance levels presented in Table A1 It was shown that at the taxonomic family level (−0.79/0.8) and genus level (−0.89/0.89), Lachnospiraceae correlated significantly negatively with C. difficile cell and spore counts (Figures 6 and 7). This is consistent with findings of Reeves et al. (2012) with experiments using aseptic mice, where it was shown that administration of a single bacterium of the family Lachnospiraceae could reduce the cell density of *C. difficile*. Lachnospiraceae can convert primary bile acids into secondary bile acids and thus inhibit the growth of *C. difficile* (Figure 8A, step 1). In addition, Lachnospiraceae can produce butyric acid, which is also negatively correlated with the growth of *C. difficile*.

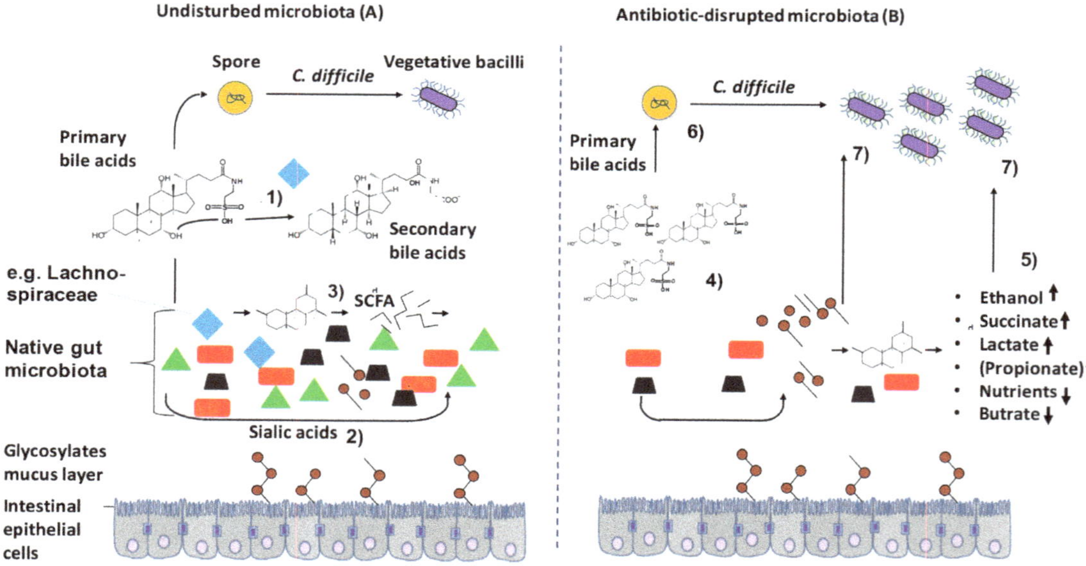

Figure 8. The role of the indigenous gut microbiota on CDI. Microbiota-mediated defense with native microbiota (**A**), omission of defense mechanism after antibiotic caused disruption of microbiota (**B**), modified from [17] and supplemented with our own correlation data.

In addition, indigenous intestinal bacteria express sialidases that cleave sugars from glycosylated proteins bound to epithelial cells, which, in turn, release free sialic acid into the intestinal lumen [18] (Figure 8A, step 2). In addition, carbohydrates enter the colon via food, and fermenting gut bacteria break down the split carbohydrates and convert them into short chain fatty acids (SCFAs) [19] (Figure 8A, step 3). Succinate is a typical SCFA [16]. Among others, the metabolites glucose, galactose, sialic acid and succinate are used as energy sources for other commensal gut bacteria.

However, treatment with antibiotics, especially broad-spectrum antibiotics, significantly changes the intestinal microbiota and inactivates, for example, Lachnospiraceae, as shown by our results. The altered relative composition of the intestinal microbiome led to higher concentrations of metabolites, which correlate significantly positive with *C. difficile* in the case of sialic acid [16] succinate (r = 0.77) lactate (r = 0.67), ethanol (r = 0.82) and propionate (r = 0.41) (Figure 8B, step 5). This was likely due to the lack of organisms breaking these molecules down or because of the increased growth of organisms producing these metabolites. This indicates that a more hospitable environment for the growth of *C. difficile* is produced by these metabolites, as was also shown for succinate [20]. In addition, the dietary restriction, i.e., a low concentration of glucose (r = −0.92) and galactose (r = −0.68 favors the growth of *C. difficile* (Figure 8B, step 5). *C. difficile* can metabolize these molecules (Figure 8B step 7), followed by toxin production and CDI symptoms.

Our results contribute to a better understanding of the role of intestinal microbiome in CDI by correlating different metabolic by-products with *C. difficile* cell and spore counts. High concentrations of nutrients such as glucose and galactose, as well as butyric acid, inhibit the growth of *C. difficile*, whereas high concentrations of ethanol, lactic acid and succinate support the growth of *C. difficile*. The results also confirm that the specific approach using bovine antibodies does not interfere with the natural microbial balance and, therefore, is a sustainable alternative to the antibiotics used so far. As a follow-up, it is suggested that this knowledge could possibly be used to support the selection and cultivation of a so-called minimal consortium of intestinal bacteria, which may in the future be an alternative to FMT and would ideally complement our specific approach for CDI treatment.

3. Materials and Methods

3.1. Study Design

The study design is described in detail by Heidebrecht et al. (2019) [5]. Briefly, anti-*Clostridium difficile* whey protein isolate (anti-CD-WPI) powder was prepared from the milk or colostrum of specifically vaccinated cows. Cows were multiple vaccinated with inactivated TcdA and TcdB (accountable for CDI pathogenesis) and *C. difficile* cell/spore material to induce antigen-specific secretory immunoglobulin A (sIgA) and IgG antibodies in the milk (animal study approval number AZ 55.2-1-54-2532.6-17-12). Six groups of ten healthy hamsters each were infected orally with 100 spores of *C. difficile* strain 630 (tgcBiomics, Bingen, Germany) one day after the susceptibility antibody Clindamycin was provided. Three different concentrations were used based on their neutralization capacity (NC) against toxin A (anti-CD-WPI 10,000, anti-CD-WPI 1000, anti-CD-WPI 100) as described by [5]. Reference groups were treated with control WPI from the same cows before immunization, the standard of care antibiotic Vancomycin and liquidation buffer only. Hamsters were dosed with 1 mL WPI-solution/100 g body weight by oral gavage. Preparations were administered 3 h before and 3 h after bacterial challenge and then every 8 h during the consecutive days for 75 h in total. All procedures were conducted in accordance with the approved protocol of the 'Institutional Animal Care and Use Committee' (IACUC-2016-0015).

3.2. Sample Collection

A single fecal pellet was collected from individual cages of all hamsters. Samples were collected on day one, i.e., after five days of acclimation and before administration of Clindamycin, on day zero, i.e., after administration of Clindamycin and before first treatment, and thereafter on day 3, 6, 10, 14 and 21 from surviving hamsters. In addition, about 10 mL of caecal fluid was taken from all 60 hamsters either on the day of death due to the disease or at the study end (day 21) after euthanization of surviving hamsters. Samples were stored and shipped on dried ice and subsequently stored at −20 °C for further analysis.

3.3. Microbiome Analysis by Sequencing of 16S rRNA

Microbiome analysis was done as described by [21]. Paired end sequencing was performed by using specific primer (341 forward and 785 reverse) targeting the V3–V4 region of the hypervariable region of the 16S rRNA gene [22,23]. Amplicons were generated by a two-step (25 cycles) polymerase chain reaction (PCR), purified and pooled. The DNA quality and quantity of all samples were in the calibration range and were checked by water samples. The 2nM PCR-fragment was sequenced on a MiSeq (Illumina) at the Technical University of Munich (TUM) Microbiome Core Facility. The negative controls' sole DNA stabilization buffer and water on every 96-well plate were inconspicuous and removed for further data processing.

3.4. Data Processing

Raw FASTQ files were demultiplexed using the pipeline 'Integrated Microbial Next Generation Sequencing' (IMNGS) [24], which is based on UPARSE approach [25]. Two errors in barcode sequences were the maximal allowed number. Reads were trimmed to the position of the first base with a quality factor <3 and then paired. The resulting sequences were size filtered, except those of assembled size <300 and >600 nucleotides. Paired reads with expected error >3 were further filtered out and the remaining reads were trimmed at each end by 10 nucleotides to prevent analysis of the distorted base composition regions at the beginning of the sequences. Operational taxonomic units (OTUs) were grouped with a sequence similarity of 97%, keeping only those with a relative abundance of >0.25% in at least one sample of the 412 samples (352 fecal samples and 60 ceacal samples). OTU tables of all study groups are provided in the Appendix A. The Rhea pipeline [26], a set of scripts of the statistical computing software R, was used for data processing. In brief, sequences were normalized to the minimum count of sequences observed. Samples with less than 2500 reads counts were excluded [26]. Microbial diversity between groups was calculated by generalized Unifrac distances [27]. The Ribosomal Database Project (RDP v.9) classifier (Wang et al., 2007) was used to assign taxonomies at 80% confidence level. Important unidentified OTUs were classified using ExTaxon. p values were corrected for multiple comparisons according to the Benjamini-Hochberg method. Only taxa with a prevalence of 10% (proportion of samples positive for the given taxa) in at least one group were considered for statistical testing.

3.5. Determination of Intestinal Metabolites with Reversed-Phase High-Performance Liquid Chromatography (RP-HPLC)

A new HPLC method was established to measure the different metabolites. The intestinal fluid was sterile-filtered directly into a vial using a 0.2 µm syringe filter. An Aminex HPX-87H 300 × 7.8 mm (Bio-Rad, Hercules, CA, USA) and a guard column were used for separation, in which 20 µL were injected and isocratically eluted with 0.005 M sulfuric acid at a flow rate of 0.450 mL/min and a temperature of 35 °C. The detection was done by measuring refractive index. With this method the metabolites glucose, galactose, succinic acid, lactic acid, acetic acid, propionic acid, ethanol, butyric acid and iso-valeric acid could be quantified simultaneously. Phosphate and citrate elute at the same time with this method and therefore could not be differentiated.

4. Conclusions

From the comparison of the groups among themselves and with the group treated with Vancomycin and integrating our previous data (8) published in Heidebrecht et al. (2019), several conclusions can be drawn. As described above, an active and antibody-induced mechanism must take place in the intestine which causes the survival of the animals. Our antibodies can inactivate foreign *C. difficile* antigens through various mechanisms of action. These include opsonization, activation of the complement system, agglutination, prevention of adhesion and direct neutralization. It is unlikely, or at least not the primary mechanism of action, that cell adhesion is prevented, and direct neutralization of the *C. difficile* cells occurs. Had this been the case, there would not have been initial spore germination and cell growth [5], but the cells would have been directly eliminated. The later decline in cell growth between days six and eight indicates that the host's own immune system was activated (which is a delayed process), either by activation of the complement system or by direct labelling of the cells for the host's own defense cells. However, since cell decline was also observed in some control groups (e.g., control WPI), the deduced conclusion is that both indirect regeneration of intestinal microbial diversity (as observed in all groups except the antibiotics group) and direct antibody-induced inactivation were crucial for cell and spore decline of *C. difficile*. In other words, prevention of recurrences (only observed in the groups treated with active antibodies) can only be achieved if both mechanisms are given the chance to work, which is the case for Ig-based CDI treatment instead of antibiotics.

Author Contributions: Conceptualization: H.-J.H., U.K., M.W.P.; methodology, formal, analysis: H.-J.H., I.L., S.R., C.H., interpretation of results: H.-J.H., U.K., M.W.P., I.L., S.R., C.H.; writing—original draft preparation: H.-J.H., writing—review and editing: all authors; supervision, U.K., M.W.P.; funding acquisition U.K. All authors have read and agreed to the published version of the manuscript.

Funding: This study was partly funded by our industry partner, Biosys Health, who provided input into study design, but had no role in data collection and analysis, interpretation or decision to pub-lish or preparation of the manuscript.

Institutional Review Board Statement: The animals were acclimatized for five days prior to the study in the biosafety level laboratories at University of North Texas Health Science Center in accordance with NIH guidelines. All procedures were carried out in accordance with the approved protocol of the Institutional Animal Care and Use Committee (IACUC-2016-0015).

Informed Consent Statement: Not applicable.

Data Availability Statement: The data is available in this manuscript.

Acknowledgments: We thank everybody who supported this study for their helpful contributions, especially the Microbiome core facility members Angela Sachsenhauser, Caroline Ziegler and Klaus Neuhaus.

Conflicts of Interest: The authors declare no conflict of interest.

Appendix A

Table A1. Concentration of Different Metabolites in Intestinal Fluid Measured by RP-HPLC.

	Phosphate [mg/mL]	Glucose [mg/mL]	Galactose [mg/mL]	Succinic Acid [mg/mL]	Lactic Acid [mg/mL]	Acetic Acid [mg/mL]	Propionic Acid [mg/mL]	Ethanol [mg/mL]	Butyric Acid [mg/mL]	Iso-Valeric Acid [mg/mL]
Placebo	2.68	1.23	0.23	0.09	0.34	1.77	0.42	0.18	0.40	0.60
	1.44	0.00	0.21	2.05	0.25	3.90	1.15	0.76	0.25	0.70
	0.96	0.00	0.02	0.84	1.30	1.11	0.29	1.66	0.48	0.77
	1.36	0.00	0.13	2.01	0.97	2.37	1.11	1.43	0.24	0.50
	1.03	0.00	0.09	2.29	0.74	2.51	1.23	2.10	0.52	0.16
	1.06	0.00	0.18	1.37	1.10	2.03	0.96	3.57	0.48	0.14
	1.23	0.00	0.04	1.48	0.13	3.83	1.25	2.28	0.49	0.24
	1.54	0.24	0.24	1.87	1.53	4.04	1.18	1.89	0.82	0.32
WPI 1000	3.28	2.89	0.27	0.11	0.11	2.25	0.31	0.45	1.50	0.03
	3.29	1.45	0.31	0.04	0.13	1.29	0.20	0.08	0.63	0.02
	2.84	1.74	0.27	0.03	0.16	1.29	0.17	0.05	0.90	0.70
	3.25	1.87	0.26	0.79	0.14	1.86	0.29	0.00	1.06	0.46
	1.60	0.67	0.16	0.03	0.13	0.76	0.11	0.02	0.49	0.01
WPI100	2.83	1.08	0.36	0.09	0.19	1.68	0.27	0.03	0.81	0.53
	3.91	2.88	0.44	0.11	0.31	3.02	0.27	0.07	2.04	1.02
	1.02	0.04	0.11	0.19	0.25	0.64	0.03	0.96	0.28	0.02
	2.91	1.37	0.19	0.01	0.29	1.53	0.15	0.10	1.03	0.49
	3.06	1.47	0.23	0.04	0.18	1.66	0.18	0.03	1.05	0.39
	3.04	1.85	0.28	0.22	0.15	1.58	0.42	0.03	0.84	0.82
	3.34	1.98	0.32	0.05	0.09	1.86	0.27	0.28	1.05	0.61
	2.45	1.28	0.18	0.03	0.21	1.11	0.30	0.01	0.61	0.64
	3.08	1.52	0.51	0.05	0.12	1.60	0.31	0.06	0.99	0.53

Table A1. *Cont.*

	Phosphate [mg/mL]	Glucose [mg/mL]	Galactose [mg/mL]	Succinic Acid [mg/mL]	Lactic Acid [mg/mL]	Acetic Acid [mg/mL]	Propionic Acid [mg/mL]	Ethanol [mg/mL]	Butyric Acid [mg/mL]	Iso-Valeric Acid [mg/mL]
WPI10000	3.00	1.85	0.29	0.27	0.31	1.73	0.27	0.12	1.12	0.04
	3.02	1.44	0.59	0.02	0.10	1.68	0.20	0.07	1.00	0.04
	3.17	2.30	0.25	0.09	0.08	1.62	0.17	0.10	1.10	0.46
	3.06	1.76	0.18	0.01	0.09	1.09	0.12	0.01	0.77	0.44
	2.96	1.78	0.20	0.17	0.07	1.61	0.57	0.00	0.86	0.04
	3.08	1.64	0.27	0.05	0.13	1.34	0.25	0.09	0.75	0.62
	2.91	1.09	0.43	0.48	0.08	1.33	0.21	0.12	0.86	0.76
	2.81	1.80	0.28	0.04	0.11	1.44	0.15	0.02	0.89	0.44
	3.22	1.79	0.36	0.10	0.07	1.31	0.19	0.05	0.86	0.58
	3.48	2.00	0.29	0.05	0.16	1.51	0.20	0.04	1.25	0.61
Vancomycin	1.73	0.00	0.14	0.82	0.80	2.56	1.09	0.64	1.21	0.33
	1.67	0.00	0.06	1.36	0.41	2.03	0.26	1.07	0.98	0.33
	1.24	0.07	0.08	0.84	0.19	2.59	0.94	5.71	0.97	0.24
	2.61	0.77	0.20	0.03	0.22	0.84	0.13	0.14	0.63	0.02
	1.62	0.00	0.09	1.35	0.77	3.28	1.05	0.34	1.03	0.28
Vehicle	1.02	0.00	0.09	0.43	0.44	0.71	0.09	0.25	0.43	0.58
	0.90	0.00	0.13	0.89	0.00	1.39	0.47	1.88	0.35	0.07
	1.04	0.00	0.18	0.62	0.21	1.26	0.35	1.70	0.58	0.62
	0.80	0.10	0.07	0.13	0.20	1.20	0.07	0.74	0.44	0.04
	0.97	0.06	0.14	0.38	0.07	0.63	0.23	0.09	0.23	0.04
	1.28	0.15	0.23	1.41	0.25	3.34	1.30	1.92	1.07	0.24

Table A2. Individual pairwise correlation coefficients and *p*-values.

Variable 1	Variable 1	Correlation	*p*-Value	Number of Supporting Data
Phosphate/Citrate	Log value of vegetative *C. difficile* count	−0.86	2.9×10^{-13}	43
Phosphate/Citrate	Log value of *C. difficile* spore count	−0.89	8.88×10^{-16}	43
Glucose	Log value of vegetative *C. difficile* count	0.85	1.67×10^{-09}	31
Glucose	Log value of *C. difficile* spore count	−0.92	1.05×10^{-13}	31
Galactose	Log value of vegetative *C. difficile* count	−0.67	8.79×10^{-7}	43
Galactose	Log value of *C. difficile* spore count	−0.68	5.89×10^{-7}	43
Butyric acid	Log value of vegetative *C. difficile* count	−0.54	1.78×10^{-4}	43
Butyric acid	Log value of *C. difficile* spore count	−0.51	4.83×10^{-4}	43
Ethanol	Log value of vegetative *C. difficile* count	0.79	9.44×10^{-10}	41
Ethanol	Log value of *C. difficile* spore count	0.82	4.03×10^{-11}	41
Succinic acid	Log value of vegetative *C. difficile* count	0.74	1.61×10^{-8}	43
Succinic acid	Log value of *C. difficile* spore count	0.77	1.11×10^{-9}	43
Lactic acid	Log value of vegetative *C. difficile* count	0.61	2.10×10^{-5}	42
Lactic acid	Log value of *C. difficile* spore count	0.67	1.24×10^{-6}	42
Richness	Log value of vegetative *C. difficile* count	−0.80	9.33×10^{-15}	60
Richness	Log value of *C. difficile* spore count	−0.81	5.55×10^{-15}	60
Shannon effective Index	Log value of vegetative *C. difficile* count	−0.61	2.22×10^{-7}	60
Shannon effective Index	Log value of *C. difficile* spore count	−0.63	8.06×10^{-8}	60
Simpson effective Index	Log value of vegetative *C. difficile* count	−0.41	1.04×10^{-3}	60
Simpson effective Index	Log value of *C. difficile* spore count	−0.44	4.86×10^{-4}	60
Simpson effective Index	Log value of *C. difficile* spore count	−0.80	9.33×10^{-15}	60

References

1. Lessa, F.C.; Mu, Y.; Bamberg, W.M.; Beldavs, Z.G.; Dumyati, G.K.; Dunn, J.R.; Farley, M.M.; Holzbauer, S.M.; Meek, J.I.; Phipps, E.C.; et al. Burden of Clostridium difficile infection in the United States. *N. Engl. J. Med.* **2015**, *372*, 825–834. [CrossRef]
2. Sartelli, M.; Malangoni, M.A.; Abu-Zidan, F.M.; Griffiths, E.A.; Di Bella, S.; McFarland, L.V.; Eltringham, I.; Shelat, V.G.; Velmahos, G.C.; Kelly, C.P.; et al. WSES guidelines for management of Clostridium difficile infection in surgical patients. *World J. Emerg. Surg.* **2015**, *10*, 38. [CrossRef]
3. Hensgens, M.P.M.; Goorhuis, A.; Dekkers, O.M.; Kuijper, E.J. Time interval of increased risk for Clostridium difficile infection after exposure to antibiotics. *J. Antimicrob. Chemother.* **2012**, *67*, 742–748. [CrossRef]
4. McFarland, L.V. Alternative treatments for Clostridium difficile disease: What really works? *J. Med. Microbiol.* **2005**, *54*, 101–111. [CrossRef] [PubMed]

5. Heidebrecht, H.-J.; Weiss, W.; Pulse, M.; Lange, A.; Gisch, K.; Kliem, H.; Mann, S.; Pfaffl, M.; Kulozik, U.; von Eichel-Streiber, C. Treatment and prevention of recurrent Clostridium difficile infection with functionalized bovine antibody-enriched whey in a hamster primary infection model. *Toxins* **2019**, *11*, 98. [CrossRef] [PubMed]
6. Van Dissel, J.T.; de Groot, N.; Hensgens, C.M.; Numan, S.; Kuijper, E.J.; Veldkamp, P.; van't Wout, J. Bovine antibody-enriched whey to aid in the prevention of a relapse of Clostridium difficile-associated diarrhoea: Preclinical and preliminary clinical data. *J. Med. Microbiol.* **2005**, *54*, 197–205. [CrossRef] [PubMed]
7. Lyerly, D.M.; Bostwick, E.; Binion, S.; Wilkins, T.D. Passive immunization of hamsters against disease caused by Clostridium difficile by use of bovine immunoglobulin G concentrate. *Infect. Immun.* **1991**, *56*. [CrossRef] [PubMed]
8. Sponseller, J.K.; Steele, J.A.; Schmidt, D.J.; Kim, H.B.; Beamer, G.; Sun, X.; Tzipori, S. Hyperimmune bovine colostrum as a novel therapy to combat Clostridium difficile infection. *J. Infect. Dis.* **2015**, *211*, 1334–1341. [CrossRef]
9. Hutton, M.L.; Cunningham, B.A.; Mackin, K.E.; Lyon, S.A.; James, M.L.; Rood, J.I.; Lyras, D. Bovine antibodies targeting primary and recurrent Clostridium difficile disease are a potent antibiotic alternative. *Sci. Rep.* **2017**, *7*, 3665. [CrossRef]
10. Mattila, E.; Anttila, V.-J.; Broas, M.; Marttila, H.; Poukka, P.; Kuusisto, K.; Pusa, L.; Sammalkorpi, K.; Dabek, J.; Koivurova, O.-P.; et al. A randomized, double-blind study comparing Clostridium difficile immune whey and metronidazole for recurrent Clostridium difficile-associated diarrhoea: Efficacy and safety data of a prematurely interrupted trial. *Scand. J. Infect. Dis.* **2008**, *40*, 702–708. [CrossRef]
11. Numan, S.C.; Veldkamp, P.; Kuijper, E.J.; van den Berg, R.J.; van Dissel, J.T. Clostridium difficile-associated diarrhoea: Bovine anti-Clostridium difficile whey protein to help aid the prevention of relapses. *Gut* **2007**, *56*, 888–889. [CrossRef]
12. Antonopoulos, D.A.; Huse, S.M.; Morrison, H.G.; Schmidt, T.M.; Sogin, M.L.; Young, V.B. Reproducible community dynamics of the gastrointestinal microbiota following antibiotic perturbation. *Infect. Immun.* **2009**, *77*, 2367–2375. [CrossRef]
13. Clavel, T.; Lagkouvardos, I.; Hiergeist, A. Microbiome sequencing: Challenges and opportunities for molecular medicine. *Expert Rev. Mol. Diagn.* **2016**, *16*, 795–805. [CrossRef]
14. Theriot, C.M.; Young, V.B. Microbial and metabolic interactions between the gastrointestinal tract and Clostridium difficile infection. *Gut Microbes.* **2014**, *5*, 86–95. [CrossRef] [PubMed]
15. Trzasko, A.; Leeds, J.A.; Praestgaard, J.; Lamarche, M.J.; McKenney, D. Efficacy of LFF571 in a hamster model of Clostridium difficile infection. *Antimicrob. Agents Chemother.* **2012**, *56*, 4459–4462. [CrossRef]
16. Abt, M.C.; McKenney, P.T.; Pamer, E.G. Clostridium difficile colitis: Pathogenesis and host defence. *Nat. Rev. Microbiol.* **2016**, *14*, 609–620. [CrossRef] [PubMed]
17. Loo, V.G.; Bourgault, A.-M.; Poirier, L.; Lamothe, F.; Michaud, S.; Turgeon, N.; Toye, B.; Beaudoin, A.; Frost, E.H.; Gilca, R.; et al. Host and pathogen factors for Clostridium difficile infection and colonization. *N. Engl. J. Med.* **2011**, *365*, 1693–1703. [CrossRef] [PubMed]
18. Sonnenburg, J.L.; Xu, J.; Leip, D.D.; Chen, C.-H.; Westover, B.P.; Weatherford, J.; Buhler, J.D.; Gordon, J.I. Glycan foraging in vivo by an intestine-adapted bacterial symbiont. *Science* **2005**, *307*, 1955–1959. [CrossRef] [PubMed]
19. Wong, J.M.W.; de Souza, R.; Kendall, C.W.C.; Emam, A.; Jenkins, D.J.A. Colonic health: Fermentation and short chain fatty acids. *J. Clin. Gastroenterol.* **2006**, *40*, 235–243. [CrossRef]
20. Theriot, C.M.; Koenigsknecht, M.J.; Carlson, P.E.; Hatton, G.E.; Nelson, A.M.; Li, B.; Huffnagle, G.B.; Li, J.Z.; Young, V.B. Antibiotic-induced shifts in the mouse gut microbiome and metabolome increase susceptibility to Clostridium difficile infection. *Nat. Commun.* **2014**, *5*, 3114. [CrossRef]
21. Bazanella, M.; Maier, T.V.; Clavel, T.; Lagkouvardos, I.; Lucio, M.; Maldonado-Gòmez, M.X.; Autran, C.; Walter, J.; Bode, L.; Schmitt-Kopplin, P.; et al. Randomized controlled trial on the impact of early-life intervention with bifidobacteria on the healthy infant fecal microbiota and metabolome. *Am. J. Clin. Nutr.* **2017**, *106*, 1274–1286. [CrossRef]
22. Lagkouvardos, I.; Kläring, K.; Heinzmann, S.S.; Platz, S.; Scholz, B.; Engel, K.-H.; Schmitt-Kopplin, P.; Haller, D.; Rohn, S.; Skurk, T.; et al. Gut metabolites and bacterial community networks during a pilot intervention study with flaxseeds in healthy adult men. *Mol. Nutr. Food Res.* **2015**, *59*, 1614–1628. [CrossRef]
23. Kozich, J.J.; Westcott, S.L.; Baxter, N.T.; Highlander, S.K.; Schloss, P.D. Development of a dual-index sequencing strategy and curation pipeline for analyzing amplicon sequence data on the MiSeq Illumina sequencing platform. *Appl. Environ. Microbiol.* **2013**, *79*, 5112–5120. [CrossRef] [PubMed]
24. Lagkouvardos, I.; Joseph, D.; Kapfhammer, M.; Giritli, S.; Horn, M.; Haller, D.; Clavel, T. IMNGS: A comprehensive open resource of processed 16S rRNA microbial profiles for ecology and diversity studies. *Sci. Rep.* **2016**, *6*, 33721. [CrossRef] [PubMed]
25. Edgar, R.C. UPARSE: Highly accurate OTU sequences from microbial amplicon reads. *Nat. Methods* **2013**, *10*, 996–998. [CrossRef] [PubMed]
26. Lagkouvardos, I.; Fischer, S.; Kumar, N.; Clavel, T. Rhea: A transparent and modular R pipeline for microbial profiling based on 16S rRNA gene amplicons. *PeerJ* **2017**, *5*, e2836. [CrossRef] [PubMed]
27. Chen, J.; Bittinger, K.; Charlson, E.S.; Hoffmann, C.; Lewis, J.; Wu, G.D.; Collman, R.G.; Bushman, F.D.; Li, H. Associating microbiome composition with environmental covariates using generalized UniFrac distances. *Bioinformatics* **2012**, *28*, 2106–2113. [CrossRef] [PubMed]

antibiotics

Article

Protective Effect of Baicalin against *Clostridioides difficile* Infection in Mice

Abraham Joseph Pellissery [1], Poonam Gopika Vinayamohan [2], Deepa Ashwarya Kuttappan [1], Neha Mishra [3], Breno de Oliveira Fragomeni [1], Kendra Maas [4], Shankumar Mooyottu [5] and Kumar Venkitanarayanan [1,*]

1 Department of Animal Science, University of Connecticut, Storrs, CT 06269, USA; abraham.pellissery@uconn.edu (A.J.P.); deepa.kuttappan@uconn.edu (D.A.K.); breno.fragomeni@uconn.edu (B.O.F.)
2 Department of Veterinary Preventive Medicine, Ohio State University, Columbus, OH 43210, USA; vinayamohan.1@osu.edu
3 Department of Pathobiology and Veterinary Science, University of Connecticut, Storrs, CT 06269, USA; neha.mishra@uconn.edu
4 Microbial Analysis, Resources, and Services, University of Connecticut, Storrs, CT 06269, USA; kendra.maas@uconn.edu
5 Department of Veterinary Pathology, Iowa State University, Ames, IA 50011, USA; shaan@iastate.edu
* Correspondence: kumar.venkitanarayanan@uconn.edu; Tel.: +1-(860)-486-1957

Abstract: This study investigated the prophylactic and therapeutic efficacies of baicalin (BC), a plant-derived flavone glycoside, in reducing the severity of *Clostridioides difficile* infection (CDI) in a mouse model. In the prophylactic trial, C57BL/6 mice were provided with BC (0, 11, and 22 mg/L in drinking water) from 12 days before *C. difficile* challenge through the end of the experiment, whereas BC administration started day 1 post challenge in the therapeutic trial. Both challenge and control groups were infected with 10^6 CFU/mL of hypervirulent *C. difficile* BAA 1803 spores or sterile PBS, and the clinical and diarrheal scores were recorded for 10 days post challenge. On day 2 post challenge, fecal and tissue samples were collected from mice prophylactically administered with BC for microbiome and histopathologic analysis. Both prophylactic and therapeutic supplementation of BC significantly reduced the severity of colonic lesions and improved CDI clinical progression and outcome compared with control ($p < 0.05$). Microbiome analysis revealed a significant increase in Gammaproteobacteria and reduction in the abundance of protective microbiota (Firmicutes) in antibiotic-treated and *C. difficile*-infected mice compared with controls ($p < 0.05$). However, baicalin supplementation favorably altered the microbiome composition, as revealed by an increased abundance in beneficial bacteria, especially *Lachnospiraceae* and *Akkermansia*. Our results warrant follow-up investigations on the use of BC as an adjunct to antibiotic therapy to control gut dysbiosis and reduce *C. difficile* infection in humans.

Keywords: *Clostridioides difficile*; baicalin; microbiome; gut dysbiosis; mouse model

Citation: Pellissery, A.J.; Vinayamohan, P.G.; Kuttappan, D.A.; Mishra, N.; Fragomeni, B.O.; Maas, K.; Mooyottu, S.; Venkitanarayanan, K. Protective Effect of Baicalin against *Clostridioides difficile* Infection in Mice. *Antibiotics* **2021**, *10*, 926. https://doi.org/10.3390/antibiotics10080926

Academic Editors: Guido Granata and Seok-Hoon Jeong

Received: 15 May 2021
Accepted: 27 July 2021
Published: 30 July 2021

1. Introduction

Clostridioides difficile is an important cause of nosocomial, antibiotic-associated diarrhea around the world [1,2]. The pathogen causes a toxin-mediated colitis in individuals of all age groups, with more severity observed in elderly and immunocompromised patients [3]. In the United States, more than 453,000 cases of *C. difficile* infection (CDI) with 29,000 deaths are reported annually, which incur an economic burden ranging between USD 0.4 to 3.0 billion as healthcare-associated costs [4,5]. The increased incidence of CDI in humans is primarily attributed to the emergence of NAP1/ribotype 027, a highly toxigenic and hypervirulent *C. difficile* strain [1,6–8].

Generally, individuals requiring long-term antibiotic therapy and gastric acid suppressing agents are highly predisposed to CDI [9–11]. Broad-spectrum antibiotics and acid suppressants alter the diversity and abundance of the normal gut microbial communities, resulting in a condition known as gut dysbiosis [12–15]. The dysbiotic gut environment facilitates *C. difficile* spore germination, outgrowth, colonization, and toxin productions in the distal gut [16]. *C. difficile* exotoxins—namely, toxin A and toxin B—disrupt the actin cytoskeleton and interepithelial tight junctions of the colonic epithelium, leading to severe diarrhea and suppurative inflammation that could culminate in pseudomembranous colitis and toxic megacolon in extreme cases [1,8,17,18].

Although extended antibiotic therapy predisposes individuals to CDI, antibiotics are still considered as the primary line of treatment for this disease, and the most commonly prescribed drugs include metronidazole, vancomycin, and fidaxomicin [4,7,19,20]. However, *C. difficile* has been continuously acquiring resistance to different classes of antibiotics, including those currently in clinical use against CDI [7,21]. With global emergence of antibiotic resistant and hypervirulent *C. difficile* strains, the Centers for Disease Control and Prevention (CDC) categorized the pathogen a few years ago as one among the three urgent threats to public health [22]. Therefore, there is an emergent need to identify alternative therapeutic agents that could reduce *C. difficile* virulence without adversely affecting the gut microbiota.

Phytochemicals represent a natural group of molecules that have been used for treating various diseases in traditional medicine [23]. Baicalin (5,6-dihydroxy-7-O-glucuronide flavone) is a flavone glycoside present in the plant *Scutellaria baicalensis* Georgi, known to possess antimicrobial, antioxidant, and anti-inflammatory properties [24–30]. Previously, our laboratory demonstrated the use of baicalin as a potential anti-*C. difficile* therapeutic agent owing to its inhibitory effect on *C. difficile* toxin production with minimal effects on the growth of selected beneficial microbiota in vitro [31]. As a logical next step, this study investigated the prophylactic and therapeutic effects of baicalin against CDI in an in vivo model by focusing on the clinical course and host microbiome changes in mice. Mouse models for CDI are well established, and antibiotic-induced gut dysbiosis in mice can be simulated by administering antibiotics orally and intraperitoneally, followed by inoculation of *C. difficile* spores [32,33].

2. Results

2.1. *Effect of Baicalin Supplementation on the Incidence of Diarrhea and Severity of* C. difficile *Infection in Mice*

The prophylactic efficacy of baicalin against CDI in mice was assessed by supplementing the phytochemical in drinking water at two different concentrations (11 and 22 mg/L). Oral administration of 10^6 CFU/mL *C. difficile* spores (ATCC BAA 1803) resulted in high morbidity with low mortality in infected mice. In *C. difficile*-infected control groups (CD), 61% and 85% of animals showed severe diarrhea on the first- and second-day post infection (DPI) ($n = 13$), respectively (Figure 1a). On 7 DPI, one animal from the CD group died, and no further mortality was recorded in this group (Supplementary Figure S3a). Although diarrhea continued for five days in the CD group, there was no increase in the percentage incidence of diarrhea thereafter (data not shown). However, the incidence of diarrhea was significantly lower in the CD+BC1 (challenged mice treated with 11 mg/L of BC) group, with 38% and 31% incidence on 1 DPI and 2 DPI, respectively, and with the absence of diarrhea on the subsequent days (Figure 1a). Moreover, diarrhea was not observed in the CD+BC2 group (challenged mice treated with 22 mg/L of BC) ($p < 0.05$), although there were two mortalities recorded in this group, one each on days 2 and 3 post infection (Supplementary Figure S3a).

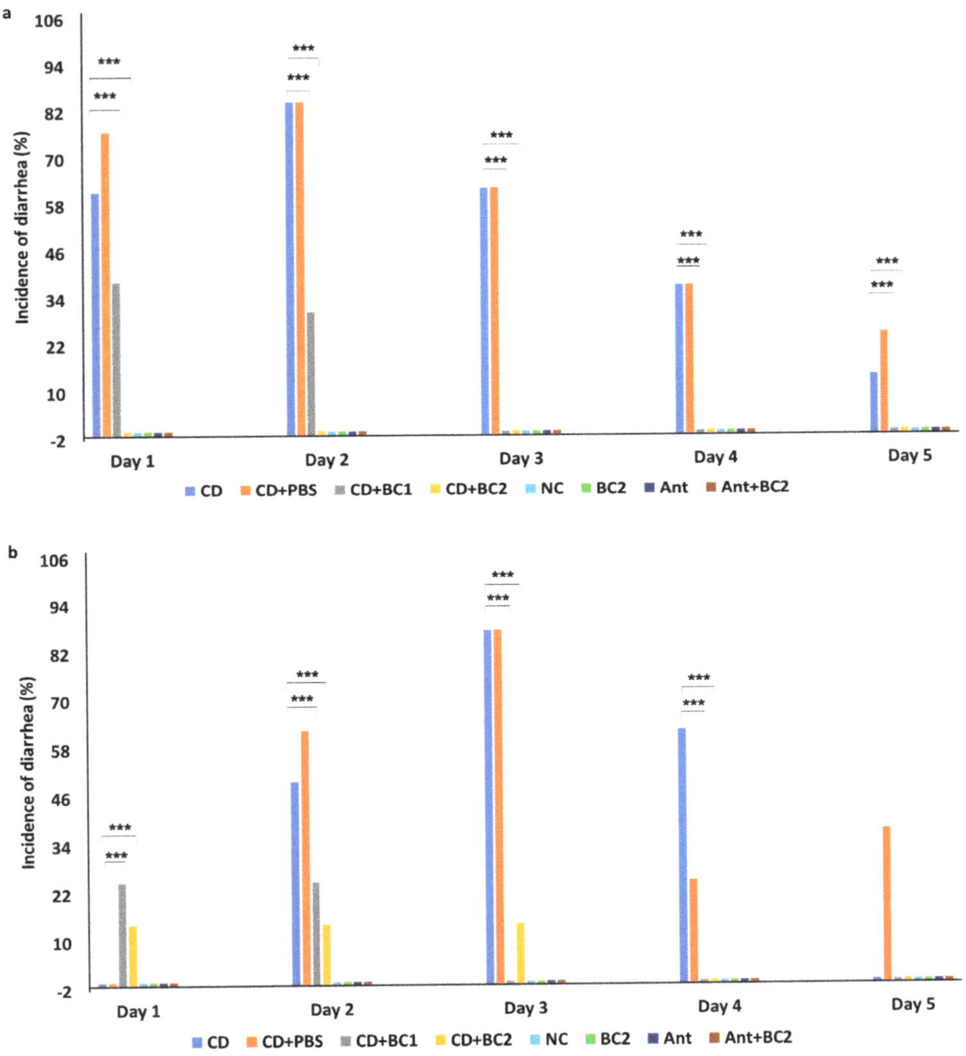

Figure 1. Effect of baicalin supplementation on the incidence of diarrhea in mice after CDI. Percentage incidence of diarrhea was recorded from 1 DPI to 5 DPI in the different treatment groups in the prophylactic BC study (**a**) therapeutic BC study (**b**). *** indicates a statistically significant difference ($p < 0.0001$) relative to challenged, positive control (CD) vs. the baicalin-treated challenged mice (CD+BC1 or CD+BC2). Error bars represent SEM. Treatment groups: NC (unchallenged negative control), Ant (unchallenged antibiotic control), Ant+BC (unchallenged antibiotic + 22 mg/L BC control), BC2 (unchallenged 22 mg/L BC control), CD (Ant+*C. difficile*-challenged control), CD+PBS (Ant+*C. difficile*-challenged control, PBS solvent control), CD+BC1 (Ant+ CD + 11 mg/L BC), CD+BC2 (Ant+ CD + 22 mg/L BC).

In the therapeutic trial, baicalin was supplemented in drinking water similar to the prophylactic trial but was initiated from day 1 post challenge. Interestingly, the *C. difficile* positive control group (Ant+CD) did not show any diarrhea on 1 DPI; however, diarrhea was observed in 62.5% and 87.5% animals on 2 DPI ($n = 13$) and 3 DPI ($n = 5$), respectively (Figure 1b). Diarrhea was observed until the fifth day post infection in this group, with no additional increase in percentage incidence after 3 DPI. Diarrhea was observed from

1 DPI in the CD+BC1 and CD+BC2 groups, although a significantly reduced incidence was observed for both BC-treated groups compared with the positive control ($p < 0.05$). An incidence of 25% was observed on both 2 DPI and 3 DPI in CD+BC1 group, with no diarrhea thereafter. In the CD+BC2 group, the incidence of diarrhea stayed at 14% for days 1–3 post infection, with no more diarrhea observed for the remainder of experiment duration (Figure 1b). In addition, there was only one mortality recorded in the *C. difficile*-positive control group on 6 DPI (Supplementary Figure S3b).

No diarrhea was observed in the control groups (i.e., negative control (NC), baicalin control (BC2), antibiotic control (Ant), and antibiotic with baicalin control (Ant+BC2)) in both the prophylactic and therapeutic BC studies.

2.2. Effect of Baicalin Supplementation on Clinical Score and Body Weight of C. difficile-Infected Mice

Clinical scores of animals from different treatment groups were individually recorded using a standard score chart, from 1 DPI to 10 DPI (Supplementary Table S1) (Chen et al., 2008). Groups receiving prophylactic supplementation of baicalin (CD+BC1 and CD+BC2) had a significantly reduced average clinical score compared with the challenge control (CD) ($p < 0.05$) (Figure 2a). The recovery of surviving morbid animals in the *C. difficile* control group was much slower compared with baicalin-treated groups ($p < 0.05$), with apparent clinical resolution observed by 9 DPI. However, the baicalin-supplemented groups showed a dose-dependent reduction in disease severity, with complete recovery observed by 6 DPI ($p < 0.05$). Although not statistically significant, the clinical score of the CD+BC2 group was lower compared with that of CD+BC1 group. Interestingly, a similar trend in the average clinical scores was also observed in the baicalin therapeutic trial. The clinical scores in CD+BC1 and CD+BC2 groups also followed a dose-dependent reduction in disease severity (Figure 2b). However, the recovery rate was much slower compared with the prophylactic study, where no complete resolution of clinical disease was observed until the end of the experiment (day 10 post-*C. difficile* challenge).

Body weights were recorded on a daily basis post infection, and the relative percentage weight with respect to the initial weight prior to the *C. difficile* challenge was calculated. In the prophylactic study, the baicalin control group (BC2) and Ant+BC2 group showed no significant weight loss compared with negative control. However, mice in the *C. difficile*-positive control (CD) showed a significant and progressive weight loss from 1 DPI to 5 DPI compared with unchallenged control ($p < 0.05$), with animals regaining their pre-challenge body weights by 9 DPI. Although there was no significant difference in the average body weights of mice from the BC-treated challenge groups (CD+BC1 and CD+BC2) compared with positive control, baicalin-treated animals were able to rapidly regain their pre-challenge body weights by 5 DPI compared with the *C. difficile*-positive control (9 DPI) (Figure 2c).

In the therapeutic trial, *C. difficile*-challenge control (CD) showed significant weight loss compared with negative controls ($p < 0.05$). Mice in the *C. difficile*-challenge control group showed progressive weight reduction 3 DPI through 6 DPI, returning to their initial body weights by 8 DPI. In addition, there was no significant difference in average percentage body weights between the CD group and CD+BC1 group. However, a significant difference was observed in the average percentage body weights of the CD+BC2 groups compared with the CD group on days 3 and 4 post challenge ($p < 0.05$) (Figure 2d). Moreover, the CD+BC2 group attained their pre-challenge body weight by 4 DPI; however, a slight delay was observed in the CD+BC1 group, with animals attaining their initial body weight by 6 DPI (Figure 2d).

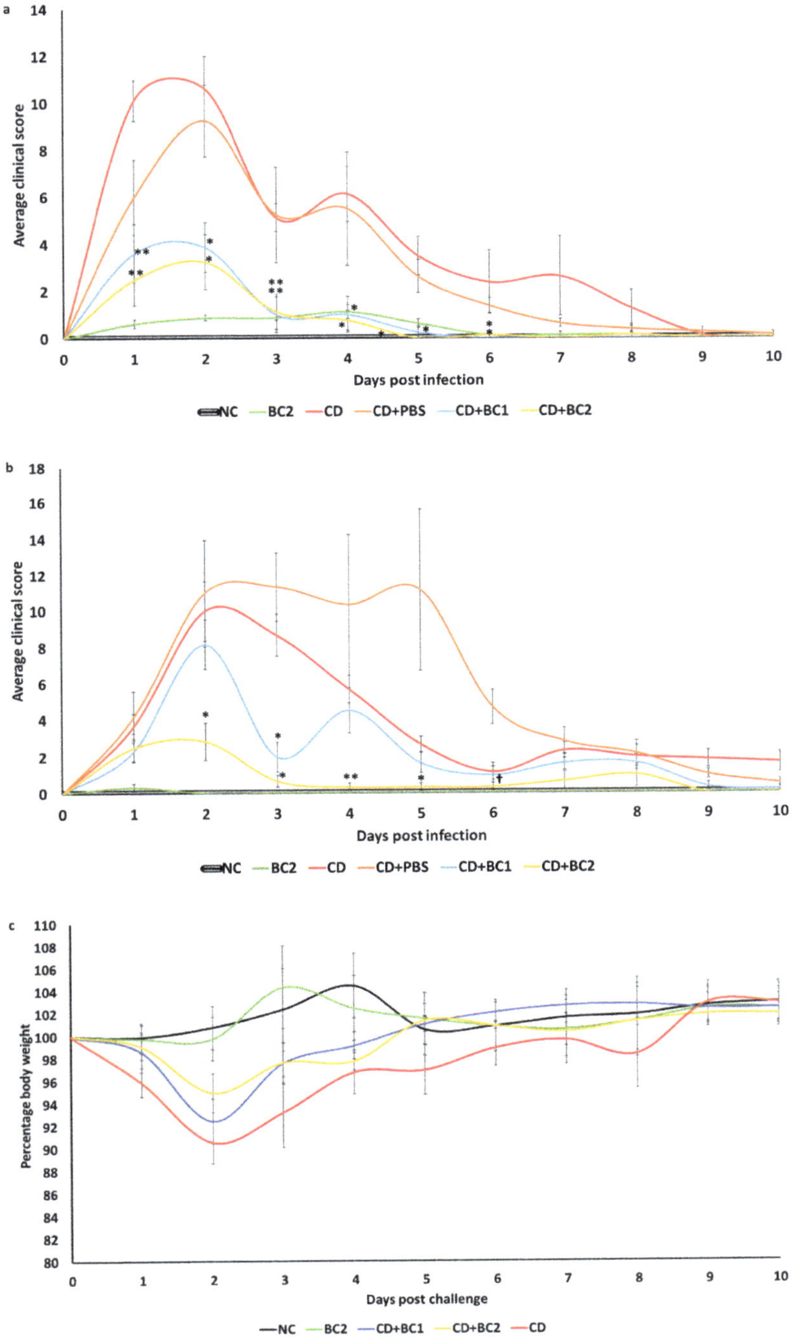

Figure 2. *Cont.*

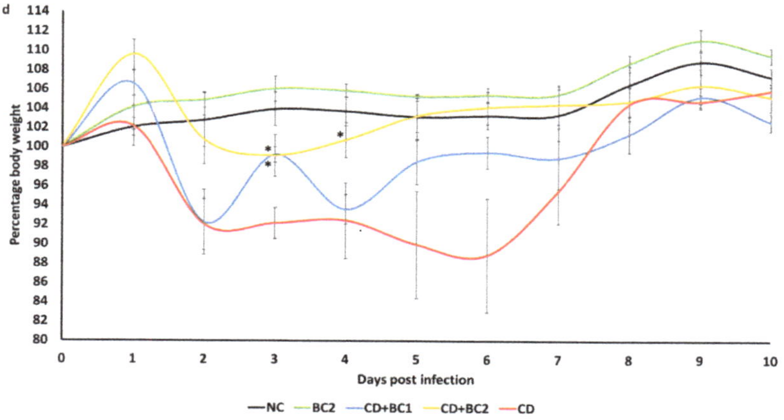

Figure 2. Effect of baicalin supplementation on clinical severity and change in body weight in mice after CDI. Average clinical scores and percentage body weights were recorded from 1 DPI to 10 DPI for the different treatment groups in the prophylactic BC study (**a**,**c**) and therapeutic BC study (**b**,**d**). **, * indicates a statistically significant difference ($p < 0.001$, $p < 0.05$, respectively) relative to the untreated challenge group (CD); † symbol indicates a statistically significant difference ($p < 0.05$) relative to CD+PBS. Percentage body weights among treatment groups (in (c,d) were compared within the same day time point. Error bars represent SEM. Treatment groups: NC (unchallenged negative control), Ant (unchallenged antibiotic control), Ant+BC (unchallenged antibiotic + 22 mg/L BC control), BC2 (unchallenged 22 mg/L BC control), CD (Ant+*C. difficile*-challenged control), CD+PBS (Ant+*C. difficile*-challenged control, PBS solvent control), CD+BC1 (Ant+CD + 11 mg/L BC), CD+BC2 (Ant+CD + 22 mg/L BC).

2.3. *Effect of Baicalin Supplementation on the Gut Microbiome of C. difficile-Challenged and Non-Challenged Mice*

The results from the prophylactic trial revealed distinctive patterns in the composition of bacterial communities in the different treatment groups. In the unchallenged control group (NC), the predominant phyla groups consisted of Firmicutes and Bacteroidetes in a ratio of 1.05:1, with a minimal proportion of other taxa related to opportunistic pathogens such as Gammaproteobacteria and *Enterococcaceae* (Figure 3a). In the baicalin control group (BC2), a higher proportion of Firmicutes was observed, compared with Bacteroidetes having a ratio of 1.79:1. Although, the phyla comparisons seemingly had a greater degree of difference in their proportion across groups, it was statistically insignificant. The antibiotic control group (Ant) had a higher proportion of Gammaproteobacteria and *Enterococcaceae* compared with the negative control and baicalin control group. The supplementation of baicalin along with the antibiotic (Ant+BC2) seemed to reduce the proportion of *Enterococcaceae* but was not able to reverse the increase in Gammaproteobacteria. However, there was an increase in the proportion of the phylum Verrucomicrobia (represented as genus *Akkermansia*) compared with the antibiotic control group (Figure 3a). The baicalin untreated challenge groups (CD and CD+PBS) had a predominantly higher proportion of Firmicutes and Gammaproteobacteria compared with uninfected controls. However, baicalin administration to *C. difficile*-challenged groups (CD+BC1 and CD+BC2) reduced the abundance of Firmicutes and increased the proportion of Proteobacteria compared with the antibiotic control and positive control groups (CD and CD+PBS). A notably distinct phylum that prevailed among baicalin-treated, spore-challenged (CD+BC1 and CD+BC2), and unchallenged (BC2 and Ant+BC2) groups was Verrucomicrobia, specifically the genus *Akkermansia* (Figure 3a).

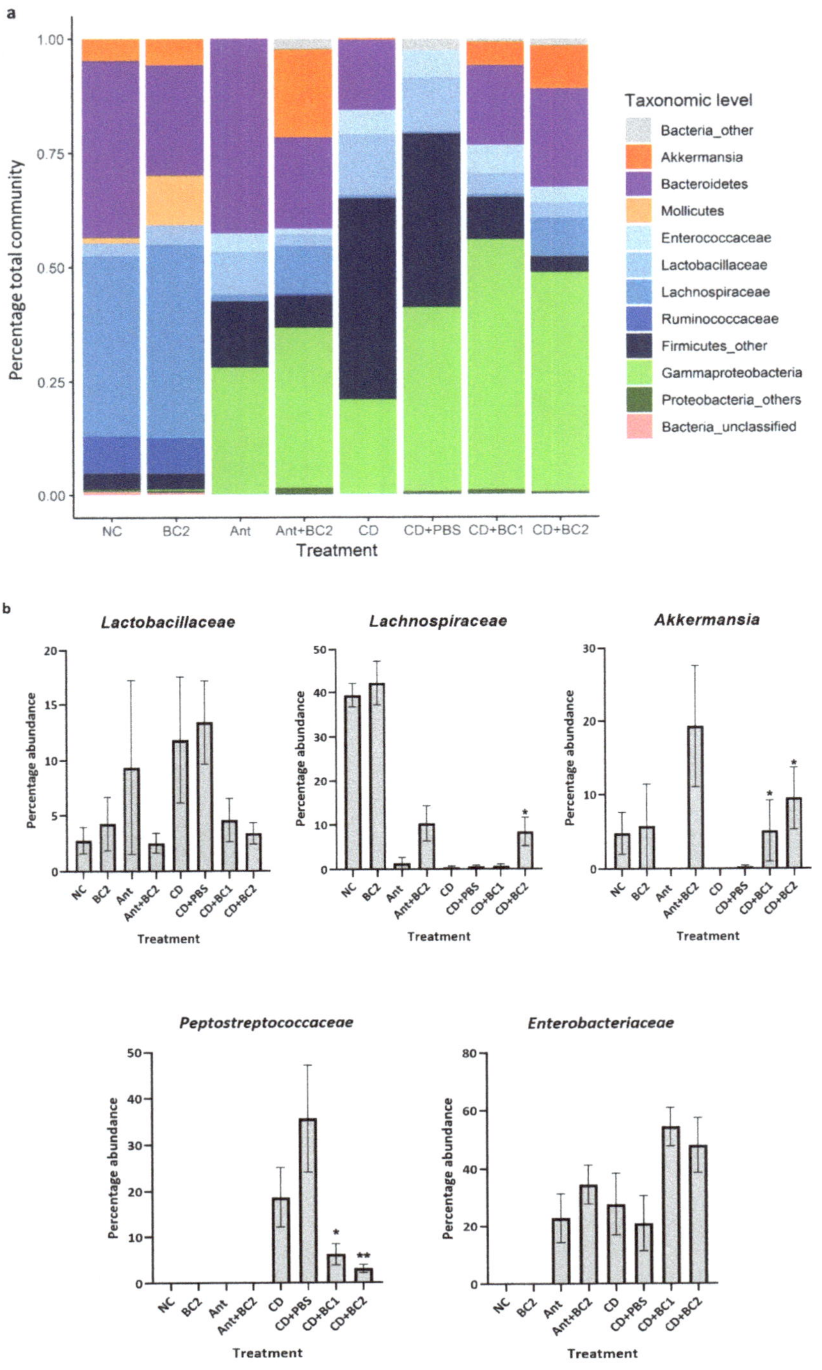

Figure 3. *Cont.*

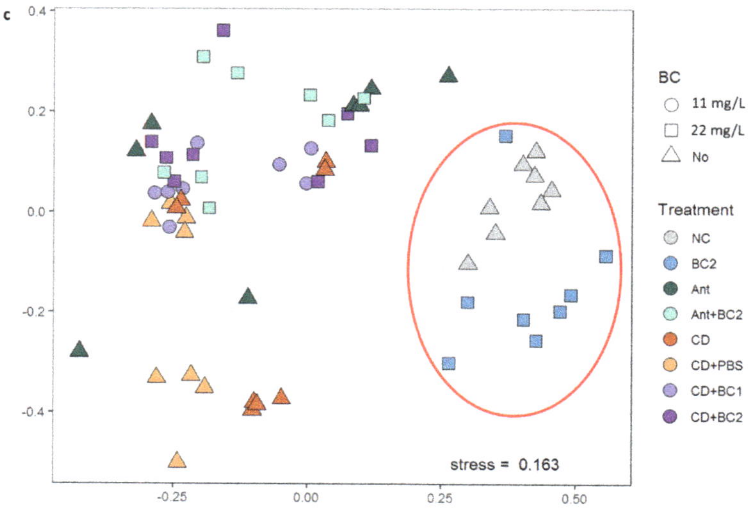

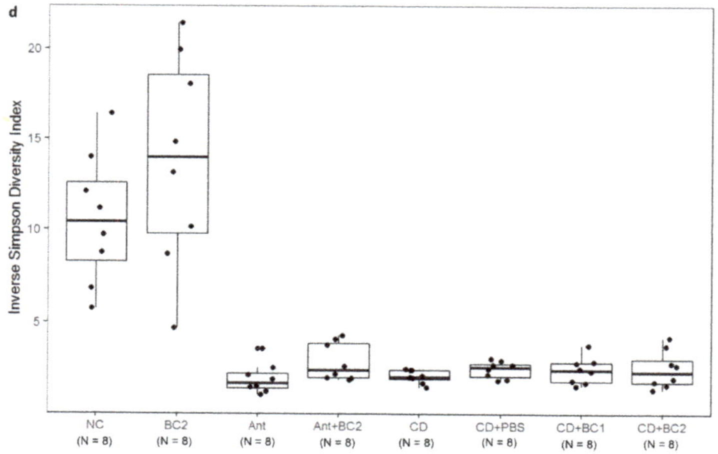

Figure 3. Effect of baicalin supplementation on the abundance of major gut microbiome taxa and microbiome diversity in the antibiotic-treated and *C. difficile*-challenged mice. (**a**) Relative taxa abundance of OTUs: Fecal samples were collected 2 DPI from the prophylactic BC study. DNA was extracted for microbiome analysis using Illumina MiSeq platform, and the relative abundance of OTUs of major phyla, order, family, and genera was determined. (**b**) Abundance of major bacterial family taxa. Percentage abundances of major families—*Lactobacillaceae*, *Lachnospriaceae*, *Akkermansia*, *Peptostreptococcaceae*, and *Enterobacteriaceae*—in the mice treatment groups of the prophylactic BC study. **, * indicates a statistically significant difference ($p < 0.001$, $p < 0.05$, respectively) relative to the untreated challenge group (CD). Error bars represent SEM. (**c**) Bray–Curtis plot: Relationships between treatment groups based on the abundance of species present in each sample were plotted. NMS ordinations were run in R (v 3.3.0) using metaMDS in the vegan (v 2.3-5) package after calculating the stress scree plots to determine the number of axes required to achieve stress below 0.2, plotted using ggplot2 (v 2.1.0). (**d**) Inverse Simpson Plot: Fecal samples were collected 2 DPI of the prophylactic BC study. DNA was extracted for microbiome analysis

using Illumina MiSeq platform, and Alpha diversity was calculated using inverse Simpson to measure the richness and evenness of the OTUs. Treatment groups: NC (unchallenged negative control), Ant (unchallenged antibiotic control), Ant+BC (unchallenged antibiotic + 22 mg/L BC control), BC2 (unchallenged 22 mg/L BC control), CD (Ant+*C. difficile*-challenged control), CD+PBS (Ant+*C. difficile*-challenged control, PBS solvent control), CD+BC1 (Ant+CD + 11 mg/L BC), CD+BC2 (Ant+CD + 22 mg/L BC).

At the family/genus level, the relative abundance of *Lactobacillaceae* did not show any significant difference amongst the negative control (NC), baicalin control (BC2), and baicalin-treated antibiotic control groups (Ant+BC2) ($p > 0.05$). In contrast, the antibiotic control and untreated spore challenge groups (CD and CD+PBS) had a higher abundance of *Lactobacillaceae* compared with the aforementioned controls; however, it was not statistically significant. However, although not significant, baicalin-treated spore challenge groups had a much lower abundance of *Lactobacillaceae* compared with positive controls (Figure 3b). With regards to *Lachnospiraceae* and *Akkermansia*, although not significant, baicalin-treated control (BC2) marginally increased their relative abundance compared with the negative control ($p > 0.05$) (Figure 3b). In untreated spore challenge groups (CD and CD+PBS), the abundance of both *Lachnospiraceae* and *Akkermansia* was significantly reduced compared with the negative control (NC), baicalin control (BC2), and the baicalin-treated antibiotic control (Ant+BC2) ($p < 0.05$). However, with the exception of the CD+BC1 group, there was a significant increase in the relative abundance of *Lachnospiraceae* in the CD+BC2 group compared with untreated spore challenge groups (CD and CD+PBS) ($p < 0.05$). In terms of the relative abundance of *Akkermansia*, there was a significant increase in both baicalin-treated challenge groups compared with untreated spore challenge groups ($p < 0.05$) (Figure 3b). The relative abundance of *Peptostreptococcaceae* was negligible and showed no significant difference in the negative control (NC), baicalin control (BC2), and antibiotic controls (Ant and Ant+BC2 groups) ($p > 0.05$) (Figure 3b). However, in baicalin-treated spore-challenged groups (CD+BC1 and CD+BC2), *Peptostreptococcaceae* was significantly reduced compared with the CD+PBS group (not CD group), which had a higher abundance ($p < 0.05$). The abundance of *Enterobacteriaceae* was higher in antibiotic control (Ant), baicalin-treated antibiotic control group (Ant+BC2), *C. difficile*-positive control and PBS control (CD and CD+PBS) groups compared with negative control and baicalin control (BC2) groups (Figure 3b).

The non-metric multi-dimensional scaling (NMDS) plot indicating the differential pattern of bacterial diversity revealed a close clustering of baicalin control (BC2) and negative control, suggesting that the species abundance in the BC2 group is comparable with the untreated negative control. However, the other treatment groups (antibiotic-treated groups, challenged or unchallenged with *C. difficile*, and with or without BC treatment) did not indicate a typical relationship pattern for the abundance of species present in each sample (Figure 3c). The inverse Simpson plot representing the differential pattern of bacterial diversity revealed that the BC2 group did not alter the diversity of the gut bacterial community compared with the negative control (NC) ($p > 0.05$). However, irrespective of the baicalin treatment, there was a marked reduction in the diversity of bacterial communities in *C. difficile*-infected groups and antibiotic controls (Figure 3d).

2.4. Effect of Baicalin Supplementation on Histopathologic Lesion Score of *C. difficile*-Infected and Non-Infected Mice

In both the prophylactic and therapeutic studies, the *C. difficile*-positive control (CD) and CD+PBS group showed significantly severe colitis compared with the unchallenged negative controls ($p < 0.0001$). The representative histopathological slides shown in the figure are from the treatment groups NC (Figure 4a(i)), CD+BC1 (Figure 4a(ii)), CD+BC2 (Figure 4a(iii,iv)), and CD (Figure 4a(v,vi)) and from the histopathological scores for all the treatment groups provided in Figure 4b(i,ii)). The microscopic observations and histopathological scores indicate that the model was a severe disease challenge model, and the positive and negative control treatment groups worked accordingly.

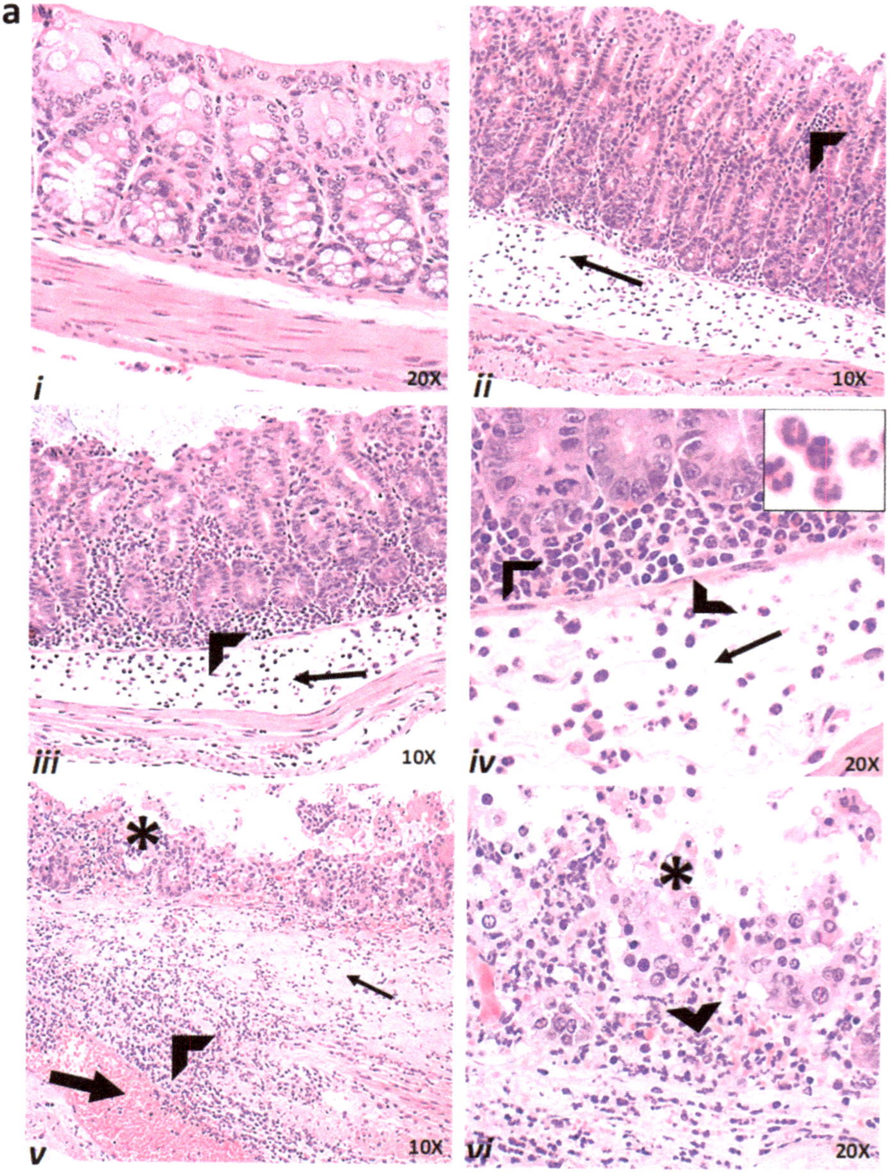

Figure 4. *Cont.*

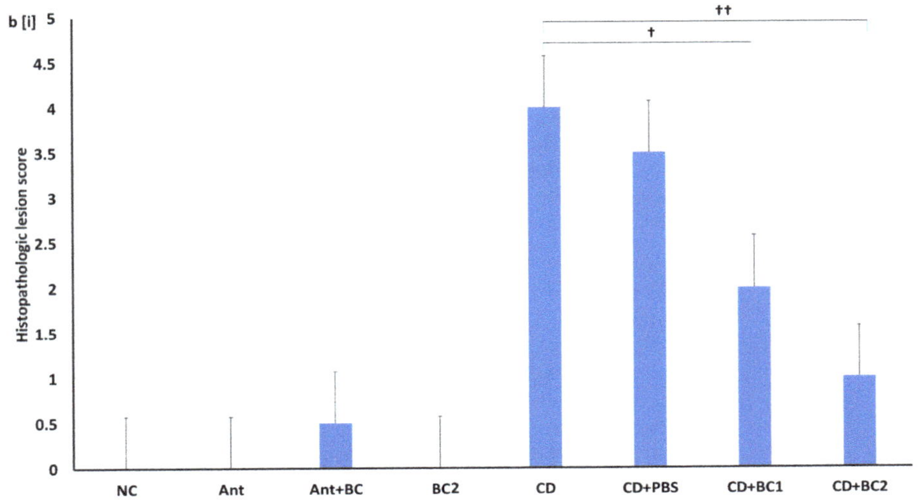

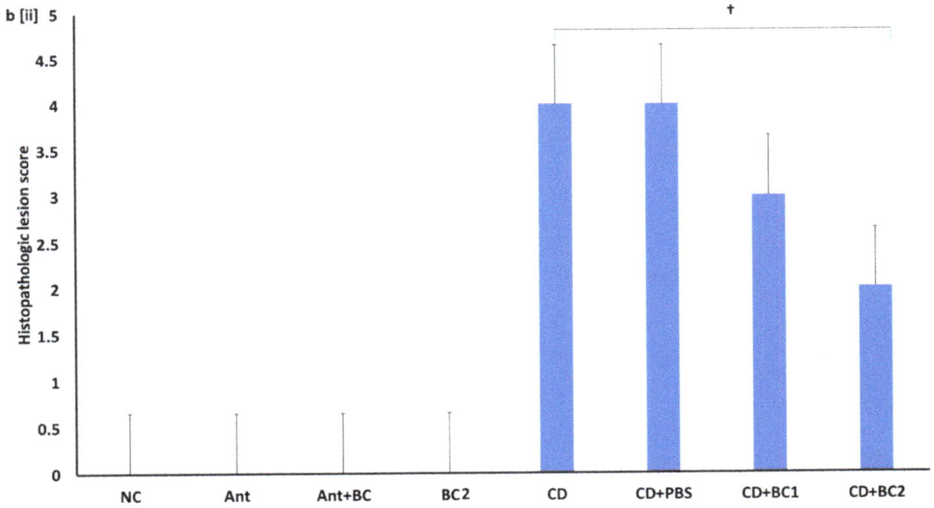

Figure 4. Colon histology and lesion scores. (**a**) Histologic examination of representative colonic tissues; (i) NC group—normal colon appearance; (ii) CD+BC1 group—colitis with submucosal and lamina propria inflammation (arrowhead) and moderate submucosal edema with dilated lymphatics (arrow); (iii,iv) CD+BC2 group—moderate colitis with submucosal edema (arrow), inflammation composed predominantly of neutrophils (arrowhead), and inset in (iv) shows neutrophils in higher magnifications (60×), which are predominantly inflammatory cells observed in the lamina propria and submucosa; (v,vi) CD group—severe colitis with marked submucosal protein-rich edema (arrow) congestion (thick arrow) and hemorrhage, enterocyte necrosis (asterisk) and erosion, and marked neutrophil infiltration (arrowhead). (**b**) Histopathologic scoring was based on (1) epithelial tissue damage; (2) congestion, edema, and hemorrhage; and (3) neutrophil infiltration. A score of 0–4 was assigned to each animal, denoting 0 for the absence of lesion, 1 for minimal, 2 for mild, 3 for moderate, and 4 for the severe histopathologic lesion. Mean of individual category scores were calculated to provide an overall histopathologic lesion score for each mouse and then for each group. Error bars represent SEM. (i) Prophylactic study; (ii) therapeutic study. ††, † symbol indicates a statistically significant difference ($p < 0.001$, $p < 0.05$, respectively) relative to challenged, positive control (CD) vs. the baicalin-treated challenged mice (CD+BC1 or CD+BC2).

Interestingly, mice groups receiving the prophylactic supplementation of baicalin (CD+BC1 and CD+BC2) had a significantly reduced histopathologic lesion score compared with *C. difficile*-positive control (CD) ($p < 0.05$ and $p < 0.001$) (Figure 4a(ii–iv),b(i)). However, in the therapeutic study, only high baicalin dose treatment (CD+BC2) had significantly reduced histopathologic lesion score ($p < 0.05$) compared with *C. difficile*-positive control (CD) (Figure 4b(ii)). However, in both study designs, i.e., the prophylactic and therapeutic studies, the higher doses in the CD+BC2 group had decreased histopathologic lesions as compared with the low dose CD+ BC1, although this reduction was not statistically significant.

2.5. Effect of Baicalin Supplementation on Fecal C. difficile Counts and Fecal Toxin-Mediated Cytotoxicity on Vero Cells

qPCR-based fecal *C. difficile* counts in the untreated, challenged mice groups, CD and CD+PBS, were 4.25 and 4.10 log CFU/mL, respectively. However, there was a mild reduction in counts by ~0.5 log CFU/mL in both the CD+BC1 and CD+BC2 treatment groups when compared with the untreated challenged mice groups (Figure 5a(i)). Fecal *C. difficile* spore enumeration was performed by serial dilution and plating on samples collected from day 4 and 6 post infection. Although there was approximately a 2-log reduction in *C. difficile* spore counts in the day 4 fecal samples of challenged, BC-treated mice compared with the positive control (CD) ($p < 0.001$), the *C. difficile* counts were almost the same level by day 6 post infection ($p > 0.05$) (Figure 5b(ii,iii)). In addition, the fecal slurry supernatants from the BC-treated, challenged mice showed a reduction in Vero cell cytotoxicity compared with the untreated, challenged mice. Vero cell cytotoxicity with day 4 and day 6 fecal samples from CD+BC1 and CD+BC2 mice groups showed 96% ($p < 0.05$) and 99% ($p < 0.05$), and 64% ($p = 0.18$) and 96% ($p < 0.05$) reduction, respectively when compared with the untreated, *C. difficile*-challenged mice (Figure 5b(i,ii)).

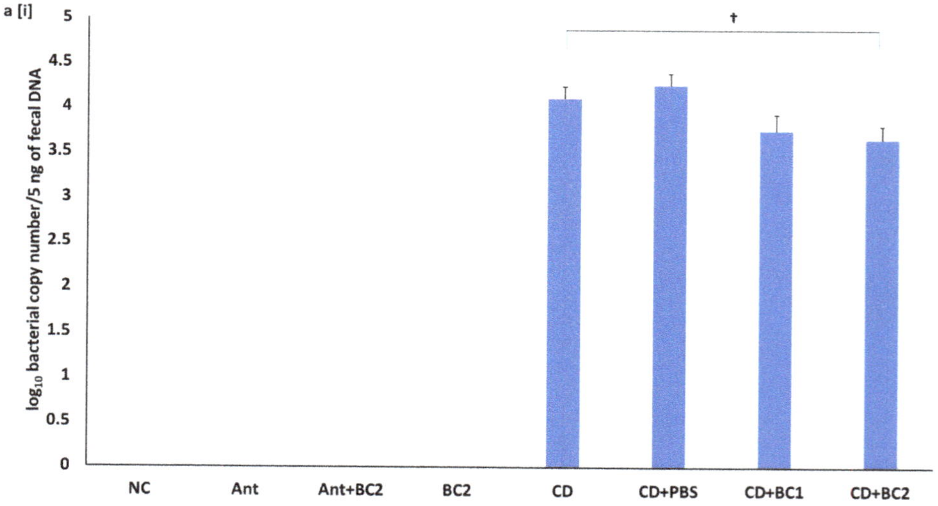

Figure 5. *Cont.*

a [ii]

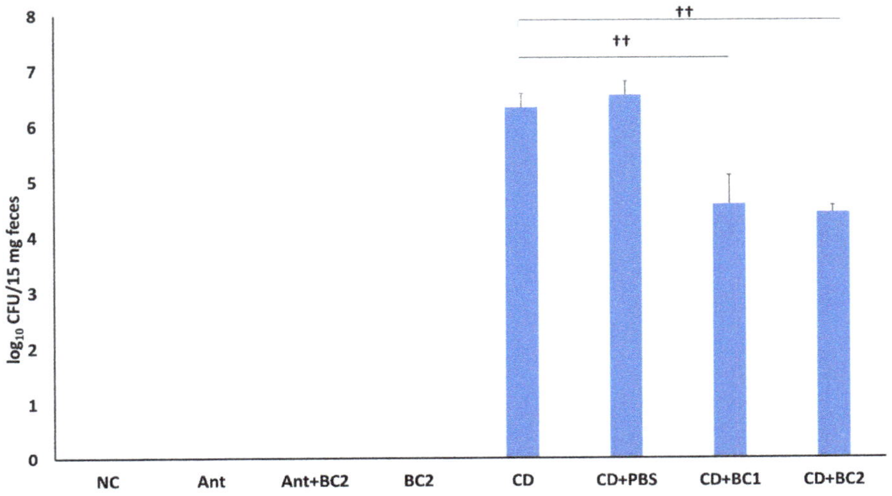

a [iii]

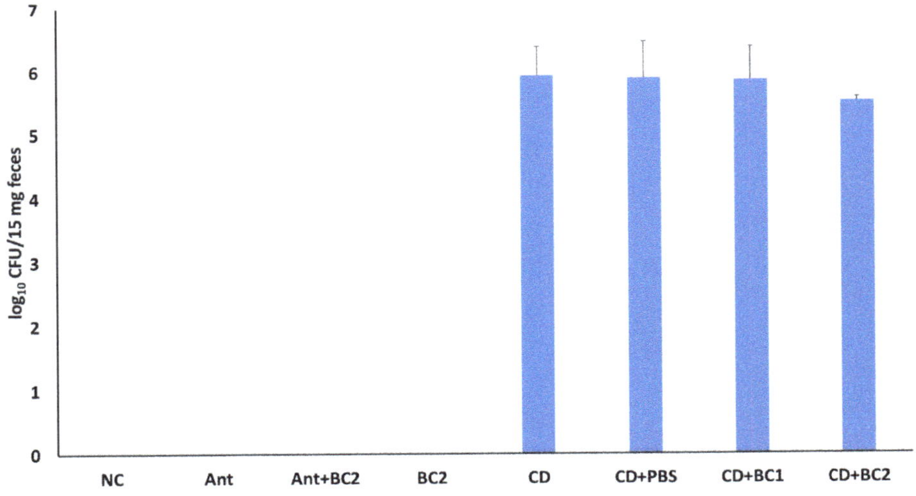

Figure 5. *Cont.*

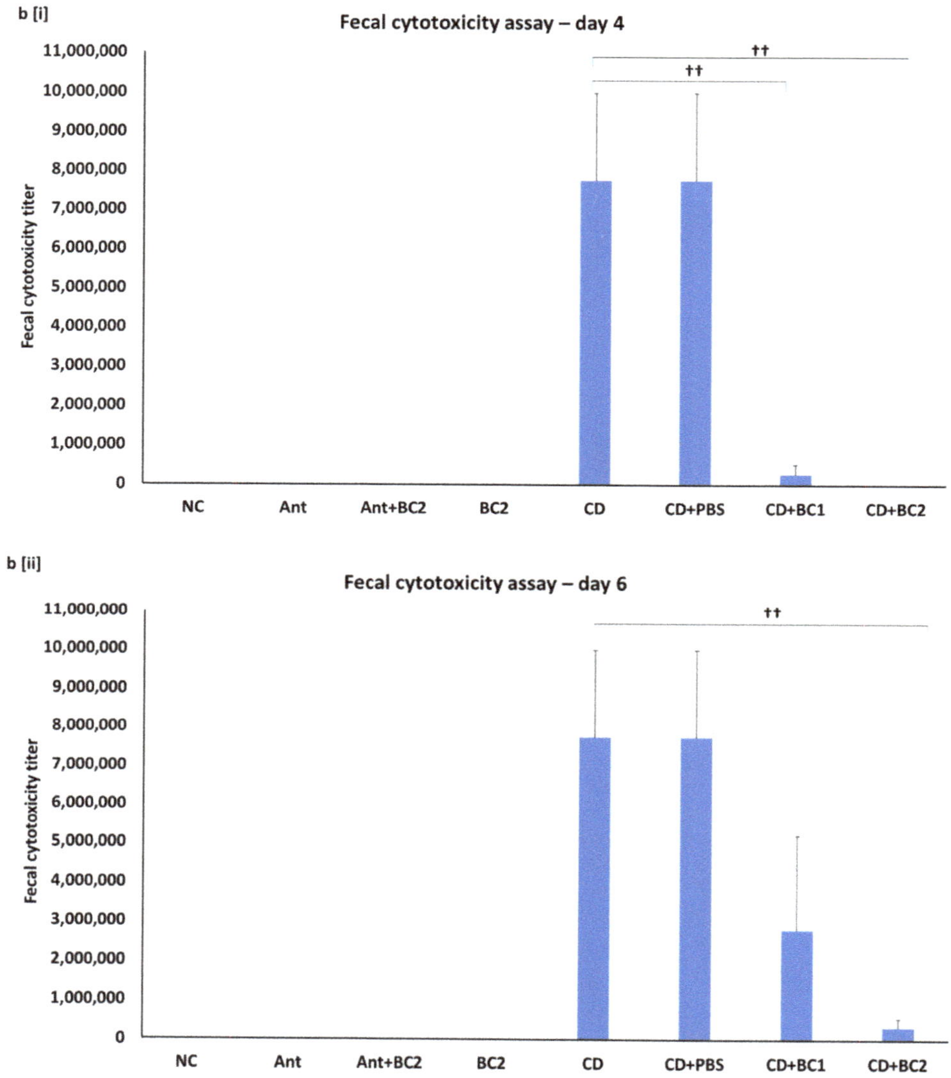

Figure 5. Effect of prophylactic baicalin supplementation on *C. difficile* counts and Vero cell cytotoxicity using fecal slurry supernatants. (**a**) Enumeration of *C. difficile* from fecal samples using (i) qPCR-based quantification using fecal DNA (5 ng content) from day 2 post infection, and (**a** (ii,iii)) serial dilution and plating of fecal samples on cycloserine-cefoxitin fructose containing 0.1% sodium taurocholate (CCFA-T) agar plates from day 4 and 6 post infection. (**b**(i,ii)) Fecal cytotoxicity assay using fecal samples collected during day 4 and 6 of the prophylactic study. Error bars represent SEM. ††, † symbol indicates a statistically significant difference ($p < 0.001$, $p < 0.05$, respectively) relative to challenged positive control (CD) vs. the baicalin-treated challenged mice (CD+BC1 or CD+BC2).

3. Discussion

In the current study, we investigated the prophylactic and therapeutic efficacies of baicalin as an alternative agent to ameliorate CDI without compromising the normal gut microbial population. Previous research conducted in our laboratory revealed that sub-inhibitory concentration of baicalin reduced *C. difficile* toxin production and cytotoxicity in vitro. Additionally, baicalin inhibited *C. difficile* spore germination and outgrowth [31]. The results from the current study translate our previous findings in vivo by demonstrating a dose-dependent reduction of CDI severity in BC-supplemented mice. Concurring with the reduced incidence of diarrhea in baicalin-treated *C. difficile*-infected mice ($p < 0.05$) (Figure 2a,b), a significant reduction in average clinical scores, fecal toxin-mediated Vero cell cytotoxicity, and histopathologic lesion scores were also observed compared with the challenge control group (CD) ($p < 0.05$) (Figure 2c,d, Figures 4b and 5b). Although the fecal *C. difficile* counts on day 6 were comparable across the challenged mice groups treated with or without BC (5a (iii)), there was a significant reduction in the fecal toxin-mediated Vero cell cytotoxicity in the CD+BC2 mouse group (Figure 5b(ii)). The reduced CDI severity in baicalin-treated mice could be attributed to the inhibitory effect of baicalin on *C. difficile* toxin production, as observed in our in vitro studies [31]. In addition, baicalin is known to possess anti-inflammatory and anti-diarrheal properties [34–36], which could also have contributed to the improved clinical outcome in BC-administered mice.

A normal and healthy gastrointestinal microbiota is key for preventing pathogen colonization, including *C. difficile* [37]. Disruption of host gut microbiota as a result of antibiotic therapy is the most important predisposing factor for CDI [1]. Antibiotic administration significantly alters microbiome diversity and composition, the effects of which can persist even after the withdrawal of antibiotics [38,39]. The increased risk for CDI susceptibility in the elderly is attributed to the reduction of the protective bacterial population such as Firmicutes and undesirable Proteobacteria groups in the gut [40–42].

In this study, baicalin did not reduce the bacterial diversity of the mouse gut microbiome compared with the untreated negative control (Figure 3c,d). Baicalin treatment alone significantly increased the abundance of Firmicutes, especially the members of *Lachnospiraceae* and, to a modest extent, the *Lactobacillaceae* group, compared with the negative control (Figure 3b). Microbiome analyses of human CDI patients by previous researchers have identified that *Ruminococcaceae* and *Lachnospiraceae*, as well as butyrate-producing bacteria were significantly depleted in patients with CDI compared with healthy subjects, whereas *Enterococcus* and *Lactobacillus* were more abundant in CDI patients [43]. In addition, a decrease in *Enterococcaceae* along with an increase in *Peptostreptococcaceae*, *Lactobacillaceae*, and *Enterobacteriaceae* have also been reported in *C. difficile*-positive patients [44–49]. An abundance of *Lachnospiraceae*, *Ruminococcaceae*, and *Bacteroidaceae* families mainly contribute to *C. difficile* colonization resistance in humans [43,47,50]. Similar observations in the gut microbiome of mice were also observed, wherein an increase in *Lactobacillaceae* and *Enterobacteriaceae* families was noted in susceptible mice that were treated with antibiotics, whereas *Lachnospiraceae* dominated in animals that remained resistant to CDI [51]. In addition, it has been collectively implicated from several research findings that that a decrease in *Lachnospiraceae* and Barnesiella with an increase in *Lactobacillaceae* and *Enterobacteriaceae* is responsible for the loss of colonization resistance against *C. difficile* [50]. Antibiotic-induced microbiome dynamics observed in the current study are in agreement with the findings reported by previous researchers. Antibiotic pre-treatment significantly increased the abundance of the *Lactobacillaceae* and Proteobacteria, with a drastic reduction in the *Lachnospiraceae* (Figure 3b). This change in the microbial composition could be correlated with an increased susceptibility of mice to *C. difficile* challenge. *Akkermansia* genus (phylum Verrucomicrobia) is a strictly anaerobic, Gram-negative bacterium that has been detected in the intestine of most healthy individuals, representing 1–4% of the total microbiota, and is capable of utilizing gut-secreted mucin as a sole source of carbon and nitrogen [52,53]. The only species in this genus, *Akkermansia muciniphila*, has beneficial effects on metabolism and gut health by exhibiting anti-inflammatory and immunostimulant properties [53,54]. Recent studies have revealed that co-administration of *A. muciniphila* with polyphenols or prebiotics resulted in improvement of gut barrier function and reduced endotoxemia [55]. Although co-administration of baicalin with antibiotics (Ant+BC2) was not able to reverse the abundance of *Enterobacteriaceae*, a significant increase in *Lachnospiraceae* and *Akkermansia* was observed ($p < 0.05$) (Figure 3b). Therefore, in the CD+BC1 and CD+BC2 groups, the microbiome shift observed during co-administration of baicalin and antibiotics may have contributed to the colonization resistance against *C. difficile* on days 2 and 4 post infection. The untreated spore-challenged mice groups (CD and CD+PBS) had invariably shown an increased abundance of *Lactobacillus* and Proteobacteria due to antibiotic administration, along with an increase in the abundance of *Peptostreptococcaceae*, the family under which the pathogenic *C. difficile* are classified [56]. However, in baicalin-treated spore challenge groups, we observed a dose-dependent increase in the abundance of *Lachnospiraceae* and *Akkermansia*, along with a significant reduction in *Peptostreptococcaceae* ($p < 0.05$) (Figure 3b). These results suggest that the reduced clinical symptoms and infection in baicalin-treated animals could be attributed in part to the beneficial shift in the gut microbiome, especially with the improved abundance of *Lachnospiraceae* and *Akkermansia*.

4. Materials and Methods

4.1. Ethics Statement, Animals, and Housing

The study was performed with the approval of the Institutional Animal Care and Use Committee (IACUC) at the University of Connecticut, following the endorsed guidelines for animal care and use. Five- to six-week-old C57BL/6 mice were obtained from Charles River (Boston, MA), housed in a biohazard level II AALAC-accredited facility, and monitored for health status twice daily. Mice were provided with irradiated feed, autoclaved water, and bedding, along with 12 h light/dark cycles. The procedures that required animal handling (spore administration, cage changes, and sample collection) were done under a biosafety cabinet (class II) using proper personal protective equipment. Decontamination and sterilization of the biosafety cabinet was done using 10% bleach to prevent cross-contamination between experimental treatment groups. The mice were singly housed in a cage, and twelve cages were included for each treatment in each of the experiments.

4.2. Prophylactic and Therapeutic Administration of Baicalin in a Mouse Model of C. difficile Infection

The in vivo infection model was based on a previously established protocol with minor modifications [32]. Five- to six-week-old female animals were randomly assigned to one of the following eight treatment groups of thirteen animals each (Table 1). In the prophylactic model, animals were provided irradiated pellet feed and incorporated baicalin in drinking water containing 0, 11, and 22 mg/L of the compound for a period of twenty-two days (Supplementary Figure S1). As equated from the average daily water consumed by each mouse (~5–7 mL per day), baicalin-treated water was expected to deliver approximately 250 mg/kg and 500 mg/kg of the compound per day in the 11 and 22 mg/L treatments, respectively. Previous researchers have indicated that baicalin dosage of 400 mg/kg is well tolerated by mice [57]. Subsequently, an antibiotic cocktail comprising kanamycin (0.4 mg/mL), gentamicin (0.03 mg/mL), colistin (850 U/mL), metronidazole (0.215 mg/mL), and vancomycin (0.045 mg/mL) was added in drinking water for 3 days. After antibiotic supplementation, the mice were switched back to their prior treatment regimens, and all animals in the challenge groups (CD, CD+PBS, CD+BC1, and CD+BC2) and the antibiotic control group (Ant) received a single intraperitoneal injection of clindamycin (10 mg/kg, with a maximum of 0.5 mL/mouse using a 27G needle and syringe) a day prior to *C. difficile* challenge. Pre-treatment of mice with antibiotics was intended to induce gastrointestinal dysbiosis and enable *C. difficile* colonization following the spore challenge. Mice proposed for *C. difficile* infection were orally administered 10^6 spores (CFU) per 0.1 mL total volume of hypervirulent *C. difficile* ATCC BAA 1803 using a straight 18G gavage needle (1″ shaft length) and were observed for signs of CDI, including diarrhea, wet tail, and hunched posture using a mouse clinical score sheet (Supplementary Figure S2 and Supplementary Table S1).

Table 1. Different treatment groups used in the experiment. Abbreviations: Ant (antibiotic); CD (*C. difficile*); BC (baicalin); PBS (phosphate buffered saline).

Group	Antibiotic	BC	Spore Challenge
NC (Unchallenged negative control)	-	-	-
Ant (Unchallenged antibiotic control)	+	-	-
Ant+BC (Unchallenged antibiotic + 22 mg/L BC control)	+	+	-
BC2 (Unchallenged 22 mg/L BC control)	-	+	-
CD (Ant + C. difficile challenged control)	+	-	+
CD+PBS (Ant + CD challenged, PBS solvent control)	+	-	+
CD+BC1 (Ant + CD + 11 mg/L BC)	+	+	+
CD+BC2 (Ant + CD + 22 mg/L BC)	+	+	+

The individual weight of each mouse was measured every day, fecal samples were collected on alternate days post infection (DPI; days 4 and 6 for the prophylactic study only), and all animals were observed twice daily for ten days for morbidity and mortality. At the end of the experiment (10th day after challenge), all animals were euthanized. In the therapeutic model, the only difference from the aforementioned procedure is that baicalin was administered from day 1 post-*C. difficile* spore challenge (1 DPI). In addition, microbiome analysis was not performed in the therapeutic study (Supplementary Figure S1).

4.3. Histopathologic Analysis

Colon and cecum were collected from each mouse from the prophylactic study ($n = 8$), and the tissues were fixed in 10% formalin. Formalin-fixed tissues were then embedded in paraffin, and slides were made and stained with hematoxylin and eosin. A board-certified veterinary pathologist performed blinded histopathological analysis on all sections. Histopathologic grading was based on a scoring system reported previously [32,58]. Briefly, scoring was based on (1) epithelial tissue damage; (2) edema, congestion, and hemorrhage; and (3) neutrophil infiltration. A score of 0–4 was assigned to each animal, with 0 denoting the absence of lesion, 1 for minimal, 2 for mild, 3 for moderate, and 4 for severe. Mean of individual category scores were calculated to provide an overall histopathologic lesion score for each mouse and then for each group.

4.4. DNA Extraction, PCR Amplification, and Sequencing of Taxonomic Markers

Fecal samples from day 2 post infection from all treatment groups (from eight animals per treatment group) of the prophylactic baicalin study were subjected to DNA extraction using the MoBio PowerMag Soil 96 well kit (MoBio Laboratories, Inc., Carlsbad, CA, USA), according to the manufacturer's protocol for the Eppendorf ep Motion liquid-handling robot. Quantification of DNA was performed using the Quant-iT PicoGreen kit (Invitrogen, ThermoFisher Scientific, Waltham, MA, USA), and DNA was subjected to amplification of partial bacterial 16S rRNA genes (V4 region) from 30 ng of extracted DNA as template, using 515F and 806R primers bound with Illumina adapters and dual indices (8 basepair golay in 3′ and 5′) [59,60]. Amplification was performed in triplicates with the addition of 10 µg BSA (New England BioLabs, Ipswich, MA, USA) using Phusion High-Fidelity PCR master mix (New England BioLabs, Ipswich, MA, USA). The reaction mixes were incubated at 95 °C for 3.5 min and then subjected to PCR reaction for 30 cycles of 30 s at 95.0 °C, 30 s at 50.0 °C, and 90 s at 72.0 °C, followed by a final extension at 72.0 °C for 1 min. Quantification and visualization of pooled PCR products were performed using the QIAxcel DNA Fast Analysis (Qiagen, Germantown, MD, USA). DNA concentrations of the PCR products were normalized to 250–400 bp and pooled using the QIAgility liquid handling robot. Pooled PCR products were cleaned up using the Gene Read Size Selection kit (Qiagen, Germantown, MD, USA) according to the manufacturer's protocol, and the cleaned pool was subjected to sequencing on MiSeq using a v2 2 × 250 base pair kit (Illumina, Inc., San Diego, CA, USA).

4.5. Sequence Analysis

Microbiome analysis was set up as a completely randomized design with treatments done in replicates of eight. Filtering and clustering of sequences were performed using Mothur 1.36.1 based on a published protocol [60]. The operational taxonomic units (OTUs) of samples were clustered at 97% sequence similarity, and downstream analysis was done using R version 3.2. The richness and evenness of sample OTUs were calculated by estimating alpha diversity using inverse Simpson diversity index, which were then analyzed using Tukey's test. Permutational multivariate analysis (PERMANOVA, adonis function, 75 permutations) was performed to analyze differences in bacterial community composition in the various treatment groups. Test for significance in alpha diversity was determined by ANOVA followed by Tukey's honest significant differences, adjusting for multiple comparisons ($p = 0.05$). NMS ordinations were run in R (v 3.3.0) using metaMDS in the vegan (v 2.3-5) package after calculating the stress scree plots to determine the number of axes required to achieve stress below 0.2, plotted using ggplot2 (v 2.1.0). In addition, the relative abundance of OTUs of major phyla, order, and genera was determined to assess the effect of treatment. Tukey's test was used to identify changes in groups of bacteria based on treatment, and the significance was detected at $p < 0.05$.

4.6. Fecal *C. difficile* Enumeration and Cytotoxicity Assay

DNA extracted from day 2 post-infection fecal samples in the previous section (prophylactic study; $n = 8$) was subjected to qPCR-based enumeration of *C. difficile*. The Ct values obtained were compared against the standard curve for the *tcd*A gene of BAA 1803. The bacterial counts for the standard curve ranged from 0.5 log CFU/mL to 6 log CFU/mL. The trendline from the scatter plot of the standard curve generated the regression equation $y = -3.8456x = 36.4$ ($R^2 = 0.9899$), wherein y denotes the Ct values of the respective samples and x would provide the counts in $\log_{10}$ bacterial copy number/qPCR. Fecal material obtained from days 4 and 6 of the prophylactic study ($n = 4$) was subjected to *C. difficile* enumeration using serial dilution and plating. An amount of 15 mg of fecal material was weighed and transferred into an Eppendorf tube containing 500 µL of PBS. The samples were mixed thoroughly by vortexing and subjected to heat shock at 60 °C for 20 min (in a water bath) to kill the vegetative bacteria and favor sporulation of *C. difficile* in the fecal slurry. To enumerate *C. difficile* spores, the samples were serially diluted and plated on to cycloserine-cefoxitin fructose agar containing 0.1% sodium taurocholate (CCFA-T)) and incubated in an anaerobic chamber (A35, Don Whitley Scientific Ltd., Bingley, UK) at 37 °C for 48 h. In addition, fecal samples collected from day 4 and 6 post infection were also subjected to Vero cell cytotoxicity. In this method, 15 mg of fecal material was weighed and mixed thoroughly by vortexing with 200 µL of sterile PBS and subsequently centrifuged at 14,000× g at 4 °C for 10 min (samples were stored at −80 °C if not used immediately). The supernatants of the fecal slurry were subjected to Vero cell cytotoxicity assay [31]. Fecal slurry supernatants were serially diluted by 1:10 up to a dilution of 1:100,000,000 onto confluent Vero cell monolayers in 96-well microtiter plates. The cell culture plates were incubated in a carbon dioxide incubator (5% CO_2) at 37 °C for 24 h and observed for cytopathic changes under an inverted microscope. Cytopathic changes were observed as Vero cell rounding, and the cytotoxicity titer was considered as the highest microtiter well dilution showing 80% cell rounding. The identified titer values were expressed as the reciprocal of the identified dilution.

4.7. Statistical Analysis

Data were analyzed using R and GraphPad Prism 8.4.2. Chi-squared test was used to compare diarrhea incidence rate between to different treatments. For analyzing the percentage body weight and average clinical scores, the differences between means between experimental groups across the days were compared by two-way mixed ANOVA using Tukey's test. For analyzing the qPCR based fecal *C. difficile* counts and fecal cytotoxicity assay, the differences between means were compared using one-way ANOVA. Percentage abundance of major family taxa in the microbiome was analyzed using one-way analysis using the Mann–Whitney test. A two-sided Cochran–Armitage test was used to compare the histopathologic lesion scores between the groups, with the Benjamini and Hochberg correction being applied to p values. The statistical significance level was set at $p < 0.05$. Survival curve comparisons were analyzed using the log-rank (Mantel–Cox) test.

5. Conclusions

The results from this study suggest that oral BC supplementation protects mice from antibiotic-induced gut dysbiosis and CDI. Baicalin supplementation significantly reduced the incidence of diarrhea as well as the severity of CDI clinical symptoms and enteric lesions in mice. In addition, BC favorably modulated the composition of gut microbiota without detrimentally affecting the gut microbiome diversity. However, further mechanistic and clinical investigations are warranted to validate and extrapolate these results for controlling CDI in human patients.

Supplementary Materials: The following are available online at https://www.mdpi.com/article/10.3390/antibiotics10080926/s1, Figure S1: Antibiotic-induced murine CDI model, Figure S2: Mouse body condition chart, Table S1: Mouse clinical score sheet, Figure S3: Mouse survival curves.

Author Contributions: Conceptualization, K.V. and A.J.P.; methodology, A.J.P., S.M. and K.V.; software, A.J.P., B.O.F. and K.M.; validation, A.J.P., N.M., B.O.F. and K.M.; formal analysis, A.J.P.; investigation, A.J.P., P.G.V., D.A.K. and N.M.; resources, K.V.; data curation, A.J.P., N.M., B.O.F. and K.M.; writing—original draft preparation, A.J.P.; writing—review and editing, A.J.P., P.G.V., N.M., S.M. and K.V.; visualization, K.M. and A.J.P.; supervision, K.V.; project administration, A.J.P. and K.V.; funding acquisition, K.V. All authors have read and agreed to the published version of the manuscript.

Funding: This research was supported by the University of Connecticut, Office of Vice President for Research, under the Research Excellence Program 2019–20.

Institutional Review Board Statement: The study was approved by the Institutional Animal Care and Use Committee (IACUC) of the University of Connecticut (Protocol #: A16-022, June 2018).

Informed Consent Statement: Not applicable.

Conflicts of Interest: The authors declare no conflict of interest.

References

1. Hookman, P.; Barkin, J.S. Clostridium difficile associated infection, diarrhea and colitis. *World J. Gastroenterol.* **2009**, *15*, 1554–1580. [CrossRef] [PubMed]
2. McFarland, L.V. Antibiotic-associated diarrhea: Epidemiology, trends and treatment. *Future Microbiol.* **2008**, *3*, 563–578. [CrossRef]
3. Weese, J.S.; Rousseau, J.; Deckert, A.; Gow, S.; Reid-Smith, R.J. Clostridium difficile and methicillin-resistant Staphylococcus aureus shedding by slaughter-age pigs. *BMC Vet. Res.* **2011**, *7*, 41. [CrossRef] [PubMed]
4. Leffler, D.A.; Lamont, J.T. Clostridium difficile infection. *N. Engl. J. Med.* **2015**, *372*, 1539–1548. [CrossRef]
5. Napolitano, L.M.; Edmiston, C.E., Jr. Clostridium difficile disease: Diagnosis, pathogenesis, and treatment update. *Surgery* **2017**, *162*, 325–348. [CrossRef]
6. Blossom, D.B.; McDonald, L.C. The challenges posed by reemerging Clostridium difficile infection. *Clin. Infect. Dis.* **2007**, *45*, 222–227. [CrossRef]
7. Spigaglia, P. Recent advances in the understanding of antibiotic resistance in Clostridium difficile infection. *Ther. Adv. Infect. Dis.* **2016**, *3*, 23–42.
8. Sunenshine, R.H.; McDonald, L.C. Clostridium difficile-associated disease: New challenges from an established pathogen. *Cleve. Clin. J. Med.* **2006**, *73*, 187–197. [CrossRef]
9. Bartlett, J.G. Antibiotic-associated diarrhea. *Clin. Infect. Dis.* **1992**, *15*, 573–581. [CrossRef]
10. Dial, S.; Delaney, J.A.; Schneider, V.; Suissa, S. Proton pump inhibitor use and risk of community-acquired Clostridium difficile-associated disease defined by prescription for oral vancomycin therapy. *CMAJ* **2006**, *175*, 745–748. [CrossRef]
11. Kelly, C.P.; LaMont, J.T. Clostridium difficile infection. *Annu. Rev. Med.* **1998**, *49*, 375–390. [CrossRef] [PubMed]

12. Ling, Z.; Liu, X.; Jia, X.; Cheng, Y.; Luo, Y.; Yuan, L.; Wang, Y.; Zhao, C.; Guo, S.; Li, L.; et al. Impacts of infection with different toxigenic Clostridium difficile strains on faecal microbiota in children. *Sci. Rep.* **2014**, *4*, 7485. [CrossRef] [PubMed]
13. Seekatz, A.M.; Young, V.B. Clostridium difficile and the microbiota. *J. Clin. Investig.* **2014**, *124*, 4182–4189. [CrossRef] [PubMed]
14. Shahinas, D.; Silverman, M.; Sittler, T.; Chiu, C.; Kim, P.; Allen-Vercoe, E.; Weese, S.; Wong, A.; Low, D.E.; Pillai, D.R. Toward an understanding of changes in diversity associated with fecal microbiome transplantation based on 16S rRNA gene deep sequencing. *MBio* **2012**, *3*, e00338-12. [CrossRef]
15. Theriot, C.M.; Koenigsknecht, M.J.; Carlson, P.E.; Hatton, G.E.; Nelson, A.M.; Li, B.; Huffnagle, G.B.; Li, J.Z.; Young, V.B. Antibiotic-induced shifts in the mouse gut microbiome and metabolome increase susceptibility to Clostridium difficile infection. *Nat. Commun.* **2014**, *5*, 3114. [CrossRef]
16. Voth, D.E.; Ballard, J.D. Clostridium difficile toxins: Mechanism of action and role in disease. *Clin. Microbiol. Rev.* **2005**, *18*, 247–263. [CrossRef]
17. McDonald, L.C. Clostridium difficile: Responding to a new threat from an old enemy. *Infect. Control Hosp. Epidemiol.* **2005**, *26*, 672–675. [CrossRef] [PubMed]
18. McDonald, L.C.; Killgore, G.E.; Thompson, A.; Owens, R.C., Jr.; Kazakova, S.V.; Sambol, S.P.; Johnson, S.; Gerding, D.N. An epidemic, toxin gene-variant strain of Clostridium difficile. *N. Engl. J. Med.* **2005**, *353*, 2433–2441. [CrossRef]
19. Cohen, S.H.; Gerding, D.N.; Johnson, S.; Kelly, C.P.; Loo, V.G.; McDonald, L.C.; Pepin, J.; Wilcox, M.H. Clinical practice guidelines for Clostridium difficile infection in adults: 2010 update by the Society for Healthcare Epidemiology of America (SHEA) and the Infectious Diseases Society of America (IDSA). *Infect. Control* **2010**, *31*, 431–455. [CrossRef]
20. Debast, S.B.; Bauer, M.P.; Kuijper, E.J. European Society of Clinical Microbiology and Infectious Diseases: Update of the treatment guidance document for Clostridium difficile infection. *Clin. Microbiol. Infect.* **2014**, *20*, 1–26. [CrossRef]
21. Peng, Z.; Ling, L.; Stratton, C.W.; Li, C.; Polage, C.R.; Wu, B.; Tang, Y.-W. Advances in the diagnosis and treatment of Clostridium difficile infections. *Emerg. Microbes Infect.* **2018**, *7*, 15. [CrossRef]
22. US Department of Health and Human Services. Antibiotic resistance threats in the United States, 2013. *Cent. Dis. Control Prev.* **2013**. Available online: https://www.cdc.gov/drugresistance/threat-report-2013/pdf/ar-threats-2013-508.pdf (accessed on 20 March 2021).
23. Wollenweber, E. Occurrence of flavonoid aglycones in medicinal plants. *Prog. Clin. Biol. Res.* **1988**, *280*, 45–55. [PubMed]
24. Chen, Y.-C.; Shen, S.-C.; Chen, L.-G.; Lee, T.J.F.; Yang, L.-L. Wogonin, baicalin, and baicalein inhibition of inducible nitric oxide synthase and cyclooxygenase-2 gene expressions induced by nitric oxide synthase inhibitors and lipopolysaccharide. *Biochem. Pharmacol.* **2001**, *61*, 1417–1427. [CrossRef]
25. Liu, I.X.; Durham, D.G.; Richards, R.M.E. Baicalin Synergy with β-Lactam Antibiotics Against Methicillin-resistant Staphylococcus aureus and Other β-Lactam-resistant Strains of S. aureus. *J. Pharm. Pharmacol.* **2000**, *52*, 361–366. [CrossRef] [PubMed]
26. Novy, P.; Urban, J.; Leuner, O.; Vadlejch, J.; Kokoska, L. In vitro synergistic effects of baicalin with oxytetracycline and tetracycline against Staphylococcus aureus. *J. Antimicrob. Chemother.* **2011**, *66*, 1298–1300. [CrossRef]
27. Tsou, L.K.; Lara-Tejero, M.; RoseFigura, J.; Zhang, Z.J.; Wang, Y.-C.; Yount, J.S.; Lefebre, M.; Dossa, P.D.; Kato, J.; Guan, F. Antibacterial flavonoids from medicinal plants covalently inactivate type III protein secretion substrates. *J. Am. Chem. Soc.* **2016**, *138*, 2209–2218. [CrossRef]
28. Wang, H.; Liu, D. Baicalin inhibits high-mobility group box 1 release and improves survival in experimental sepsis. *Shock* **2014**, *41*, 324–330. [CrossRef]
29. Zhang, Y.; Qi, Z.; Liu, Y.; He, W.; Yang, C.; Wang, Q.; Dong, J.; Deng, X. Baicalin Protects Mice from Lethal Infection by Enterohemorrhagic Escherichia coli. *Front. Microbiol.* **2017**, *8*, 395. [CrossRef] [PubMed]
30. Zhu, J.; Wang, J.; Sheng, Y.; Zou, Y.; Bo, L.; Wang, F.; Lou, J.; Fan, X.; Bao, R.; Wu, Y. Baicalin improves survival in a murine model of polymicrobial sepsis via suppressing inflammatory response and lymphocyte apoptosis. *PLoS ONE* **2012**, *7*, e35523. [CrossRef]
31. Pellissery, A.J.; Vinayamohan, P.G.; Venkitanarayanan, K. In vitro antivirulence activity of baicalin against Clostridioides difficile. *J. Med. Microbiol.* **2020**, *69*, 631–639. [CrossRef]
32. Chen, X.; Katchar, K.; Goldsmith, J.D.; Nanthakumar, N.; Cheknis, A.; Gerding, D.N.; Kelly, C.P. A mouse model of Clostridium difficile-associated disease. *Gastroenterology* **2008**, *135*, 1984–1992. [CrossRef]
33. Sun, X.; Wang, H.; Zhang, Y.; Chen, K.; Davis, B.; Feng, H. Mouse relapse model of Clostridium difficile infection. *Infect. Immun.* **2011**, *79*, 2856–2864. [CrossRef]
34. Chen, J.; Zhang, R.; Wang, J.; Yu, P.; Liu, Q.; Zeng, D.; Song, H.; Kuang, Z. Protective effects of baicalin on LPS-induced injury in intestinal epithelial cells and intercellular tight junctions. *Can. J. Physiol. Pharmacol.* **2014**, *93*, 233–237. [CrossRef]
35. Dou, W.; Mukherjee, S.; Li, H.; Venkatesh, M.; Wang, H.; Kortagere, S.; Peleg, A.; Chilimuri, S.S.; Wang, Z.-T.; Feng, Y. Alleviation of gut inflammation by Cdx2/Pxr pathway in a mouse model of chemical colitis. *PLoS ONE* **2012**, *7*, e36075.
36. Ishimaru, K.; Nishikawa, K.; Omoto, T.; Asai, I.; Yoshihira, K.; Shimomura, K. Two flavone 2′-glucosides from Scutellaria baicalensis. *Phytochemistry* **1995**, *40*, 279–281. [CrossRef]
37. Britton, R.A.; Young, V.B. Role of the intestinal microbiota in resistance to colonization by Clostridium difficile. *Gastroenterology* **2014**, *146*, 1547–1553. [CrossRef]
38. Antonopoulos, D.A.; Huse, S.M.; Morrison, H.G.; Schmidt, T.M.; Sogin, M.L.; Young, V.B. Reproducible community dynamics of the gastrointestinal microbiota following antibiotic perturbation. *Infect. Immun.* **2009**, *77*, 2367–2375. [CrossRef]

39. Dethlefsen, L.; Huse, S.; Sogin, M.L.; Relman, D.A. The pervasive effects of an antibiotic on the human gut microbiota, as revealed by deep 16S rRNA sequencing. *PLoS Biol.* **2008**, *6*, e280. [CrossRef]
40. Biagi, E.; Nylund, L.; Candela, M.; Ostan, R.; Bucci, L.; Pini, E.; Nikkila, J.; Monti, D.; Satokari, R.; Franceschi, C.; et al. Through ageing, and beyond: Gut microbiota and inflammatory status in seniors and centenarians. *PLoS ONE* **2010**, *5*, e10667. [CrossRef]
41. Claesson, M.J.; Cusack, S.; O'Sullivan, O.; Greene-Diniz, R.; de Weerd, H.; Flannery, E.; Marchesi, J.R.; Falush, D.; Dinan, T.; Fitzgerald, G.; et al. Composition, variability, and temporal stability of the intestinal microbiota of the elderly. *Proc. Natl. Acad. Sci. USA* **2011**, *108*, 4586–4591. [CrossRef]
42. Hopkins, M.J.; Sharp, R.; Macfarlane, G.T. Age and disease related changes in intestinal bacterial populations assessed by cell culture, 16S rRNA abundance, and community cellular fatty acid profiles. *Gut* **2001**, *48*, 198–205. [CrossRef] [PubMed]
43. Antharam, V.C.; Li, E.C.; Ishmael, A.; Sharma, A.; Mai, V.; Rand, K.H.; Wang, G.P. Intestinal dysbiosis and depletion of butyrogenic bacteria in Clostridium difficile infection and nosocomial diarrhea. *J. Clin. Microbiol.* **2013**, *51*, 2884–2892. [CrossRef]
44. Buffie, C.G.; Jarchum, I.; Equinda, M.; Lipuma, L.; Gobourne, A.; Viale, A.; Ubeda, C.; Xavier, J.; Pamer, E.G. Profound alterations of intestinal microbiota following a single dose of clindamycin results in sustained susceptibility to Clostridium difficile-induced colitis. *Infect. Immun.* **2012**, *80*, 62–73. [CrossRef] [PubMed]
45. Perez-Cobas, A.E.; Artacho, A.; Ott, S.J.; Moya, A.; Gosalbes, M.J.; Latorre, A. Structural and functional changes in the gut microbiota associated to Clostridium difficile infection. *Front. Microbiol.* **2014**, *5*, 335. [CrossRef]
46. Rea, M.C.; O'Sullivan, O.; Shanahan, F.; O'Toole, P.W.; Stanton, C.; Ross, R.P.; Hill, C. Clostridium difficile carriage in elderly subjects and associated changes in the intestinal microbiota. *J. Clin. Microbiol.* **2012**, *50*, 867–875. [CrossRef]
47. Schubert, A.M.; Rogers, M.A.; Ring, C.; Mogle, J.; Petrosino, J.P.; Young, V.B.; Aronoff, D.M.; Schloss, P.D. Microbiome data distinguish patients with Clostridium difficile infection and non-*C. difficile*-associated diarrhea from healthy controls. *MBio* **2014**, *5*, e01021-14. [CrossRef]
48. Skraban, J.; Dzeroski, S.; Zenko, B.; Mongus, D.; Gangl, S.; Rupnik, M. Gut microbiota patterns associated with colonization of different Clostridium difficile ribotypes. *PLoS ONE* **2013**, *8*, e58005.
49. Zhang, L.; Dong, D.; Jiang, C.; Li, Z.; Wang, X.; Peng, Y. Insight into alteration of gut microbiota in Clostridium difficile infection and asymptomatic C. difficile colonization. *Anaerobe* **2015**, *34*, 1–7. [CrossRef]
50. Schubert, A.M.; Sinani, H.; Schloss, P.D. Antibiotic-Induced Alterations of the Murine Gut Microbiota and Subsequent Effects on Colonization Resistance against Clostridium difficile. *MBio* **2015**, *6*, e00974-15. [CrossRef]
51. Reeves, A.E.; Koenigsknecht, M.J.; Bergin, I.L.; Young, V.B. Suppression of Clostridium difficile in the gastrointestinal tracts of germfree mice inoculated with a murine isolate from the family Lachnospiraceae. *Infect. Immun.* **2012**, *80*, 3786–3794. [CrossRef]
52. Collado, M.C.; Derrien, M.; Isolauri, E.; de Vos, W.M.; Salminen, S. Intestinal integrity and Akkermansia muciniphila, a mucin-degrading member of the intestinal microbiota present in infants, adults, and the elderly. *Appl. Environ. Microbiol.* **2007**, *73*, 7767–7770. [CrossRef] [PubMed]
53. Derrien, M.; Van Baarlen, P.; Hooiveld, G.; Norin, E.; Muller, M.; de Vos, W. Modulation of mucosal immune response, tolerance, and proliferation in mice colonized by the mucin-degrader Akkermansia muciniphila. *Front. Microbiol.* **2011**, *2*, 166. [CrossRef] [PubMed]
54. Naito, Y.; Uchiyama, K.; Takagi, T. A next-generation beneficial microbe: Akkermansia muciniphila. *J. Clin. Biochem. Nutr.* **2018**, 18–57. [CrossRef]
55. Anhê, F.F.; Pilon, G.; Roy, D.; Desjardins, Y.; Levy, E.; Marette, A. Triggering Akkermansia with dietary polyphenols: A new weapon to combat the metabolic syndrome? *Gut Microbes* **2016**, *7*, 146–153. [CrossRef] [PubMed]
56. Yutin, N.; Galperin, M.Y. A genomic update on clostridial phylogeny: G ram-negative spore formers and other misplaced clostridia. *Environ. Microbiol.* **2013**, *15*, 2631–2641. [PubMed]
57. Xi, Y.; Wu, M.; Li, H.; Dong, S.; Luo, E.; Gu, M.; Shen, X.; Jiang, Y.; Liu, Y.; Liu, H. Baicalin Attenuates High Fat Diet-Induced Obesity and Liver Dysfunction: Dose-Response and Potential Role of CaMKKbeta/AMPK/ACC Pathway. *Cell. Physiol. Biochem.* **2015**, *35*, 2349–2359. [CrossRef]
58. Shelby, R.D.; Tengberg, N.; Conces, M.; Olson, J.K.; Navarro, J.B.; Bailey, M.T.; Goodman, S.D.; Besner, G.E. Development of a standardized scoring system to assess a murine model of Clostridium difficile colitis. *J. Investig. Surg.* **2019**, *33*, 887–895. [CrossRef] [PubMed]
59. Caporaso, J.G.; Lauber, C.L.; Walters, W.A.; Berg-Lyons, D.; Huntley, J.; Fierer, N.; Owens, S.M.; Betley, J.; Fraser, L.; Bauer, M.; et al. Ultra-high-throughput microbial community analysis on the Illumina HiSeq and MiSeq platforms. *ISME J.* **2012**, *6*, 1621–1624. [CrossRef]
60. Kozich, J.J.; Westcott, S.L.; Baxter, N.T.; Highlander, S.K.; Schloss, P.D. Development of a dual-index sequencing strategy and curation pipeline for analyzing amplicon sequence data on the MiSeq Illumina sequencing platform. *Appl. Environ. Microbiol.* **2013**, *79*, 5112–5120. [CrossRef]

antibiotics

MDPI

Article

Cationic Peptidomimetic Amphiphiles Having a *N*-Aryl- or *N*-Naphthyl-1,2,3-Triazole Core Structure Targeting *Clostridioides* (*Clostridium*) *difficile*: Synthesis, Antibacterial Evaluation, and an In Vivo *C. difficile* Infection Model

Muni Kumar Mahadari [1], Sreenu Jennepalli [1], Andrew J. Tague [1], Papanin Putsathit [2], Melanie L. Hutton [3], Katherine A. Hammer [4], Daniel R. Knight [4,5], Thomas V. Riley [2,4,5,6], Dena Lyras [3], Paul A. Keller [1,*] and Stephen G. Pyne [1,*]

1 School of Chemistry and Biomolecular Science, University of Wollongong, Wollongong, NSW 2522, Australia; mkm933@uowmail.edu.au (M.K.M.); jennepal@ohsu.edu (S.J.); atague@uow.edu.au (A.J.T.)
2 School of Medical and Health Sciences, Edith Cowan University, Perth, WA 6027, Australia; papanin.putsathit@uwa.edu.au (P.P.); thomas.riley@uwa.edu.au (T.V.R.)
3 Infection and Immunity Program, Monash Biomedicine Discovery Institute and Department of Microbiology, Monash University, Clayton, VIC 3800, Australia; melanie.hutton@monash.edu (M.L.H.); dena.lyras@monash.edu (D.L.)
4 School of Biomedical Sciences, The University of Western Australia, Perth, WA 6009, Australia; katherine.hammer@uwa.edu.au (K.A.H.); Daniel.Knight@murdoch.edu.au (D.R.K.)
5 Biosecurity and One Health Research Centre, Harry Butler Institute, Murdoch University, Perth, WA 6150, Australia
6 PathWest Laboratory Medicine, Queen Elizabeth II Medical Centre, Perth, WA 6009, Australia
* Correspondence: keller@uow.edu.au (P.A.K.); spyne@uow.edu.au (S.G.P.)

Citation: Mahadari, M.K.; Jennepalli, S.; Tague, A.J.; Putsathit, P.; Hutton, M.L.; Hammer, K.A.; Knight, D.R.; Riley, T.V.; Lyras, D.; Keller, P.A.; et al. Cationic Peptidomimetic Amphiphiles Having a *N*-Aryl- or *N*-Naphthyl-1,2,3-Triazole Core Structure Targeting *Clostridioides* (*Clostridium*) *difficile*: Synthesis, Antibacterial Evaluation, and an In Vivo *C. difficile* Infection Model. *Antibiotics* **2021**, *10*, 913. https://doi.org/10.3390/antibiotics10080913

Academic Editor: Guido Granata

Received: 22 June 2021
Accepted: 21 July 2021
Published: 26 July 2021

Publisher's Note: MDPI stays neutral with regard to jurisdictional claims in published maps and institutional affiliations.

Abstract: *Clostridioides* (also known as *Clostridium*) *difficile* is a Gram-positive anaerobic, spore producing bacterial pathogen that causes severe gastrointestinal infection in humans. The current chemotherapeutic options are inadequate, expensive, and limited, and thus inexpensive drug treatments for *C. difficile* infection (CDI) with improved efficacy and specificity are urgently needed. To improve the solubility of our cationic amphiphilic 1,1′-binaphthylpeptidomimetics developed earlier that showed promise in an in vivo murine CDI model we have synthesized related compounds with an *N*-arytriazole or *N*-naphthyltriazole moiety instead of the 1,1′-biphenyl or 1,1′-binaphthyl moiety. This modification was made to increase the polarity and thus water solubility of the overall peptidomimetics, while maintaining the aromatic character. The dicationic *N*-naphthyltriazole derivative **40** was identified as a *C. difficile*-selective antibacterial with MIC values of 8 μg/mL against *C. difficile* strains ATCC 700057 and 132 (both ribotype 027). This compound displayed increased water solubility and reduced hemolytic activity (32 μg/mL) in an in vitro hemolysis assay and reduced cytotoxicity (CC_{50} 32 μg/mL against HEK293 cells) relative to lead compound **2**. Compound **40** exhibited mild efficacy (with 80% survival observed after 24 h compared to the DMSO control of 40%) in an in vivo murine model of *C. difficile* infection by reducing the severity and slowing the onset of disease.

Keywords: antibacterial; *Clostridioides* (*Clostridium*) *difficile*; peptidomimetic; triazole

1. Introduction

Clostridioides (also known as *Clostridium*) *difficile* is a Gram-positive, anaerobic spore-forming bacterium that causes mild to serious infections in the gastrointestinal tract (GIT) due to the production of potent exotoxins (TcdA, TcdB, and CDT) that cause severe gastrointestinal damage [1–3]. The resilient endospores contaminate healthcare environments and facilitate disease initiation, dissemination, and re-infection. In the GIT, spores require glycine and cholate derivatives for germination. In a healthy GIT, the microbiota metabolizes cholate derivatives preventing germination of *C. difficile* spores. CDI occurs when the normal GIT microbiota is disrupted or killed by conventional broad-spectrum antimicrobials [1]. Under these conditions the metabolism of cholate is significantly compromised, facilitating the germination of spores into *C. difficile* vegetative cells [4,5].

CDI has a mortality rate of up to 8% [2] with the reoccurrence of infections occurring in up to 20% of cases treated with vancomycin or metronidazole [6]. A 2019 Antibiotic Resistance Threat Report from the US Centers for Disease Control and Prevention indicated that in the USA in 2017 an estimated 223,900 cases of CDI in hospitalized patients resulted in 12,800 deaths and $1 billion in attributed healthcare costs [7]. Thus, there is a significant and important incentive to develop novel therapeutics that show selectivity for *C. difficile* over other gut bacteria to effectively combat CDI. While fecal microbiota transplantation can be effective for recurrent CDI, there can be adverse effects and the long-term impacts are unknown [1,2,8].

Fidaxomicin was specifically approved by the FDA in 2011 for treating CDI [9]; resulting in approximately 50% less CDI recurrence compared to vancomycin [10] most likely due to its greater selectivity for *C. difficile,* less impact on commensal enteric microflora (i.e., *Bacteroides* spp.), and its ability to reduce *C. difficile* sporulation [11]. There are many potential chemotherapeutics undergoing clinical trials for the treatment of CDI [12]. Other small molecule chemotherapeutics currently under investigation for use against *C. difficile,* include antimicrobial peptidomimetics [13–15], glycopeptides [16], bis-indoles [17], purine derivatives [18], tetramic acids [19], nitroheterocycles [20], macrolides [21], and nylon-3 polymers [22]. Two vaccines are being investigated in clinical trials (Pfizer and Intercell [23]), whereas bezlotoxumab (a monoclonal antibody targeting *C. difficile* TcdB) was given FDA approval in 2016 as adjunctive therapy for patients undergoing antimicrobial treatment who were at high risk of recurrent infection [24].

In our earlier work on the development of the cationic amphiphilic 1,1′-binaphthylpeptidomimetics, we established the pharmacophoric importance of a hydrophobic head group (e.g., a binaphthyl moiety) connected to a dicationic peptide in the development of broad-spectrum antibacterial agents. This led to the identification of compound **1** with potent antibacterial activity against drug resistant Gram-positive bacteria with potential for topical applications (Figure 1) [25]. More recent work in our laboratory has identified compounds **2**–**4** from a class of small molecule cationic amphiphilic 1,1′-biarylpeptidomimetics that exert antibacterial activity through cytoplasmic membrane disruption [13,14]. These compounds have IC_{50} values of 4–8 µg/mL against *C. difficile* (Figure 1). The efficacy of these compounds at treating CDI in an in vivo murine CDI model was assessed against vancomycin as a positive control with 10% DMSO as the negative control. Compound **2** appeared to protect the mice from disease at the 24 h point with a 50% survival rate (2/4 mice) vs. 0% survival in the 10% DMSO group; this was not statistically significant due to the small sample size. These results clearly showed that compound **2** exhibited a notable positive effect in the treatment of CDI. Unfortunately compound **3** showed poor solubility with precipitation during preparation in a 10% DMSO solution, and high in vitro hemolytic activity against HEK293 cells. While compound **4** showed promising in vitro properties, it performed poorly in the *C. difficile* murine model with a survival rate of 60% after 24 h, but a 0% rate after 48 h [13], despite its low hemolytic activity. Despite some positive results, more water-soluble derivatives with lower hemolytic activity for further in vivo murine CDI model studies needed to be developed. To achieve this aim, we replaced the hydrophobic binaphthyl group found in **2** and **3** with an *N*-arytriazole or *N*-naphthyltriazole moiety as shown in Figure 2. These modifications should retain the aromatic character of these molecules while inducing a better polarity profile and thereby increasing the water solubility of the overall peptidomimetics. It was not clear at the start what effect these modifications would have on the antibacterial activities of these newly proposed compounds or their specificity for *C. difficile* over other pathogenic bacteria. Herein, we disclose the results of this investigation.

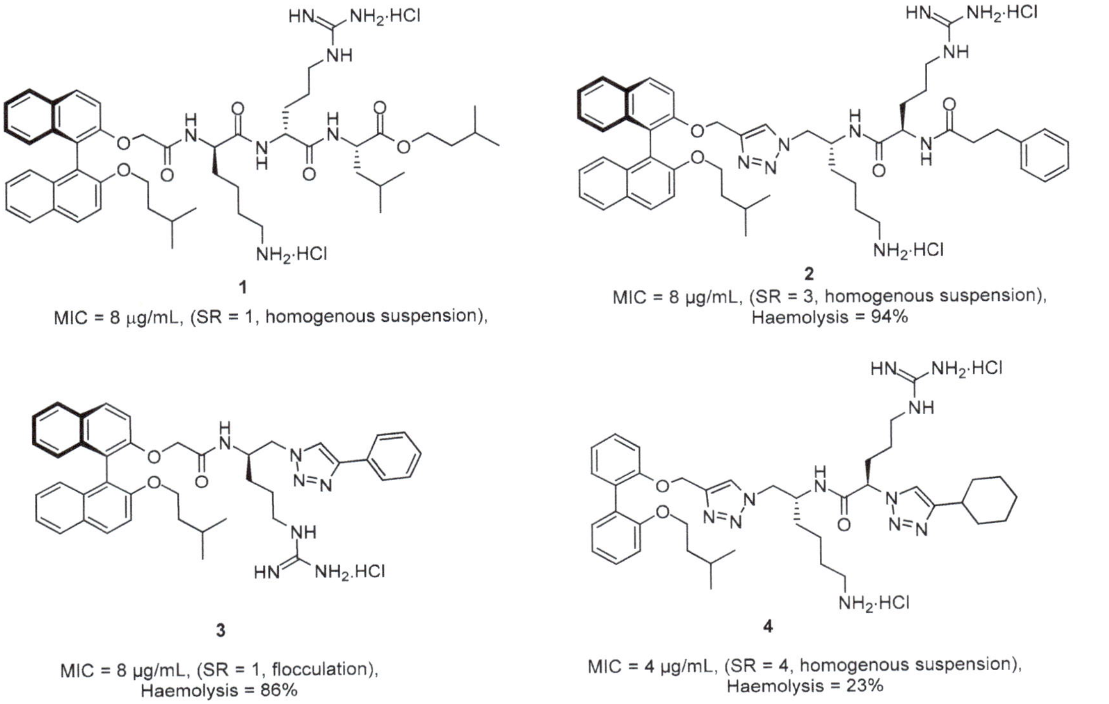

Figure 1. Previously published cationic amphiphilic hydrophobic anchored peptidomimetic antimicrobial agents. MIC values against *C. difficile* in μg/mL. SR = solubility ratio relative to that of compound **1**–see Ref [13].

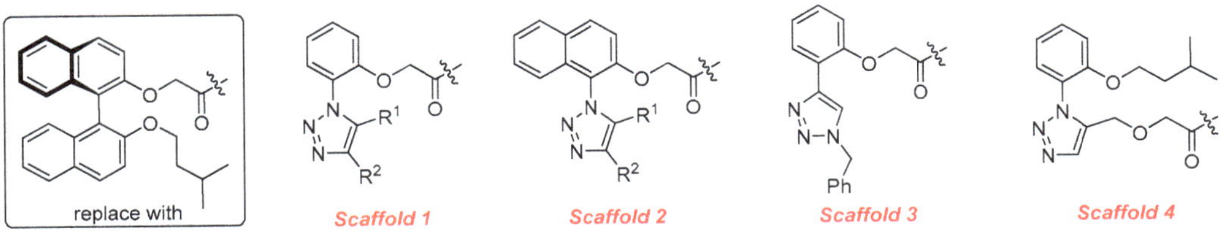

Figure 2. Hydrophobic scaffold replacements of the binaphthyl moiety for the target peptidomimetics.

2. Results and Discussion

Preparation of the target *N*-arytriazole or *N*-naphthyltriazole peptidomimetics required the synthesis of the carboxylic acid derivatives **5**, **6**, **17**, **18**, **27**, and **28** based on scaffolds 1–4 (Figure 2); the syntheses of acid **17** is described in the experimental section with the other acid syntheses described in the Supporting Information.

The synthesis of the new peptidomimetic derivatives is described in Schemes 1–3. In a typical example, derivative **40** (Scheme 3) was generated starting from acid **17** coupling with the protected azidodipetide **29** under standard peptide coupling conditions (EDCI/HOBt) [26,27] to give amide **32** in 67% yield. This was followed by a standard copper-catalyzed azide-alkyne cycloaddition reactions [28] with ethenylcyclohexane to give the corresponding 1,4-disubstituted 1,2,3-triazole product which was deprotected using TFA/CH_2Cl_2/H_2O followed by treatment with ethereal HCl to yield the dicationic amphiphile **40** in 46% yield over two steps. The synthesis of the additional mono- and dicationic peptidomimetic amphiphiles **10–16**, **21–26**, and **36–50** followed an analogous strategy and is summarized in Schemes 1–3 with experimental and characterization details provided in the Supporting Information.

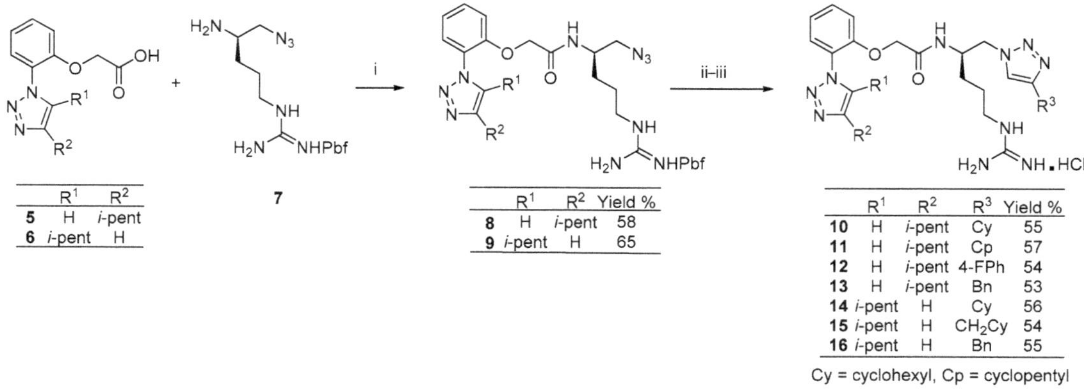

Scheme 1. Synthesis of *N*-aryltriazole monocationic peptidomimetics **10–16**. i. HOBt (1.1 eq), EDCI.HCl (1.1 eq), Et_3N (1.0 eq), CH_2Cl_2, rt, 16 h. ii. $R^3C{\equiv}CH$, $CuSO_4.5H_2O$ (0.2 eq), Na.ascorbate (0.4 eq), *t*-BuOH:H_2O (4:1), rt, 16 h. iii. TFA/H_2O/DCM, rt, 16 h; then HCl in Et_2O.

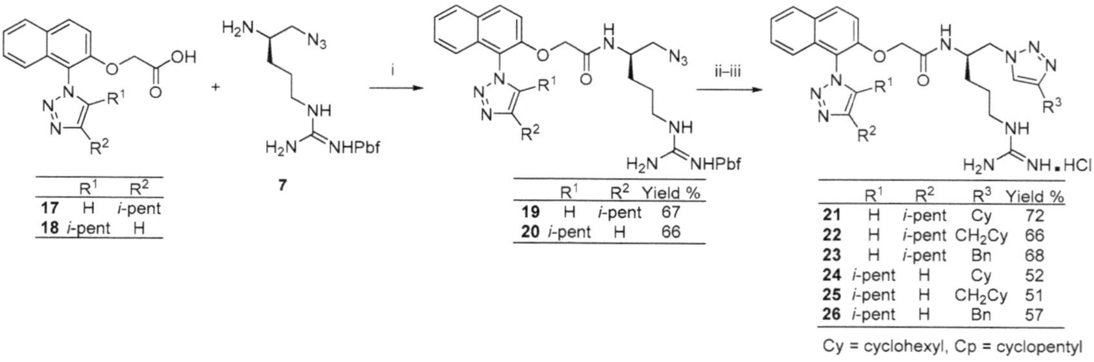

Scheme 2. Synthesis of *N*-naphthyltriazole monocationic peptidomimetics **21–26**. i. HOBt (1.1 eq), EDC.HCl (1.1 eq), Et_3N (1.0 eq), CH_2Cl_2, rt, 16 h. ii. $R^3C{\equiv}CH$, $CuSO_4.5H_2O$ (0.2 eq), Na.ascorbate (0.4 eq), *t*-BuOH:H_2O (4:1), rt, 16 h. iii. TFA/H_2O/DCM, rt, 16 h; then HCl in Et_2O.

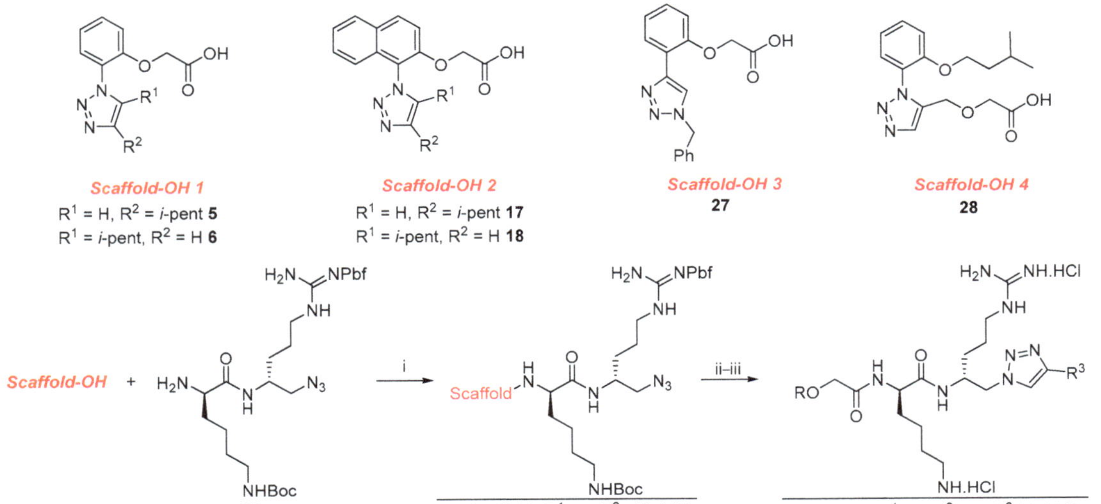

	Scaffold	R^1	R^2	Yield %
30	1	H	*i*-pent	78
31	1	*i*-pent	H	74
32	2	H	*i*-pent	67
33	2	*i*-pent	H	66
34	3	-	-	49
35	4	-	-	70

	Scaffold	R^1	R^2	R^3	Yield %
36	1	H	*i*-pent	Bn	56
37	1	*i*-pent	H	Cy	98
38	1	*i*-pent	H	CH_2Cy	64
39	1	*i*-pent	H	Bn	52
40	2	H	*i*-pent	Cy	46
41	2	H	*i*-pent	CH_2Cy	52
42	2	H	*i*-pent	Bn	52
43	2	*i*-pent	H	Cy	55
44	2	*i*-pent	H	CH_2Cy	54
45	2	*i*-pent	H	Bn	53
46	3	-	-	Bn	55
47	3	-	-	Bn	57
48	4	-	-	Cy	61
49	4	-	-	CH_2Cy	83
50	4	-	-	Bn	51

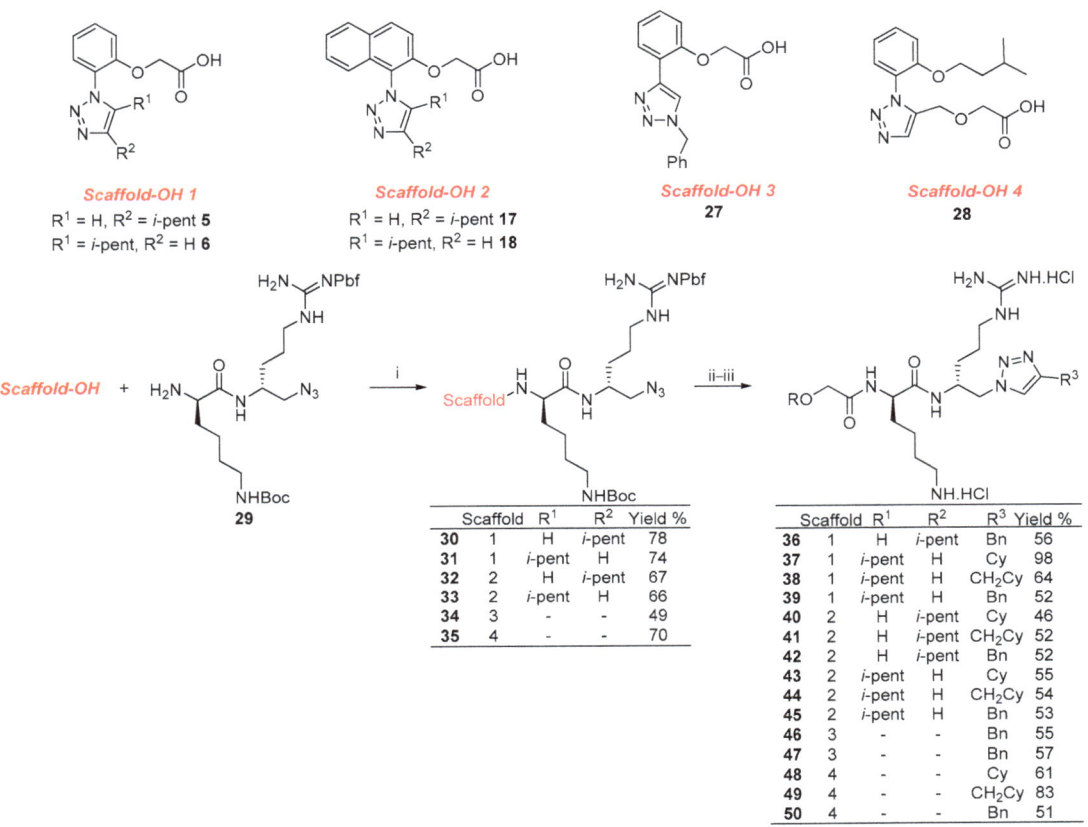

Scheme 3. Synthesis of dicationic peptidomimetics **36–50**-i. HOBt (1.1 eq), EDC.HCl (1.1 eq), Et_3N (1.0 eq), CH_2Cl_2, rt, 16 h. ii. R′C≡CH, $CuSO_4.5H_2O$ (0.2 eq), Na.ascorbate (0.4 eq), *t*-BuOH:H_2O (4:1), rt, 16 h. iii. TFA/H_2O/DCM, rt, 16 h; then HCl in Et_2O.

The *N*-arytriazole and *N*-naphthyltriazole peptidomimetics were subjected to antimicrobial screening. In the first instance, minimum inhibitory concentrations (MICs) were determined against a panel of Gram-positive (including two strains of *C. difficile*) and Gram-negative pathogenic bacteria with vancomycin and the commercially available peptide colistin as positive controls, respectively; the MICs are displayed in Table 1. The compounds were then tested against a second panel of Gram-positive and Gram-negative pathogenic bacteria and two fungi strains at the Community for Open Antimicrobial Drug Discovery (CO-ADD)-these results are reported in the Supporting Information (Table S1) [29]. A cytotoxicity concentration (CC_{50}) assay was also performed by CO-ADD; the synthesized compounds were tested at concentrations ≤32 μg/mL on human embryonic kidney cells (HEK293 cells; ATCC CRL-1573) while hemolysis assays for lysis of human erythrocytes were also performed. Vancomycin, colistin, fluconazole, and tamoxifen were used as positive controls (see Table 1 for details). The CC_{50} and HC_{50} values are also shown in Table 1.

Table 1. Preliminary antibacterial screening [a].

	Compound	*C. difficile* ATCC 700057	*C. difficile* 132 [b] (RT027)	*S. aureus* ATCC 29213	*S. aureus* NCTC 10442 [c]	*E. faecalis* ATCC 29212	*S. pneumoniae* ATCC 49619	*E. coli* ATCC 25922	CC_{50} [d]	HC_{50} [e]
1	**10**	32	64	32	32	32	16	128	>32	>32
2	**11**	32	64	32	32	32	16	128	>32	>32
3	**12**	32	64	32	32	32	16	128	>32	>32
4	**13**	32	64	32	32	32	16	128	>32	>32
5	**14**	128	128	32	32	32	32	>128	>32	>32
6	**15**	64	64	16	16	16	16	128	>32	>32
7	**16**	32	32	32	32	32	32	>128	>32	>32
8	**21**	128	>128	8	8	16	16	128	>32	>32
8	**22**	32	32	4	4	8	8	32	>32	>32
9	**23**	32	32	4	4	4	4	64	>32	>32
10	**24**	32	32	8	8	8	8	32	21.9	>32
11	**25**	32	64	4	4	8	8	16	>32	10.6
12	**26**	64	>128	8	8	16	4	64	23.5	>32
13	**36**	128	128	32	32	64	16	128	>32	>32
14	**37**	64	64	16	32	16	8	64	>32	>32
15	**38**	128	>128	128	128	>128	128	>128	32	32
16	**39**	64	32	32	64	32	16	128	>32	>32
17	**40**	8	8	16	16	32	16	64	32	32
18	**41**	16	16	8	8	8	16	128	16	32
19	**42**	8	8	8	8	8	8	32	32	32
20	**43**	128	128	16	16	64	4	64	>32	>32
21	**44**	32	32	8	4	16	4	64	>32	>32
22	**45**	128	128	16	16	64	4	128	>32	>32
23	**46**	128	128	32	32	64	16	128	>32	>32
24	**47**	128	128	32	32	64	16	128	>32	>32
25	**48**	>32	>32	>32	>32	>32	>32	>32	>32	24.5
26	**49**	>32	>32	32	>32	>32	>32	>32	>32	17.1
27	**50**	>32	>32	32	>32	>32	>32	>32	>32	19.8
	vanc	0.5	0.5	1	1	4	1	>16	-	-
	colistin				0.25	0.25	0.25	0.125		
	tamoxifen								13.1	

[a] Values are reported as MIC values in μg/mL. [b] *C. difficile* PCR Ribotype (RT027). [c] Methicillin resistant *S. aureus* (MRSA). [d] Cytotoxicity; determined on HEK293 cells. [e] Hemolysis; HC50 values determined by lysis of human erythrocytes and % hemolysis was determined by lysis of sheep erythrocytes. Vanc = vancomycin. Coloured cells refer to the same activities.

Preliminary screening revealed that compared to the previously synthesized compounds **1–4**, the new *N*-naphthyltriazole dicationic derivatives **40** and **42** showed the best activities against the two *C. difficile* RT 027 strains, ATCC 700,057 and 132 with a similar activity of 8 μg/mL compared to compounds **1**, **3**, and **4**. However, they were generally less active against the other Gram-positive and Gram-negative bacteria (Table 1). The relative solubility ratios (relative to compound **1**) [13] for **40** and **42** were 5 and 4 with CLogP values of 4.46 and 4.39, respectively, when compared to **1** with a ClogP of 7.47. Therefore, despite the better solubility profiles of these compounds, they failed to show better activity against *C. difficile*. However, the increased solubility (enhanced polarity) of derivatives **40–42** could be a factor in the reduced activities against the other bacteria, when compared to compounds **1–4** (see Table 2). None of the other derivatives synthesized in this study showed appreciable activity against *C. difficile* with MIC values ranging from 32 to 128 μg/mL (Table 1). Importantly, the remaining anti-bacterial results were generally poor, however for these specific derivatives, these reduced activities could indicate reduced capacity to interfere with normal GIT microbiota (Table 2). Compounds **40** and **42** showed a slight reduction in cytotoxicity against HEK293 cells compared to compounds **2** and **4**. The hemolytic activity of these compounds was 32 μg/mL against human erythrocytes, 2-fold more than their IC_{50} values against *C. difficile*.

Table 2. Antimicrobial, cytotoxicity, and hemolytic activities of the three most active derivatives synthesized in this study [a].

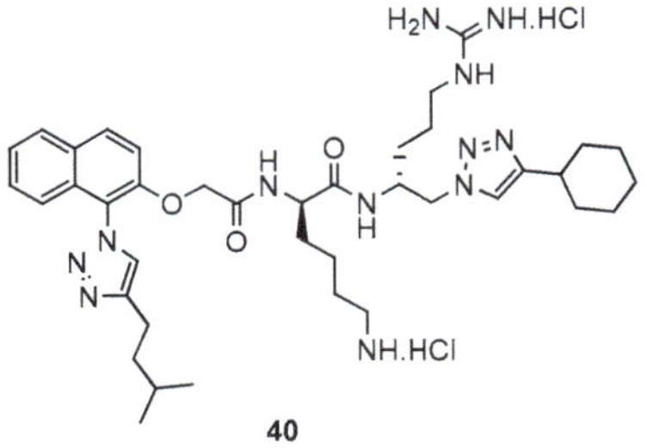

40

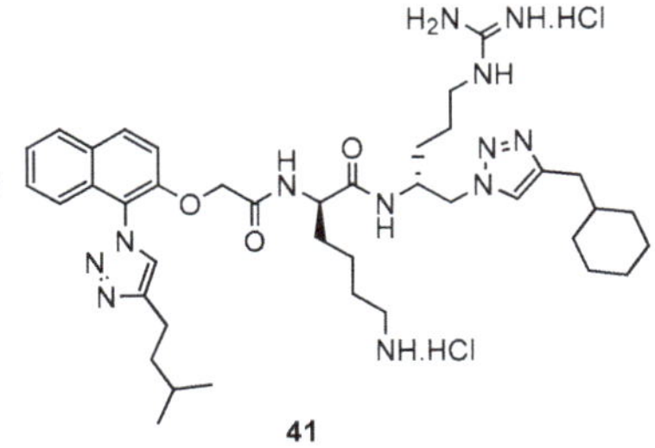

41

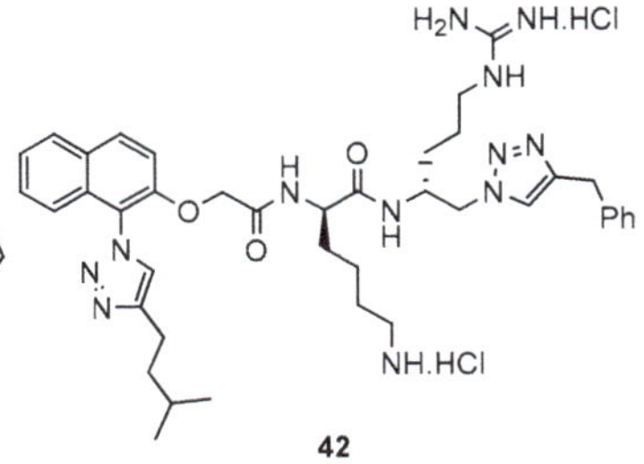

42

Compound	*C. difficile* ATCC 700057	*C. difficile* 132 [b] (RT027)	*S. aureus* ATCC 29213	*S. aureus* ATCC 43300 [c]	*S. aureus* NCTC 104422 [c,d]	*E. faecalis* ATCC 29212	*S. pneumoniae* ATCC 49619	*E. coli* ATCC 25922	CC_{50} [e]	HC_{50} [f]
40	8	8	16	8	16	32	16	64	32	32
41	16	16	8	4	8	8	16	128	16	32
42	8	8	8	8	8	8	8	32	32	32
1 [30]	8 [g]	8 [h]	2	-	-	2	2	16	-	-
2 [31]	-	32	4	2	4	4	4	8	27.4	94% [i]
3 [19]	8 [g]	8 [h]	2	-	2	4	8	>128	-	-
4 [31]	-	8	8	4	4	8	4	8	14.2	23% [i]
vanc	0.5	0.5	1	-	1	4	1	>16	-	-

[a] Values are reported as MIC values in μg/mL. [b] *C. difficile* PCR Ribotype (RT027). [c] Methicillin resistant *S. aureus* (MRSA). [d] Testing performed by the Community for Open Antimicrobial Drug Discovery (CO-ADD). [e] Cytotoxicity; determined on HEK293 cells. [f] Hemolysis; determined by lysis of sheep erythrocytes [g] *C. difficile strain* tested M7404 (RT027). [h] *C. difficile strain* tested R20291 (RT207). [i] % hemolysis at 50 μg/mL. vanc = vancomycin. Coloured cells refer to the same activities.

Analysis of the anti-bacterial activities against other bacterial species indicated that the monocationic naphthyltriazole derivatives **21–26** showed appreciable activity against *Staphylococcus aureus* (including an MRSA strain) with MIC values between 4 and 8 μg/mL (Table 1). Additionally, compound **21** had notable MIC values of 4 μg/mL against *Enterococcus faecalis* and *Streptococcus pneumoniae*. An overview of activity shown in Table 1 showed "pockets" of activities focused on the naphthyl-based derivatives (**21–26** and **40–45**, columns 1–4), with the monocationic examples (**21–26**) producing better outcomes against the Gram positive strains. The second screening results (Table S1, Supporting Information) were consistent with these results with analogous trends in activity against an additional *S. aureus* strain.

The secondary testing (Table S1, Supporting Information) also identified compounds **21**, **25**, and **40–46** as having activity against the fungal strain *Cryptococcus neoformans* var. *grubii* (ATCC208821) (MIC 4-8 μg/mL).

3. In Vivo Assay: Murine Model of CDI

Compound **40** was selected for further evaluation as an effective treatment for *C. difficile* using a murine model of CDI study because of its sustained antimicrobial potency against *C. difficile* and its better water solubility profile. The results from these studies are summarized in Figure 3.

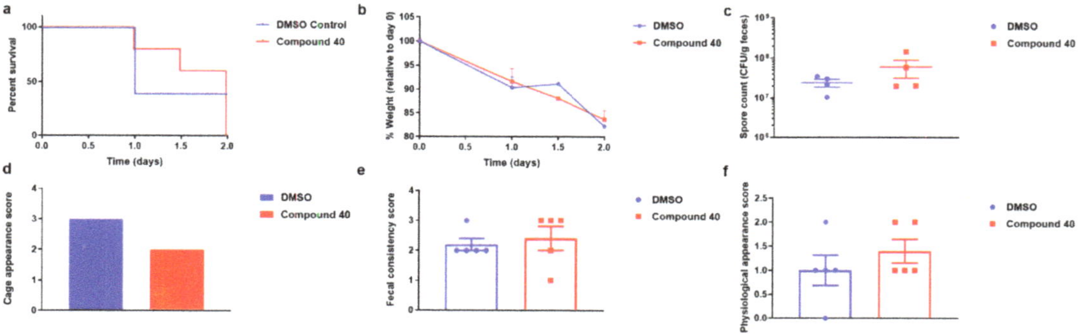

Figure 3. C57BL/6J mice (n = 5 per group) were infected with 10^5 spores of *C. difficile* strain M7404 (RT027). Six hours post-infection and then every 12 h thereafter, mice were administered either 10% DMSO (blue) or 2.5 mg (100 mg/kg in 10% DMSO) of compound **40** (red) by oral gavage. Mice were monitored daily for survival (**a**) and weight loss relative to day 0, which was the day of infection (**b**). Fecal spore load at 1-day post-infection was determined by plating (**c**). Data are presented as CFU/gram feces, with each point representing a single mouse. Mouse cages were scored on day 1 post-infection for appearance (**d**) and mice were individually assessed for fecal consistency (**e**) and physiological appearance (**f**). Data represent the mean ±S.E.M. and statistical significance was assessed using a log-rank (Mantel–Cox) test or one-way ANOVA with a post hoc Tukey's multiple comparison test.

The mice treated with compound **40** (red) showed delayed disease onset compared to mice treated with DMSO (blue; Figure 3), although they still succumbed to infection by day 2. Notably, at day 1 post-infection, mice treated with compound **40** showed 40% greater survival compared with mice treated with DMSO (Figure 3a), although there was no effect on mouse weight (Figure 3b), or spore numbers shed in the feces of these animals (Figure 3c), suggesting that compound **40** was not impacting *C. difficile* colonization. Furthermore, on day 1 post-infection, treatment with compound **40** resulted in a lower overall cage appearance score when compared to DMSO (Figure 3d), which suggested that this compound was delaying diarrheal onset although there was no significant difference in individual fecal score (Figure 3e) or physiological appearance score (Figure 3f) detected between the two groups of mice (Figure 3e). Thus, collectively these data suggest that compound **40** may reduce the severity of disease caused by *C. difficile*.

4. Materials and Methods

Synthetic methods and general characterization and analysis were as described previously [13].

Notes and other considerations. Known reagents that were not available commercially were prepared as reported using known methods and is detailed in the Supporting Information, [14,32–35].

4.1. General Synthesis Procedures

4.1.1. General Procedure I: Alkylation of Phenols (with Ethyl Bromoacetate)

A solution of the phenol (1 eq) in dry DMF (5 mL/mmol substrate) was stirred during the addition of K_2CO_3 (3 eq). Ethyl bromoacetate (1.3 eq) was added at room temperature and stirring was continued at rt for 12 h, before being diluted with EtOAc (2 × 50 mL). The resulting mixture was washed with water (2 × 50 mL), brine (2 × 50 mL), dried ($MgSO_4$), filtered, and concentrated under vacuum. The residue was subjected to silica gel flash column chromatography to afford the desired ester product.

4.1.2. General Procedure II: Ester Hydrolysis

A solution of the ester (1 eq) in ethanol (10 mL/mmol substrate) was stirred followed by the addition of 7% KOH solution (5 mL/mmol) at rt. The mixture was stirred at rt for

2 h, then acidified with 1 M HCl (25 mL). The resulting mixture was extracted with EtOAc (2 × 25 mL) and the combined extracts washed with brine (50 mL), dried ($MgSO_4$), filtered, and concentrated under vacuum to afford the acid product.

4.1.3. General Procedure III: Amide Coupling

A mixture of the amine (1.0 eq), carboxylic acid (1.0 eq), EDC.HCl (1.2 eq), HOBt (1.1 eq), and TEA (1 eq) in dichloromethane/acetonitrile solution (10 mL/mmol amine) was stirred at rt for the specified time. The mixture was concentrated (if >5.0 mL dichloromethane/acetonitrile), and then the resulting residue dissolved in EtOAc (25 mL for reactions that contained ≤1.0 mmol amine or 25 mL/mmol amine for larger scale reactions) and washed with aqueous HCl (1.0 M–2 × 25 mL), saturated aqueous $NaHCO_3$ (3 × 25 mL), and brine (1 × 25 mL). The organic solution was dried ($MgSO_4$), filtered, concentrated and subjected to further purification via flash chromatography (if required) to furnish the targeted amide product.

4.1.4. General Procedure IV: Copper-Catalyzed Azide-Alkyne Cycloaddition

To a stirred solution of the azide (1.0 eq) and alkyne (2.0–3.0 eq) in *tert*-butanol/water (4:1) at rt was added $CuSO_4{\cdot}5H_2O$ (0.2 eq), followed by sodium ascorbate (0.4 eq). The reaction was stirred at rt (unless noted otherwise) for the specified time. To the mixture was added aqueous saturated NH_4Cl solution (1 mL), and water (20 mL) with the mixture then extracted with EtOAc (20 mL for reactions that contained ≤1.0 mmol azide or 20 mL/mmol azide for larger scale reactions). The organic layers were back-washed with water (2 × 25 mL), brine (2 × 25 mL), then dried ($MgSO_4$), filtered, concentrated under vacuum and subjected to flash chromatography to afford the desired 1,4-disubstituted 1,2,3-triazole product.

4.1.5. General Procedure VII: Amine Deprotection (*N*-Boc and/or *N*-Pbf Removal)

To a solution of the *N*-protected amine (1.0 eq) in CH_2Cl_2 (30 mL/mmol substrate) (if the substrate contained an *N*-Pbf moiety, H_2O (20.0 eq) was added to the solution) was added TFA (30.0 mL/mmol substrate) and then stirred at rt overnight (>16 h). The solvent was removed and the resulting residue dissolved in CH_2Cl_2 (30 mL/mmol substrate). Excess anhydrous HCl (2.0 M in Et_2O, 15 mL/mmol substrate, 30.0 eq) was added and the solvent was then removed. The residue was then dissolved in a minimal volume of CH_2Cl_2 (or MeOH) and excess Et_2O (25 mL for ≤0.1 mmol substrate) was added, resulting in a precipitate of the hydrochloride salt of the amine. The reaction mixture was filtered; the resulting filtrate collected, concentrated, triturated with Et_2O (3 × 20 mL); and the solids then dissolved in MeOH. The solution was concentrated and dried in vacuo to yield the mono or di-hydrochloride salt as a thin, translucent film that usually required scratching with a spatula, producing a fine hygroscopic powder or amorphous gum.

4.2. Representative Synthesis of Compound ***40***

4.2.1. Ethyl 2-((1-iodonaphthalen-2-yl)oxy)acetate

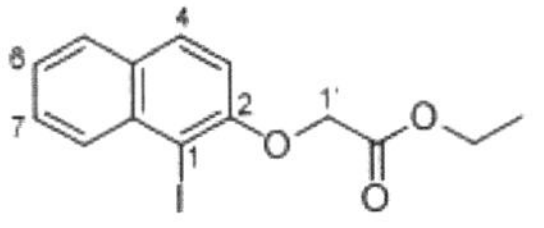

Following **General Procedure I**, 1-iodonaphthol (1.00 g, 3.70 mmol), K_2CO_3 (1.53 g, 11.11 mmol), and ethyl bromoacetate (0.80 g, 4.81 mmol) were stirred in DMF (8 mL) at rt for 16 h to give the titled ester (0.68 g, 52%) as a pale yellow waxy solid after flash chromatography over silica gel (EtOAc/*n*-hexane-10:90). TLC (EtOAc/*n*-hexane-20:80): R_f = 0.6; ^{1}H NMR (400 MHz, $CDCl_3$) δ 8.16 (d, *J* = 7.2 Hz, 1H, H8), 7.78 (d, *J* = 7.2 Hz, 1H, H5), 7.72 (d, *J* = 8.0 Hz, 1H, H4), 7.54 (t, *J* = 7.2 Hz, 1H, H7), 7.39 (t, *J* = 7.2 Hz, 1H, H6), 7.08 (d, *J* = 8.0 Hz, 1H, H3), 4.80 (s, 2H, H1′), 4.27 (q, *J* = 5.6 Hz, 2H, OCH_2CH_3),

1.29 (t, *J* = 5.6 Hz, 3H, OCH_2CH_3); ^{13}C NMR (101 MHz, $CDCl_3$) δ 168.7 (C = O), 155.6 (C2), 135.8 (C8a), 131.7 (C4a), 130.6 (C4), 130.5 (C8), 128.4 (C7), 128.3 (C5), 121.1 (C6), 114.4 (C3), 89.47 (C1), 67.6 (C1′), 61.7 (OCH_2CH_3) 14.3 (OCH_2CH_3); IR (neat) $\overline{\nu}_{max}$ 2981, 1756, 1622, 1593, 1502, 1462, 1349, 1291, 1200, 1151, 1134, 1096, 1028, 801, 764, 747 cm^{-1}; MS (ESI +ve) *m*/*z* 379 ($[M + Na]^+$, 100%); HRMS (ESI + ve TOF) calcd for $C_{14}H_{13}O_3NaI$ 378.9807, found 378.9801 ($[M + Na]^+$).

4.2.2. Ethyl 2-((1-(4-isopentyl-1*H*-1,2,3-triazol-1-yl)naphthalen-2-yl)oxy)acetate

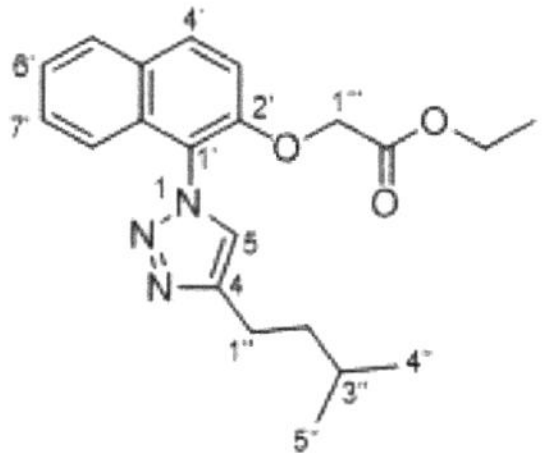

To a stirred solution of ethyl 2-(2-iodophenoxy)acetate (0.20 g, 0.54 mmol), 5-methyl-1-hexyne (0.16 g, 1.64 mmol), CuI (0.02 g, 0.11 mmol), NaN_3 (0.04 g, 0.60 mmol), and sodium ascorbate (0.04 g, 0.22 mmol) in DMSO (2.5 mL) in H_2O (0.5 mL) was added racemic *trans-N,N′*-dimethyl cyclohexane-1,2-diamine (0.016 g, 0.11 mmol) at rt under a nitrogen atmosphere. The reaction mixture was stirred and heated at 75 °C for 16 h. The reaction was cooled to rt and aqueous saturated NH_4Cl solution (3 mL) was added, and the mixture was extracted with EtOAc (2 × 25 mL). The combined extracts were washed with water (25 mL), brine (25 mL) and dried ($MgSO_4$). The solution was filtered, concentrated under vacuum and the residue was subjected to silica gel flash column chromatography (EtOAc/*n*-hexane-10:90 → 100:0) to afford the titled compound (0.05 g, 25%) as a yellow waxy solid. TLC (EtOAc/*n*-hexane-33:67); R_f = 0.4; ^{1}H NMR (400 MHz, $CDCl_3$) δ 7.97 (d, *J* = 7.2 Hz, 1H, H8′), 7.84 (d, *J* = 6.4 Hz, 1H, H5′), 7.67 (s, 1H, H5), 7.49–7.41 (m, 2H, H6′/H7′), 7.27–7.25 (m, 2H, H3′/H4′), 4.67 (s, 2H, H1‴), 4.22 (q, *J* = 5.6 Hz, 2H, OCH_2CH_3), 2.89 (t, *J* = 5.6 Hz, 2H, H1″), 1.73–1.67 (m, 3H, H2″/H3″), 1.26 (t, *J* = 5.6 Hz, 3H, OCH_2OCH_3), 0.99 (d, *J* = 4.0 Hz, 6H, H4″/H5″); ^{13}C NMR (101 MHz, $CDCl_3$) δ 168.5 (C = O), 150.5 (C2′), 148.1 (C8a′), 131.6 (C4), 131.3 (C4a′), 129.5 (C4′), 128.5 (C5′), 127.9 (C7′), 125.3 (C8′), 124.7 (C6′), 122.1 (C5), 121.3 (C3′), 114.3 (C1′), 66.7 (C1‴), 61.6 (OCH_2CH_3), 38.6 (C2″), 27.9 (C1″), 23.8 (C3″), 22.5 (C4″/C5″; Observed by gHMBC), 14.2 (OCH_2CH_3); IR (neat) $\overline{\nu}_{max}$ 2954, 2928, 2868, 1748, 1632, 1600, 1513, 1483, 1454, 1430, 1366, 1288, 1206, 1150, 1117, 1087, 1042, 806, 749 cm^{-1}; MS (ESI +ve) *m*/*z* 390 ($[M +Na]^+$, 100%); HRMS (ESI +ve TOF) calcd for $C_{21}H_{26}N_3O_3$ 368.1974, found 368.1985 ($[M + H]^+$).

4.2.3. 2-((1-(4-Isopentyl-1*H*-1,2,3-triazol-1-yl)naphthalen-2-yl)oxy)acetic acid (**17**)

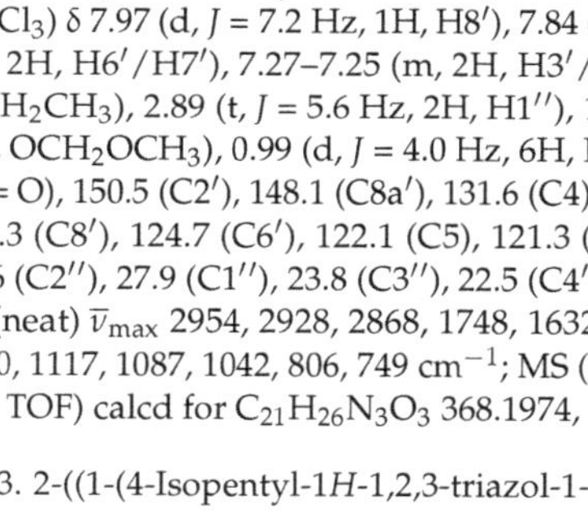

Following **General Procedure II**, ethyl 2-((1-(4-isopentyl-1*H*-1,2,3-triazol-1-yl)naphthalen-2-yl)oxy)acetate (0.07 g, 0.19 mmol) and 7% KOH solution (0.5 mL) were stirred in

ethanol (2 mL) at rt for 2 h to give after acidification the acid **17** (0.04 g, 62%) as a white solid. M.P: 152–154 °C. TLC (EtOAc/*n*-hexane-100:0): R_f = 0.2; ^{1}H NMR (500 MHz, $CDCl_3$) δ 8.00 (d, *J* = 9.0 Hz, 1H, H8′), 7.88 (d, *J* = 7.5 Hz, 1H, H5′), 7.69 (s, 1H, H5), 7.54–7.46 (m, 2H, H6′/H7′), 7.47–7.29 (m, 2H, H3′/H4′), 4.78 (s, 2H, H1‴), 2.91–2.87 (m, 2H, H1″), 1.71–1.68 (m, 3H, H2″/H3″), 0.98 (d, *J* = 6.0 Hz, 6H, H4″/H5″), COOH resonance was not observed; ^{13}C NMR (126 MHz, $CDCl_3$) δ 170.6 (C = O), 150.4 (C2′), 148.4 (C8a′), 132.2 (C4), 130.7 (C4a′), 129.6 (C4′), 128.8 (C5′), 128.2 (C7′), 125.6 (C8′), 124.9 (C6′), 121.7 (C5), 120.9 (C3′), 114.4 (C1′), 66.8 (C1‴), 38.5 (C2″), 28.0 (C1″), 23.7 (C3″), 22.6 (C4″/C5″; Observed by gHMBC); IR (neat) $\overline{\nu}_{max}$ 3147, 2954, 2929, 2868, 1731, 1631, 1600, 1514, 1483, 1429, 1366, 1284, 1213, 1151, 1118, 1087, 1062, 923, 806, 748 cm^{-1}; MS (ESI +ve) *m*/*z* 362 ([M + Na]$^+$, 40%), 340 ([M + H]$^+$, 100%); HRMS (ESI + ve TOF) calcd for $C_{19}H_{22}N_3O_3$ 340.1661, found 340.1667 ([M + H]$^+$).

4.2.4. (9*H*-Fluoren-9-yl)methyl *tert*-butyl ((*R*)-6-(((*R*)-1-azido-5-(2-((2,2-dimethyl-2,3-dihydro benzofuran-5-yl)sulfonyl)guanidino)pentan-2-yl)amino)-6-oxohexane-1,5-diyl) dicarbamate

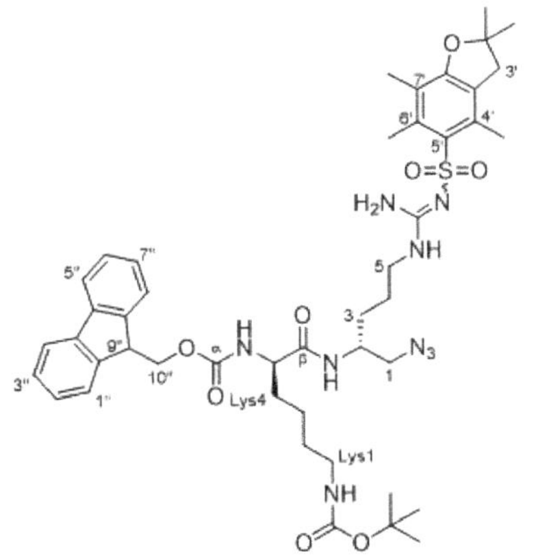

To a reaction vessel charged with azide **7** [30] (1.38 g, 3.16 mmol), Fmoc-L-Lys(Boc)-OH (1.62 g, 3.50 mmol), EDCI (0.67 g, 3.50 mmol) and HOBt (0.53 g, 3.50 mmol) was added CH_2Cl_2 (10 mL) and the mixture was stirred at rt for 12 h. The reaction mixture was concentrated and diluted with water (100 mL) and extracted with EtOAc (3 × 100 mL). The organic extracts were combined and washed with HCl (1 M–100 mL), aqueous $NaHCO_3$ (100 mL), brine (25 mL), dried ($MgSO_4$) and concentrated to give a pale-yellow residue. This residue was purified via flash chromatography over SiO_2 (MeOH/CH_2Cl_2 = 4:96) to afford the titled compound as an off-white foam (1.50 g, 54%). TLC (MeOH/CH_2Cl_2–10:90) R_f = 0.52; ^{1}H-NMR (400 MHz, $CDCl_3$) δ 7.77–7.70 (m, 2H, H4″/H5″), 7.55 (d, *J* = 7.5 Hz, 2H, H1″/H8″), 7.55 (brs, 1H, βCONH), 7.41–7.32 (m, 2H, H2″/H7″), 7.29–7.21 (m, 2H, H3″/H6″), 7.17 (brs, 1H, αCONH), 6.31–6.24 (m, 2H, NH_2 (guanidine)), 6.19–6.09 (brs, 1H, N^5-H), 4.82–4.72 (brs, 1H, LysN^1-H), 4.33 (d, *J* = 7.4 Hz, 2H, H10″), 4.25–4.07 (m, 2H, Lys5/H9″), 4.07–3.97 (m, 1H, H2), 3.41–3.23 (m, 2H, H1), 3.23–2.98 (m, 4H, H5/Lys1), 2.89 (s, 2H, H3′), 2.55 (s, 3H, C6′-CH_3), 2.48 (s, 3H, C4′-CH_3), 2.06 (s, 3H, C7′-CH_3), 1.67 (s, 6H, C2′-CH_3), 1.55–1.35 (m, 19H, H3/H4/Lys2/Lys3/Lys4/C(CH_3)$_3$); ^{13}C NMR (101 MHz, $CDCl_3$) δ 172.7 (Cβ), 158.8 (C7a′), 156.7 (Cα), 156.4 (C = N), 156.2 (COOC(CH_3)$_3$), 143.85 (C1a″or C8a″), 143.83 (C8a″ or C1a″), 143.82 (C4a″ or C5a″), 143.6 (C5a″ or C4a″), 138.3 (C3a′), 132.8 (C6′), 132.2 (C4′), 127.8 (C3″/C6″), 127.1 (C4″/C5″), 125.0 (C2″/C7″), 124.7 (C5′), 120.0 (C1″/C8″), 117.6 (C7′), 86.4 (C2′), 79.3 (C(CH_3)$_3$), 67.3 (C10″), 55.1 (Lys5), 54.8 (C1), 48.8 (C2), 47.0 (C9″), 43.2 (C3′), 40.9 (C5), 39.9 (Lys1), 31.9 (Lys2), 29.5 (Lys4), 29.3 (C3), 28.6 (C2′-(CH_3)$_2$), 28.4 (C(CH_3)$_3$), 25.5 (C4), 22.5 (Lys3), 19.3 (C6′-CH_3), 17.9

($C4'$-CH_3), 12.5 $C7'$-CH_3); IR (neat) $\overline{\nu}_{max}$ 3322, 2101, 1634, 1548, 1450, 1248, 1165, 1092, 739, 567 cm^{-1}; MS (ESI +ve) m/z 888 ([M + H]$^+$), 910 ([M + Na]$^+$); HRMS (ESI +ve TOF) calcd for $C_{45}H_{61}N_9O_8SNa$ 910.4262, found 910.4218 ([M + Na]$^+$).

4.2.5. *Tert*-butyl ((*R*)-5-amino-6-(((*R*)-1-azido-5-(2-((2,2-dimethyl-2,3-dihydrobenzofuran-5-yl)sulfonyl)guanidino)pentan-2-yl)amino)-6-oxohexyl)carbamate (**31**)

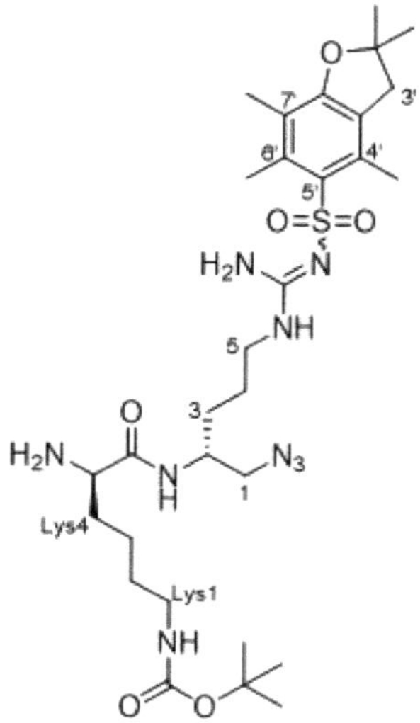

To a solution of the above Fmoc-protected amine (1.50 g, 1.69 mmol) in acetonitrile (15 mL) was added piperidine (0.25 mL, 1.5 eq.) and the reaction was stirred vigorously at rt for 12 h. The reaction mixture was diluted with MeOH (50 mL) and extracted with hexane (50 mL) multiple times until TLC analysis showed no byproduct (dibenzofulvene piperidine adduct) present in the MeOH layer. The MeOH extract was concentrated under reduced pressure to give **31** as an off-white foam (0.80 g, 71%). TLC (MeOH/CH_2Cl_2–10:90) R_f = 0.2; ^{1}H-NMR (500 MHz, $CDCl_3$) δ 7.61 (brs, 1H, N^2-H), 6.42–6.20 (m, 3H, N^5-H/NH_2 (guanidine)), 4.82–4.72 (m, 1H, LysN^1-H), 4.12–3.99 (m, 1H, Lys5), 3.46–3.29 (m, 3H, H1/H2), 3.29–3.14 (m, 2H, H5), 3.14–3.04 (m, 2H, Lys1), 2.96 (s, 2H, C3′), 2.58 (s, 3H, $C6'$-CH_3), 2.52 (s, 3H, $C4'$-CH_3), 2.10 (s, 3H, $C7'$-CH_3), 1.62–1.31 (m, 25H, H3/H4/Lys2/Lys3/Lys4/$C(CH_3)_3$/$C2'$-$(CH_3)_2$), N^5H_2 resonance was not observed; ^{13}C-NMR (126 MHz, $CDCl_3$) δ 158.8 (C7a′), 156.6 (C = O), 156.4 (C = N), 138.5 (C3a′), 133.2 (C4′), 132.4 (C6′), 124.7 (C5′), 117.6 (C7′), 86.5 (C2′), 79.4 (($C(CH_3)_3$), 55.1 (Lys5), 55.0 (C1), 46.9 (C2), 43.4 (C3′), 40.9 (C5), 40.4 (Lys1), 34.7 (Lys4), 30.1 (Lys2), 29.8 (C3), 28.8 ($C2'$-$(CH_3)_2$), 28.6 ($C(CH_3)_3$), 25.8 (C4), 22.7 (Lys3), 19.4 ($C6'$-CH_3), 18.1 ($C4'$-CH_3), 12.6 ($C7'$-CH_3), $COO(C(CH_3)_3)$ resonance was not observed; IR (neat) $\overline{\nu}_{max}$ 3327, 2101, 1685, 1620, 1551, 1454, 1366, 1278, 1250, 1168, 1094, 665, 569 cm^{-1}; MS (ESI +ve) m/z 666 ([M + H]$^+$); HRMS (ESI +ve TOF) calcd for $C_{30}H_{52}N_9O_6S$ 666.3761, found 666.3741 ([M + H]$^+$).

4.2.6. *Tert*-butyl ((*R*)-6-(((*R*)-1-azido-5-(2-((2,2,4,6,7-pentamethyl-2,3-dihydrobenzofuran-5-yl)sulfonyl)guanidino)pentan-2-yl)amino)-5-(2-((1-(4-isopentyl-1*H*-1,2,3-triazol-1-yl)naphthalen-2-yl)oxy)acetamido)-6-oxohexyl)carbamate (**32**)

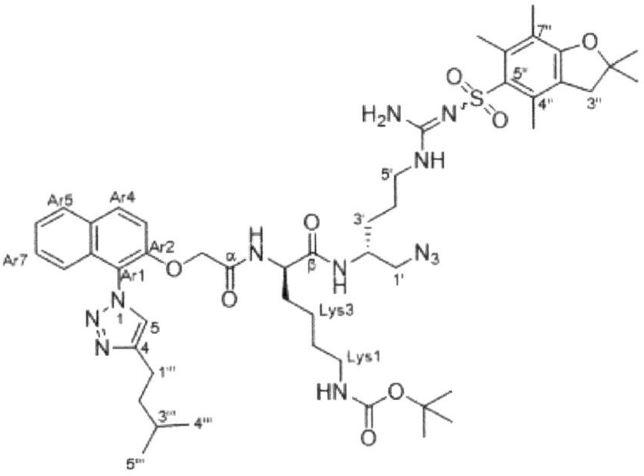

Following **General Procedure III**, 2-((1-(4-isopentyl-1*H*-1,2,3-triazol-1-yl)naphthalen-2-yl)oxy)acetic acid **17** (0.12 g, 0.35 mmol), *tert*-butyl ((*R*)-5-amino-6-(((*R*)-1-azido-5-(2-((2,2-dimethyl-2,3-dihydrobenzofuran-5-yl)sulfonyl)guanidino)pentan-2-yl)amino)-6-oxohexyl) carbamate **57** (0.24 g, 0.35 mmol), EDCI.HCl (0.08 g, 0.39 mmol), HOBt (0.06 g, 0.39 mmol), and TEA (0.03 g, 0.35 mmol) were stirred in CH_2Cl_2 (5 mL) at rt for 12 h to give the acetamide **65** (0.22 g, 64%) as an off-white solid. M.P: 236–238 °C. TLC ($MeOH/CH_2Cl_2$-10:90): $R_f = 0.5$; ^1H NMR (400 MHz, $CDCl_3$) δ 8.05 (d, J = 8.5 Hz, 1H, Ar8), 7.89 (d, J = 8.5 Hz, 1H, Ar5), 7.65 (s, 1H, H5), 7.54–7.47 (m, 2H, Ar4/βCONH), 7.37 (d, J = 8.5 Hz, 1H, Ar7), 7.26–7.19 (m, 2H, Ar6/Ar3), 6.85 (brs, 1H, αCONH), 6.36–6.08 (m, 3H, $N^{5'}$-H/NH_2 (guanidine)), 5.00 (brs, 1H, LysN^1-H), 4.69 (ABq, J = 16.5 Hz, 2H, OCH_AH_B), 4.42–4.36 (m, 1H, Lys5), 4.02–3.96 (m, 1H, H2′), 3.44–2.94 (m, 6H, H1′/H5′/Lys1), 2.88 (s, 2H, H3″), 2.88–2.84 (m, 2H, H1‴), 2.55 (s, 3H, C4″-CH_3), 2.48 (s, 3H, C6″-CH_3), 2.06 (s, 3H, C7″-CH_3), 2.00–1.86 (m, 4H, H4′/Lys4), 1.84–1.60 (m, 7H, H3′/Lys3/H2‴/H3‴), 1.44 (s, 6H, C2″(CH_3)$_2$), 1.39 (s, 9H, C(CH_3)$_3$), 1.32–1.22 (m, 2H, Lys2), 0.9 (d, J = 5.0 Hz, 6H, H4‴/H5‴); ^{13}C NMR (101 MHz, $CDCl_3$) δ 171.9 (βC = O), 168.1 (αC = O), 158.7 (C7a″), 156.4 (C = N), 150.1 (Ar2), 149.1 (COOC(CH_3)$_3$), 138.4 (Ar8a), 133.4 (C4), 132.6 (C4″), 132.46 (C6″), 132.44 (C3a″), 130.6 (C5″), 129.4 (Ar4), 129.1 (Ar4a), 128.48 (C7″), 128.47 (Ar5), 125.7 (Ar7), 124.7 (Ar8), 121.1 (C5), 120.3 (Ar6), 117.5 (Ar3), 113.8 (Ar1), 86.5 (C2″), 79.2 (C(CH_3)$_3$), 68.0 (OCH_AH_B), 54.8 (Lys5), 53.6 (C1′), 43.4 (C2′), 40.8 (C2‴), 40.2 (C5′), 38.6 (C3″), 38.5 (Lys1), 31.79 (Lys4), 31.74 (C3′), 29.4 (Lys2), 28.7 (C2″-(CH_3)$_2$), 28.6 ((CH_3)$_3$), 28.0 (C1‴), 25.5 (C4′), 23.8 (C3‴), 22.8 (C4‴/C5‴), 22.6 (Lys3), 19.4 (C4″-CH_3), 18.1 (C6″-CH_3), 12.6 (C7″-CH_3); IR (neat) $\overline{\nu}_{max}$ 3405, 3317, 3415, 3057, 2953, 2868, 2100, 1664, 1631, 1600, 1546, 1514, 1484, 1452, 1406, 1390, 1366, 1265, 1247, 1165, 1106, 1090, 1044, 994, 970, 852, 781, 733, 661, 641 cm^{-1}; MS (ESI +ve) m/z 987 ([M + H]$^+$, 100%); HRMS (ESI +ve TOF) calcd for $C_{49}H_{71}N_{12}O_8S$ 987.5239, found 987.5272 ([M + H]$^+$).

4.2.7. (*R*)-6-Amino-*N*-((*R*)-1-(4-cyclohexyl-1*H*-1,2,3-triazol-1-yl)-5-guanidinopentan-2-yl)-2-(2-((1-(4-isopentyl-1*H*-1,2,3-triazol-1-yl)naphthalen-2-yl)oxy)acetamido)hexanamide dihydrochloride (**40**)

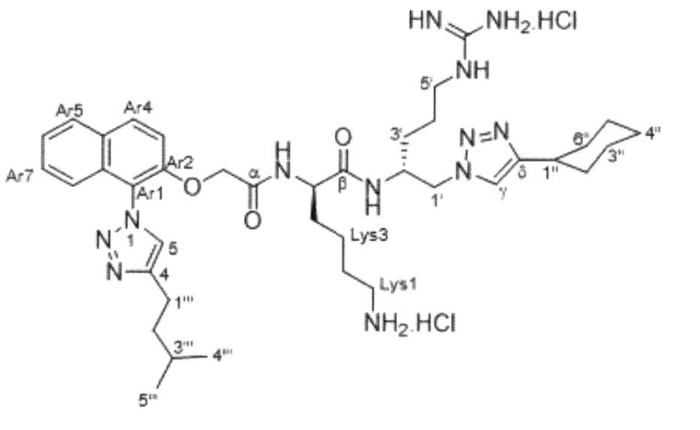

Following **General Procedure IV**, azide **32** (0.08 g, 0.08mmol), cyclohexylacetylene (0.03 g, 0.24 mmol), $CuSO_4{\cdot}5H_2O$ (0.004 g, 0.01 mmol) and sodium ascorbate (0.006 g, 0.03 mmol) were stirred in *t*-BuOH (2.0 mL) and H_2O (0.5 mL) for 16 h to give the triazole product as an off-white gum after flash chromatography over SiO_2 gel ($MeOH/CH_2Cl_2$–0:100 → 8:92). Following **General Procedure VII**, the intermediate (0.06 g, 0.05 mmol) was dissolved in CH_2Cl_2 (2 mL), treated with H_2O (0.02 g, 1.00 mmol) and CF_3COOH (1 mL) followed by work-up with ethereal HCl (3 mL) to give the amine salt **40** (0.03 g, 46% over two steps) as an off-white solid that rapidly transitioned to a sticky gum. $[\alpha]_D^{23}$ + 59.1 (*c* 0.0052, MeOH); ^{1}H NMR (400 MHz, CD_3OD) δ 8.30 (s, 1H, H5), 8.29 (s, 1H, Hγ), 8.18 (d, *J* = 9.2 Hz, 1H, Ar8), 7.98 (d, *J* = 7.5 Hz, 1H, Ar5), 7.61 (ddd, *J* = 9.2, 9.2, 1.7 Hz, 1H, Ar7), 7.57–7.49 (m, 2H, Ar6/Ar4), 7.14 (d, *J* = 8.3 Hz, 1H, Ar3), 4.93–4.89 (m, 2H, OCH_AH_B), 4.77–4.72 (m, 1H, H1′), 4.59–4.53 (m, 1H, H1′), 4.37–4.32 (m, 1H, Lys5), 4.12–4.09 (m, 1H, H2′), 3.18–3.14 (m, 2H, H5′), 2.95–2.91 (m, 2H, Lys1), 2.84–2.78 (m, 3H, H1‴/H1″), 2.00–1.96 (m, 2H, Lys4), 1.74–1.60 (m, 14H, H2‴/H3‴/Lys2/H3′/H4′/H2″/H3″/H4″/H5″/H6″), 1.48–1.21 (m, 7H, Lys3/H2″/H3″/H4″/H5″/H6″), 1.01 (d, *J* = 6.2 Hz, 6H, H4‴/H5‴); ^{13}C NMR (101 MHz, CD_3OD) δ 173.0 (βC = O), 169.1 (αC = O), 157.1 (C = N), 150.8 (Ar2), 148.7 (C4), 147.6 (Cδ), 132.5 (Ar8a), 130.3 (Ar4), 129.1 (Ar4a), 128.6 (Ar5), 128.0 (Ar7), 126.9 (Ar8), 125.5 (C5), 125.1 (Cγ), 120.2 (Ar6), 119.1 (Ar3), 113.9 (Ar1), 67.4 (OCH_AH_B), 55.7 (C1′), 53.5 (Lys5), 49.3 (C2′), 40.4 (C5′), 39.0 (Lys1), 37.9 (C2‴), 33.4 (C1″), 31.6 (C2″), 31.5 (C6″), 30.9 (Lys4), 28.1 (Lys2), 27.5 (C1‴), 26.5 (C3′), 25.2 (C4″), 25.0 (C3″/C5″), 24.8 (C3‴), 22.6 (C4′), 22.5 (C4‴/C5‴), 21.3 (Lys3); IR (neat) $\overline{\nu}_{max}$ 3348, 3265, 3202, 3066, 2932, 2860, 1662, 1544, 1514, 1483, 1451, 1384, 1366, 1349, 1279, 1220, 1168, 1117, 1081, 1049, 816, 749, 668, 585 cm^{-1}; MS (ESI + ve) *m*/*z* 743 ([M–2HCl + H]$^+$, 60%), 372 ([M–2HCl + H]$^{2+}$, 100%); HRMS (ESI + ve TOF) calcd for $C_{39}H_{59}N_{12}O_3$ 743.4833, found 743.4866 ([M–2HCl + H]$^+$).

4.3. Microbiological Assays

Primary screening (Gram-positive bacteria). Primary MIC assays were performed as described by the Clinical and Laboratory Standards Institute for aerobic [36] and anaerobic [37] bacteria. MIC values for vancomycin were within acceptable QC ranges [38].

Secondary screening (MRSA and Gram-negative bacteria) and cytotoxicity assay–performed by the Community for Open Antimicrobial Drug Discovery (CO-ADD). Samples were provided to CO-ADD [29] for antimicrobial screening by whole cell growth inhibition assays.

Bacterial Inhibition–MIC Assay. These were performed as described previously [13,29].

Cytotoxicity Assay. These were performed as described previously [13,29].

Haemolysis assay (sheep erythrocytes). These were performed as described previously [13].

Hemolysis assay (human erythrocytes)–HC_{50} determination. These were performed as described previously [13,29].

4.4. *In Vivo Murine Model of CDI Treatment*

Disease Treatment Model. These experiments were performed as previously described [39–42]. Mice were humanely killed at the onset of severe disease or at the end of the experiment (day 4), as previously described [43].

Statistical Analysis. Statistical analysis was performed using Prism 7 (GraphPad Software). The Kaplan–Meier survival curves were assessed using a log-rank (Mantel–Cox) test. Weight loss, spore shedding, fecal consistency, and physiological appearance data were analyzed by one-way ANOVA with a post hoc Tukey's multiple comparison test. Differences in data values were considered significant at a p value of <0.05.

5. Conclusions

This study reported the next generation of hydrophobic anchored cationic peptidomimetics as antibacterial agents, with a focus on targeting CDI. A major aim was to improve the solubility profile of these compounds to allow for sufficient solubility for efficient administration of the drug while maintaining gut availability and antibacterial activity. The naphthyltriazole derivates containing either a monocationic or dicationic amino acid side chain were generally the most effective, with compounds **40** and **42**, possessing terminal cyclohexyl and benzyl moieties, respectively, exhibiting MIC values of 8 μg/mL.

Naphthyltriazole **40** was selected for an in vivo murine model trials of CDI but exhibited only mild evidence of in vivo efficacy indicating that further investigation into the structural and biological parameters affecting the in vivo efficacy of these antibacterial peptidomimetics is required, as the observed in vitro efficacy did not translate directly into in vivo efficacy. We have already reported that a correlation exists between increased hemolytic activity and an increase in hydrophobic/cationic ratio [15]; unfortunately, compound **40** exhibited a slight increase in hemolytic activity relative to the majority of tested compounds in this class with an HC_{50} value of 32 μg/mL. While the selectivity ratio could be more substantial, this is acceptable for the future development of these gastrointestinal focused compounds. We have previously reported a comparative solubility assay for this class of antimicrobial agents with increasing numerical values corresponding to better aqueous solubility relative to compound **1** (which possesses a value of 1) [13]. Compound **40** showed a better solubility ratio with an assay value of 5, relative to our lead compound **2** with a value 3—this is also reflected in the CLogP values of 4.46 and 5.76 for **41** vs. **2**, respectively. These outcomes were confirmed with no issues during the mouse model trials with sufficient solubility in the dosage regimen. Variations on the triazole and *O*-naphthyl substituents could be made in future studies with the view of enhancing antibacterial activity against *C. difficile*.

Supplementary Materials: The following are available online at https://www.mdpi.com/article/10.3390/antibiotics10080913/s1, Figures S1–S85: Details of synthesis and characterization data for compounds; Table S1: Secondary antimicrobial screening [a]–(bacteria and fungi), Murine model studies experimental procedures.

Author Contributions: Conceptualization, P.A.K. and S.G.P.; methodology, P.A.K., S.G.P., D.L., and T.V.R.; validation, S.G.P., P.A.K., D.L., and T.V.R.; formal analysis, M.K.M., A.J.T., S.J., P.P., M.L.H., K.A.H., D.R.K., P.A.K., S.G.P., D.L., and T.V.R.; resources, P.A.K., S.G.P., D.L., and T.V.R.; writing—original draft preparation, M.K.M., P.P., M.L.H., P.A.K., and S.G.P.; writing—review and editing, S.G.P., P.A.K., A.J.T., D.L., T.V.R., M.L.H., and D.R.K.; supervision, P.A.K., S.G.P., D.L., and T.V.R.; project administration, P.A.K., S.G.P., D.L., and T.V.R.; funding acquisition, P.A.K., S.G.P., D.L., and T.V.R. All authors have read and agreed to the published version of the manuscript.

Funding: This research was funded by National Health and Medical Research Council of Australia, grant number #APP1124032.

Institutional Review Board Statement: The study was conducted according to the guidelines of the Declaration of Helsinki, and Victorian State Government regulations, and was approved by the Monash University Animal Ethics Committee (Monash University AEC no. MARP/2014/142).

Informed Consent Statement: Not applicable.

Data Availability Statement: The data presented in this study are available in supplementary material.

Acknowledgments: The authors thank the National Health and Medical Research Council (NHMRC) Australia for financial support (Grant #APP1145760). The authors also thank Meagan James and Chris Evans for assistance with mouse infection experiments.

Conflicts of Interest: The authors declare no conflict of interest. The funders had no role in the design of the study; in the collection, analyses, or interpretation of data; in the writing of the manuscript; or in the decision to publish the results.

References

1. Leffler, D.A.; Lamont, J.T. Treatment of *Clostridium difficile*-Associated Disease. *Gastroenterology* **2009**, *136*, 1899–1912. [CrossRef]
2. Knight, D.R.; Elliott, B.; Chang, B.J.; Perkins, T.T.; Riley, T.V. Diversity and Evolution in the Genome of *Clostridium difficile*. *Clin. Microbiol. Rev.* **2015**, *28*, 721–741. [CrossRef] [PubMed]
3. Eaton, S.R.; Mazuski, J.E. Overview of Severe *Clostridium difficile* Infection. *Crit. Care Clin.* **2013**, *29*, 827–839. [CrossRef] [PubMed]
4. Di Bella, S.; Ascenzi, P.; Siarakas, S.; Petrosillo, N.; Di Masi, A. *Clostridium difficile* Toxins A and B: Insights into Pathogenic Properties and Extraintestinal Effects. *Toxins* **2016**, *8*, 134. [CrossRef]
5. Chandrasekaran, R.; Lacy, D.B. The role of toxins in *Clostridium difficile* infection. *FEMS Microbiol. Rev.* **2017**, *41*, 723–750. [CrossRef]
6. Johnson, A.P. New antibiotics for selective treatment of gastrointestinal infection caused by *Clostridium difficile*. *Expert Opin. Ther. Pat.* **2010**, *20*, 1389–1399. [CrossRef] [PubMed]
7. Centers for Disease Control and Prevention. Clostridium Difficile Update. 2019. Available online: https://www.cdc.gov/drugresistance/pdf/threats-report/CRE-508.pdf (accessed on 26 June 2021).
8. Stanley, J.D.; Bartlett, J.G.; Dart, B.W.; Ashcraft, J. *Clostridium difficile* infection. *Curr. Probl. Surg.* **2013**, *50*, 302–337. [CrossRef] [PubMed]
9. Ritter, A.S.; Petri, W.A. New developments in chemotherapeutic options for *Clostridium difficile* colitis. *Curr. Opin. Infect. Dis.* **2013**, *26*, 461–470. [CrossRef]
10. Cornely, O.A.; Miller, M.A.; Louie, T.J.; Crook, D.W.; Gorbach, S.L. Treatment of First Recurrence of *Clostridium difficile* Infection: Fidaxomicin Versus Vancomycin. *Clin. Infect. Dis.* **2012**, *55*, S154–S161. [CrossRef]
11. Hostler, C.J.; Chen, L.F. Fidaxomicin for treatment of *Clostridium difficile*-associated diarrhea and its potential role for prophylaxis. *Expert Opin. Pharmacother.* **2013**, *14*, 1529–1536. [CrossRef]
12. Cho, J.M.; Pardi, D.S.; Khanna, S. Update on Treatment of *Clostridioides difficile* Infection. *Mayo Clin Proc.* **2020**, *95*, 758–769. [CrossRef]
13. Tague, A.J.; Putsathit, P.; Hammer, K.A.; Wales, S.M.; Knight, D.R.; Riley, T.V.; Keller, P.A.; Pyne, S.G. Cationic biaryl 1,2,3-triazolyl peptidomimetic amphiphiles targeting *Clostridioides* (*Clostridium*) *difficile*: Synthesis, antibacterial evaluation and an in vivo *C. difficile* infection model. *Eur. J. Med. Chem.* **2019**, *170*, 203–224. [CrossRef] [PubMed]
14. Wales, S.M.; Hammer, K.A.; King, A.M.; Tague, A.J.; Lyras, D.; Riley, T.V.; Keller, P.A.; Pyne, S.G. Binaphthyl-1,2,3-triazole peptidomimetics with activity against *Clostridium difficile* and other pathogenic bacteria. *Org. Biomol. Chem.* **2015**, *13*, 5743–5756. [CrossRef] [PubMed]
15. Tague, A.J.; Putsathit, P.; Riley, T.V.; Keller, P.A.; Pyne, S.G. Positional Isomers of Biphenyl Antimicrobial Peptidomimetic Amphiphiles. *ACS Med. Chem. Lett.* **2021**, *12*, 413–419. [CrossRef]
16. Zhang, S.J.; Yang, Q.; Xu, L.; Chang, J.; Sun, X. Synthesis and antibacterial activity against *Clostridium difficile* of novel demethylvancomycin derivatives. *Bioorg. Med. Chem. Lett.* **2012**, *22*, 4942–4945. [CrossRef] [PubMed]
17. Butler, M.M.; Williams, J.D.; Peet, N.P.; Moir, D.T.; Panchal, R.G.; Bavari, S.; Shinabarger, D.L.; Bowlin, T.L. Comparative In Vitro Activity Profiles of Novel Bis-Indole Antibacterials against Gram-Positive and Gram-Negative Clinical Isolates. *Antimicrob. Agents Chemother.* **2010**, *54*, 3974–3977. [CrossRef] [PubMed]
18. Dvoskin, S.; Xu, W.-C.; Brown, N.C.; Yanachkov, I.B.; Yanachkova, M.; Wright, G.E. A Novel Agent Effective against *Clostridium difficile* Infection. *Antimicrob. Agents Chemother.* **2012**, *56*, 1624–1626. [CrossRef]
19. Ueda, C.; Tateda, K.; Horikawa, M.; Kimura, S.; Ishii, Y.; Nomura, K.; Yamada, K.; Suematsu, T.; Inoue, Y.; Ishiguro, M.; et al. Anti-*Clostridium difficile* Potential of Tetramic Acid Derivatives from *Pseudomonas aeruginosa* Quorum-Sensing Autoinducers. *Antimicrob. Agents Chemother.* **2010**, *54*, 683–688. [CrossRef] [PubMed]
20. Ballard, T.E.; Wang, X.; Olekhnovich, I.; Koerner, T.; Seymour, C.; Hoffman, P.S.; Macdonald, T.L. Biological Activity of Modified and Exchanged 2-Amino-5-Nitrothiazole Amide Analogues of Nitazoxanide. *Bioorg. Med. Chem. Lett.* **2010**, *20*, 3537–3539. [CrossRef] [PubMed]

21. Kirst, H.A.; Toth, J.E.; Debono, M.; Willard, K.E.; Truedell, B.A.; Ott, J.L.; Counter, F.T.; Felty-Duckworth, A.M.; Pekarek, R.S. Synthesis and evaluation of tylosin-related macrolides modified at the aldehyde function: A new series of orally effective antibiotics. *J. Med. Chem.* **1988**, *31*, 1631–1641. [CrossRef]
22. Liu, R.; Suárez, J.M.; Weisblum, B.; Gellman, S.H.; McBride, S.M. Synthetic Polymers Active against *Clostridium difficile* Vegetative Cell Growth and Spore Outgrowth. *J. Am. Chem. Soc.* **2014**, *136*, 14498–14504. [CrossRef]
23. Jarrad, A.M.; Karoli, T.; Blaskovich, M.A.T.; Lyras, D.; Cooper, M.A. *Clostridium difficile* Drug Pipeline: Challenges in Discovery and Development of New Agents. *J. Med. Chem.* **2015**, *58*, 5164–5185. [CrossRef] [PubMed]
24. Lowes, R. FDA Approves Zinplava for Preventing Return of *C. difficile*. Available online: https://www.medscape.com/viewarticle/870887 (accessed on 26 June 2021).
25. Bremner, J.B.; Keller, P.A.; Pyne, S.G.; Boyle, T.P.; Brkic, Z.; David, D.M.; Garas, A.; Morgan, J.; Robertson, M.; Somphol, K.; et al. Binaphthyl-Based Dicationic Peptoids with Therapeutic Potential. *Angew. Chem. Int. Ed.* **2010**, *49*, 537–540. [CrossRef] [PubMed]
26. Bremner, J.B.; Keller, P.A.; Pyne, S.G.; Boyle, T.P.; Brkic, Z.; David, D.M.; Robertson, M.; Somphol, K.; Baylis, D.; Coates, J.A.; et al. Synthesis and antibacterial studies of binaphthyl-based tripeptoids. Part 1. *Bioorg. Med. Chem.* **2010**, *18*, 2611–2620. [CrossRef] [PubMed]
27. Bremner, J.B.; Keller, P.A.; Pyne, S.G.; Boyle, T.P.; Brkic, Z.; Morgan, J.; Somphol, K.; Coates, J.A.; Deadman, J.; Rhodes, D.I. Synthesis and antibacterial studies of binaphthyl-based tripeptoids. Part 2. *Bioorg. Med. Chem.* **2010**, *18*, 4793–4800. [CrossRef]
28. Mahadari, M.K.; Tague, A.J.; Keller, P.A.; Pyne, S.G. Synthesis of sterically congested 1,5-disubstituted-1,2,3-Triazoles using chloromagnesium acetylides and hindered 1-naphthyl azides. *Tetrahedron* **2021**, *81*, 131916. [CrossRef]
29. Blaskovich, M.A.T.; Zuegg, J.; Elliott, A.G.; Cooper, M.A. Helping chemists discover new antibiotics. *ACS Infect. Dis.* **2015**, *1*, 285–287. [CrossRef]
30. Wales, S.M.; Hammer, K.A.; Somphol, K.; Kemker, I.; Schröder, D.C.; Tague, A.J.; Brkic, Z.; King, A.M.; Lyras, D.; Riley, T.V.; et al. Synthesis and antimicrobial activity of binaphthylbased, functionalized oxazole and thiazole peptidomimetics. *Org. Biomol. Chem.* **2019**, *13*, 10813–10824. [CrossRef]
31. Tague, A.J.; Putsathit, P.; Hammer, K.A.; Wales, S.M.; Knight, D.R.; Riley, T.V.; Keller, P.A.; Pyne, S.G. Cationic biaryl 1,2,3-triazolyl peptidomimetic amphiphiles: Synthesis, antibacterial evaluation and preliminary mechanism of action studies. *Eur. J. Med. Chem.* **2019**, *168*, 386–404. [CrossRef]
32. Zhu, D.; Ma, J.; Luo, K.; Fu, H.; Zhang, L.; Zhu, S. Enantioselective Intramolecular C-H Insertion of Donor and Donor/Donor Carbenes by a Nondiazo Approach. *Angew. Chem. Int. Ed.* **2016**, *55*, 8452–8456. [CrossRef]
33. Maehr, H.; Smallheer, J. Total syntheses of rivularins D1 and D3. *J. Am. Chem. Soc.* **1985**, *107*, 2943–2945. [CrossRef]
34. Gamble, A.B.; Garner, J.; Gordon, C.P.; O'Conner, S.M.J.; Keller, P.A. Aryl Nitro Reduction with Iron Powder or Stannous Chloride under Ultrasonic Irradiation. *Synth. Commun.* **2007**, *37*, 2777–2786. [CrossRef]
35. Zilla, M.K.; Nayak, D.; Vishwakarma, R.A.; Sharma, P.R.; Goswami, A.; Ali, A. A convergent synthesis of alkyne-azide cycloaddition derivatives of 4-α,β-2-propyne podophyllotoxin depicting potent cytotoxic activity. *Eur. J. Med. Chem.* **2014**, *77*, 47–55. [CrossRef] [PubMed]
36. Clinical and Laboratory Standards Institute. *Methods for Dilution Antimicrobial Susceptibility Tests for Bacteria that Grow Aerobically*, 9th ed.; CLSI Document M07-A10; Clinical and Laboratory Standards Institute: Wayne, PA, USA, 2015.
37. Clinical and Laboratory Standards Institute. *Methods for Antimicrobial Susceptibility Testing of Anaerobic Bacteria*, 8th ed.; CLSI Document M11-A8; Clinical and Laboratory Standards Institute: Wayne, PA, USA, 2012.
38. Clinical Laboratory Standards Institute. *Performance Standards for Antimicrobial Susceptibility Testing*; 28th Informational Supplement; CLSI Document M100-S28; Clinical and Laboratory Standards Institute: Wayne, PA, USA, 2018.
39. Carter, G.P.; Lyras, D.; Allen, D.L.; Mackin, K.E.; Howarth, P.M.; O'Connor, J.R.; Rood, J.I. Binary toxin production in Clostridium difficile is regulated by CdtR, a LytTR family response regulator. *J. Bacteriol.* **2007**, *189*, 7290–7301. [CrossRef]
40. Hutton, M.L.; Cunningham, B.A.; Mackin, K.E.; Lyon, S.A.; James, M.L.; Rood, J.I.; Lyras, D. Bovine antibodies targeting primary and recurrent *Clostridium difficile* disease are a potent antibiotic alternative. *Sci. Rep.* **2017**, *7*, 3665. [CrossRef]
41. Lyon, S.A.; Hutton, M.L.; Rood, J.I.; Cheung, J.K.; Lyras, D. CdtR regulates TcdA and TcdB production in *Clostridium difficile*. *PLoS Pathog.* **2016**, *12*, e1005758. [CrossRef]
42. Awad, M.M.; Hutton, M.L.; Quek, A.J.; Klare, W.P.; Mileto, S.J.; Mackin, K.; Ly, D.; Oorschot, V.; Bosnjak, M.; Jenkin, G.; et al. Human Plasminogen Exacerbates *Clostridioides difficile* Enteric Disease and Alters the Spore Surface. *Gastroenterology* **2020**, *159*, 1431–1443. [CrossRef]
43. Carter, G.P.; Chakravorty, A.; Pham Nguyen, T.A.; Mileto, S.; Schreiber, F.; Li, L.; Howarth, P.; Clare, S.; Cunningham, B.; Sambol, S.P.; et al. Defining the roles of TcdA and TcdB in localized gastrointestinal disease, systemic organ damage, and the host response during *Clostridium difficile* infections. *mBio* **2015**, *6*, e00551. [CrossRef] [PubMed]

antibiotics

Review

Opportunities for Nanomedicine in *Clostridioides difficile* Infection

Pei-Wen Wang [1,2,†], Wei-Ting Lee [3,†], Ya-Na Wu [1,4] and Dar-Bin Shieh [1,2,4,5,6,*]

1 School of Dentistry and Institute of Oral Medicine, National Cheng Kung University, Tainan 701401, Taiwan; 9503049@gs.ncku.edu.tw (P.-W.W.); yana.wu@gmail.com (Y.-N.W.)
2 Center of Applied Nanomedicine, National Cheng Kung University, Tainan 701401, Taiwan
3 Department of Obstetrics and Gynecology, National Cheng Kung University Hospital, Tainan 704302, Taiwan; wesker1206@gmail.com
4 iMANI Center of the National Core Facility for Biopharmaceuticals, Ministry of Science and Technology, Taipei 701401, Taiwan
5 Department of Stomatology, National Cheng Kung University Hospital, Tainan 704302, Taiwan
6 Core Facility Center, National Cheng Kung University, Tainan 701401, Taiwan
* Correspondence: dbshieh@mail.ncku.edu.tw; Tel.: +886-6-235-3535 (ext. 5899)
† These authors contributed equally to this work.

Abstract: *Clostridioides difficile*, a spore-forming bacterium, is a nosocomial infectious pathogen which can be found in animals as well. Although various antibiotics and disinfectants were developed, *C. difficile* infection (CDI) remains a serious health problem. *C. difficile* spores have complex structures and dormant characteristics that contribute to their resistance to harsh environments, successful transmission and recurrence. *C. difficile* spores can germinate quickly after being exposed to bile acid and co-germinant in a suitable environment. The vegetative cells produce endospores, and the mature spores are released from the hosts for dissemination of the pathogen. Therefore, concurrent elimination of *C. difficile* vegetative cells and inhibition of spore germination is essential for effective control of CDI. This review focused on the molecular pathogenesis of CDI and new trends in targeting both spores and vegetative cells of this pathogen, as well as the potential contribution of nanotechnologies for the effective management of CDI.

Keywords: *Clostridioides difficile*; spores; anti-spore; spore germination; nanomaterial

Citation: Wang, P.-W.; Lee, W.-T.; Wu, Y.-N.; Shieh, D.-B. Opportunities for Nanomedicine in *Clostridioides difficile* Infection. *Antibiotics* **2021**, *10*, 948. https://doi.org/10.3390/antibiotics10080948

Academic Editor: Guido Granata

Received: 1 July 2021
Accepted: 3 August 2021
Published: 5 August 2021

1. Introduction

Clostridioides (formerly *Clostridium*) *difficile*, a Gram-positive bacterium that causes severe antibiotic-associated diarrheas and colitis, was first isolated from new-born infants in 1935 [1]. It produces oval terminal endospores [1] and is commonly acquired through community and hospital (nosocomial) infections [2]. The disease is associated with inappropriate antibiotic treatment, which causes an imbalance of the host's intestine microbial flora, in turn activating the dormant *C. difficile* [3]. Clindamycin, carbapenems and fluoroquinolones are the antibiotics most commonly associated with increasing the risk of *C. difficile* infection (CDI) [4]. Additionally, gastric acid-suppressant and older age (>65 years) are also important risk factors [5]. The symptoms of CDI include watery diarrhea, fever, abdominal pain and toxic megacolon [6]. From a recent epidemiological analysis reported by NHS trusts in England, there were a total of 13,177 CDI cases diagnosed between 2019 and 2020 [7], a small increase of 7.4% compared to the previous year (n = 12,274). The incidence of hospital-onset CDI cases mirrors the trends in the incidence of all cases, with a decline between 2007 and 2014 followed by a relatively stable state till 2018. The rate (hospital-onset cases/100,000 bed-days) of hospital-onset CDI cases increased from 12.2 to 13.6 between 2018 and 2020. In the USA, a statistical analysis revealed that CDI cases in 10 hospitals increased between 2011 and 2017, while the adjusted estimate of the burden of hospitalizations for CDI decreased by 24% [8]. Whereas the adjusted estimates of the burden of first recurrences and in-hospital deaths did not change significantly, suggesting the effectiveness of infection-prevention practices, and new more refined diagnostic techniques, it is important to eliminate false positives and to improve infection prevention. However, reducing the burden of CDI remains one of the imperative health care priorities in western countries. Different ribotypes occur according to geographic localization and time of the episodes, associated with evolutionary sophistication. Ribotype 027 and 078 strains have spread worldwide since the millennium, and this was attributed to their ability to metabolize disaccharide trehalose approved by the USA Food and Drug Administration (FDA) since 2000 [9]. Epidemic *C. difficile* ribotypes yield more toxins and have higher sporulation compared to non-epidemic ones [10,11], in spite of some controversial results [11].

The *C. difficile* spores play an important role in its pathogenesis and are well known to resist gastric acid, harsh environments and antibiotics treatment, or even survive in dry inorganic surfaces for months [12]. Hand washing has been recommended as a good practice to reduce risk of pathogen transmission, not only among health care workers but also visitors [13,14]. Hand washing with soap and water is significantly more effective at removing *C. difficile* spores than alcohol-based hand rubs [15,16]. The unique structure of the spores helps the pathogen to overcome UV-A and UV-B irradiation, heat (up to 71 °C), extreme freezing, biocides, chemical disinfectants, desiccation and nutrient deficiency [17,18]. The exosporium is the outermost layer of the spore, containing cysteine (CdeC)-rich proteins that enhance their surface adhesion and spore-host interactions [19,20] and were demonstrated to assist in resistance to heat, enzymes and macrophage-inactivation [19,21]. The next layer is the coat, which blocks oxidizing agents, hypochlorite and enzymes from damaging the microorganism [18,22]. Inside the coat is the outer membrane, and the cortex which keeps the spore in a dehydrated state [23]. The low permeability of the inner membrane prevents the core from invasion from water and other small molecules [24]. The innermost part of the spore is the dehydrated core, containing DNA, RNA, ribosomes, small acid-soluble spore proteins (SASPs) and large amounts of calcium dipicolinic acid (Ca-DPA) [18,25]. The high level of the Ca-DPA increases their resistance to environmental stressors, such as disinfectants and ultraviolet radiation [26].

Several physical methods and chemical reagents have been developed to eliminate spores. For examples, UV-C irradiation (254 nm) could be an ideal option for *C. difficile* spore elimination in a health setting [27]. Moist heat at 85 and 96 °C could effectively kill *C. difficile* spores in foods [28]. Several chemicals have also exhibited anti-spore activity. Sodium hypochlorite (NaOCl) (10%) is a disinfectant with excellent capability to eliminate spores [29]. Hydrogen peroxide (H_2O_2) (10%) also has good anti-spore properties [30]. Potassium peroxymonosulfate ($KHSO_5$) (0.2%), often used to clean water, is also effective [31]. Nevertheless, these approaches readily used in routine equipment surface and environment disinfection could not be applied for clinical treatment of *C. difficile* spores in human infection. This review provides an update on novel materials that inhibit *C. difficile* and harbor therapeutic potential.

2. Molecular Pathogenesis of *C. difficile* Infection

Transmission of *C. difficile* spores or vegetative cells occurs through the fecal—oral route, and from direct contact with contaminated items [32]. However, only spore-form *C. difficile* can pass through the gastric acid and achieve residence in the large intestine [6]. As the spores are exposed to an appropriate environment containing bile acid and co-germinant, they can be reactivated into the vegetative state [33,34]. *C. difficile* spores germinate mostly within the ileum due to the higher environment pH (around 7.4) [34]. At a molecular level, CspC serves as the bile acid germinant receptor, while CspA acts as the co-germinant receptor. Upon activation, the signal is transmitted to CspB [35–37], which converts pro-SleC into its active form to degrade the cortex [38,39]. This leads to expansion of the germ cell wall and rehydration of the core, together with the release of dipicolinic acid (DPA) [40,41]. The outgrowth of *C. difficile* spores into a vegetative cell is the result.

The vegetative form of *C. difficile* proliferates and produces toxin A (TcdA) and toxin B (TcdB), which contribute to the major pathogenesis process. TcdE protein contributes to the secretion of TcdA and TcdB whcih promotes *C. difficile* growth by obtaining nutrients from toxin-mediated collagen degradation and suppression of competitors in the gut [42–44]. Secreted TcdA binds to carbohydrates on the apical surface of colonic epithelial cells, while TcdB recognizes their Wnt receptor frizzled family (FZDs) proteins [45]. Both TcdA and TcdB toxins enter cells via endocytosis, followed by fusion with the lysosome [46,47]. Upon acidification of the organelle, protonation triggers conformation changes in TcdA and TcdB to form hairpin pores; this is followed by release of the glucosyltransferase domains of the toxins from the organelles via autoproteolysis [48,49]. These domains further glycosylate Rho and Rac in the cytosol, preventing them from being activated by guanine nucleotide exchange factors (GEFs), thereby triggering apoptosis and loss of tight junction integrity in mucosal epithelial cells [46,50].

C. difficile cells start to sporulate when nutrients are scarce in the environment, although the quorum-sensing signals to relay the environmental state are yet to be identified [25]. Stage 0 sporulation protein A (Spo0A) is a transcription factor critical for the *C. difficile* life cycle that regulates genes associated with biofilm formation, metabolism, toxin production and sporulation [51]. Phosphorylation of Spo0A is an early triggering factor for sporulation, followed by the activation of sigma factor F (σF) to control the downstream effectors σG in the forespore compartment. Activation of σG is required for spore cell wall synthesis and cortex formation [52]. Spo0A also activates σE and further activates σk to modulate coat protein expression and DPA synthesis, as well as their structural assembly after asymmetric division. At this stage, the replicated DNA is already packed into the forespore [53]. After completing the development of the membrane, spore coat and cortex proteins, the mother cell will be lysed, and the mature spore will be released (Figure 1).

Symptomatic *C. difficile* patients shed out the vegetative cells and spores leading to contamination of their environment [54]. The vegetative cells can survive 6 h in room air, while the spores may remain alive for as long as 5 months [55,56]. As the health-care workers and patients' family members contact the spore-contaminated surface, the spores tightly attach to the skin [57]. Noticeably, asymptomatic *C. difficile* carriers can shed out spores and cause another CDI outbreak [58]. Prevention of *C. difficile* spore formation is, therefore, an important strategy for CDI management and could reduce the threat of relapse [59].

Biofilm formation by vegetative cells and spores has been identified in several Clostridium species, including *Clostridium perfringens*, *C. thermocellum* and *C. acetobutylicum* [60]. Biofilm formation could play major roles in all phases of CDI, especially in their recurrence [61,62], since it helps to enhance microorganism retention, enabling them to resist the flow of luminal material in the gastrointestinal (GI) tract and to prevent the host immune system's attack. Biofilms provide a powerful shield against antibiotics and create a comfort zone for the microorganism to survive and prosper [63]. Intriguingly, biofilms could also reduce germination efficiency in *C. difficile*. Such controversy complicates the development of treatment strategies.

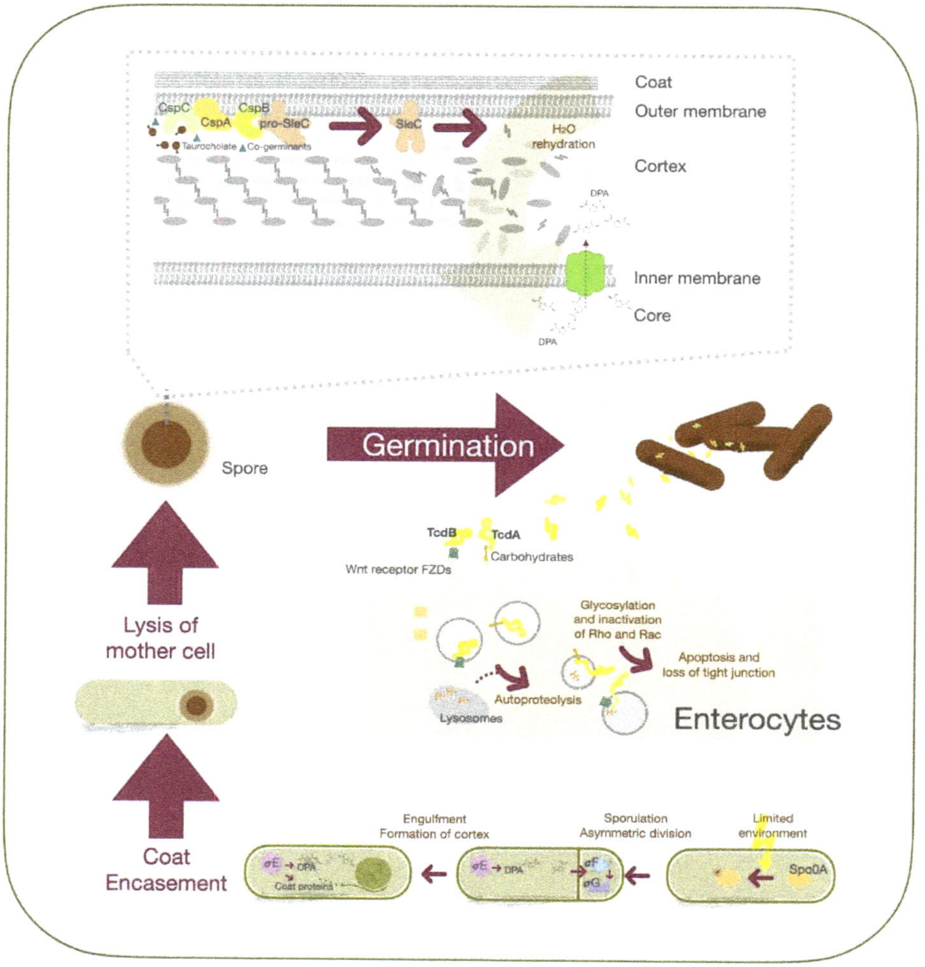

Figure 1. Schematic illustration of *C. difficile* germination, sporulation, and the molecular mechanism of toxins action in epithelial cells.

3. Advancements in the Treatment of *C. difficile* Infection

Even though antibiotic therapy is the major treatment of choice for CDI, severe side effects and resistance remain unsolved. Metronidazole and vancomycin have been considered effective treatments for CDI patients for years. However, the two antibiotics also disrupt the normal colonic flora [64] and recurrence is not uncommon [65,66]. Antibiotics also promote spore formation and shedding [67]. Moreover, strains resistant to the two antibiotics were isolated [68] and could spread widely [69]. Fidaxomicin was approved by the FDA in 2011 as a new CDI treatment option, as it showed superior efficacy with significantly less impact on normal colonic flora than vancomycin [70]. Fidaxomicin treatment also inhibits sporulation and decreases spore shedding into the environment [71,72]. Despite only one resistant isolate being reported to date [73], development of non-antibiotic therapy to prevent therapeutic resistance is urgently needed for CDI control.

Some non-antibiotic approaches were developed recently, such as the introduction of probiotics, fecal microbiota transplantation (FMT), engineered microorganisms, bacteriophages, diet control, natural active substances and nanomedicines. A microbiota-based non-antibiotic drug, RBX2660, has been developed by Rebiotix Inc. Clinical trials revealed that, although RBX2660 treatment reduced the number of antibiotic-resistant microorganisms, these still occurred [74]. FMT refers to the transference of fecal materials from healthy donors to patients and was first introduced in 1958 for the treatment of pseudomembranous colitis [75]. Further clinical studies showed that FMT successfully cured patients with recurrent CDI and attenuated CDI-associated diarrhea [76,77]. According to preclinical and clinical data, FMT in combination with vancomycin was recommended as the primary therapy for multiple recurrent CDIs (rCDIs) [78,79]. FMT not only restores healthy gut flora in CDI patients but also interferes with *C. difficile* spore germination [80]. The mechanism by which FMT battles *C. difficile* spore germination is through restoration of secondary bile acid metabolism by bile acid-metabolizing microbiota in the colon and repair of the gut barrier [80,81]. FMT is generally considered a safe treatment modality for rCDIs with only mild side effects (e.g., abdominal discomfort and transient mild fever) [82]. However, before CDI patients receive FMT therapy, both donors and recipient need to undergo rigorous checkups and tests, including evaluating the presence of metabolic syndromes and screening for fecal pathogens [83,84]. In order to improve the clinical application and safety of FMT, further studies should be performed to establish the gold standard of FMT. In addition to FMT, the use of probiotics for CDI prevention and treatment received particular attention in the clinic [85]. Delivery of appropriate probiotics into the intestinal tract could restore the balance of gut microbiota. Recently, mixed regimens containing *Lactobacillus* species, *Saccharomyces boulardii* or *C. butyricum* have been extensively explored for the prophylaxis of CDI [86]. Both probiotics and FMT are high-potential alternative strategies to rebalance the microbiota for effective clinical management of CDIs. However, FMT and probiotics still require an extended treatment course and would not be eligible for all CDI patients, rendering the unmet needs of others to be met by advanced therapeutic options.

4. Alternative Strategies for Targeting Spores

The spores of *C. difficile* can be found in food, in domestic animals, and on the surface of contaminated equipment [87] and are difficult to eliminate. Therefore, *C. difficile* endospores are the main vehicle of infection, and anti-spore strategies are undoubtedly important for both disease prevention and therapeutics. These strategies could directly aim at the structural components of the spore or their germination process, as germinating spores are very vulnerable [88]. Many chemicals inhibit *C. difficile* spores.

Ceragenins are synthetic bile acid-based mimics of antimicrobial peptides with broad-spectrum coverage [89,90]. Ceragenin (2 μM) alone significantly reduced biofilm formation by clinical *E. coli* strains, and the combination of ceragenin with LL-37 peptide (10 μM at 1:1 ratio) eliminated 79% of the *E. coli* strains [91]. Remarkably, ceragenin CSA-13 has been shown to have sporicidal activity against *Bacillus subtilis* and *C. difficile* [92,93]. CSA-13 at 75 μg/mL inhibited all *B. subtilis* spore outgrowth by disrupting the inner membrane of *B. subtilis* spores, leading to the release of Ca-DPA from the core followed by premature hydration [92]. CSA-13 affected the germination and viability of *C. difficile* spores even at a lower dose (4 μg/mL), with minimum inhibitory concentration (MIC) of 60 μg/mL [93]. Furthermore, CSA-13 (3 μM) reduced toxin A-mediated inflammation and prevented vancomycin-dependent CDI relapse (10 mg/Kg oral daily) [93]. CSA-13 has an LD_{50} of 24.74 μg/g body weight in mice [94].

Ursodeoxycholic acid (UDCA) is another spore germination inhibitor that acts through a bile acid-based mechanism. When *C. difficile* spores were spread on BHIS agar plates containing 0.1% UDCA (about 2.5 mM), the CFU recovery rate was below 0.0001% [33]. As low as 0.2 mM of the compound is effective to block *C. difficile* spore germination and, at 2 mM concentration, it could even interfere with vegetative cell growth [94]. Weingarden recently reported the successful treatment of CDI patients with UDCA (300 mg twice daily—300 mg four times daily) without relapse [95]. UDCA does not have the 12α-hydroxyl group important for sensing bile acids as a germinating signal by *C. difficile* spores [96].

More bile acid analogues have been chemically synthesized and evaluated for their ability to prevent *C. difficile* spore germination [97]. Some bile acid analogues directly bind to TcdB causing their conformation to change and lose cell binding ability [98]. These results point towards a new pathway for bile acid-based clinical management of CDI patients.

Anti-microbial peptides have also been investigated for inhibiting spore germination. Ramoplanin, a glycolipodepsipeptide antibiotic, was discovered to effectively block bacterial cell wall biosynthesis and presented antibacterial activities against methicillin-resistant *Staphylococcus aureus* and vancomycin-resistant *Enterococcus* [99]. Ramoplanin (50 mg/kg/day) treatment more prominently reduced recovery of *C. difficile* spores in the caecal contents of experimental animals, and cytotoxin production compared to vancomycin at the same dose [100]. *C. difficile* spores exposed to ramoplanin (300 μg/mL) failed to grow out to form colonies on agar plates, through interaction of the compound with the exosporium to ambush their germination [101].

Nylon-3 polymers are another artificial mimic of host-defense peptides synthesized via various β-lactams modified with cationic and lipophilic units [102]. Nylon-3 polymers demonstrated antimicrobial activities against both fungi and bacteria through cell membrane disruption [102,103]. In CDI, nylon-3 polymers not only killed the vegetative cells (MIC: 12.5–25 μg/mL) but also blocked *C. difficile* spore outgrowth (outgrowth inhibitory concentration: 3.13–12.5 μg/mL) [104] rather than directly damage the spores.

An FDA approved bacteriocin called nisin has been used to preserve food for decades [105,106]. Nisin and its analogues have been reported to show anti-bacterial activity against both Gram-positive and Gram-negative bacteria and had additive and synergistic interactions with antibiotics [107,108]. Furthermore, nisin inhibited *C. botulinum* and *B. anthracis* spore outgrowth [109,110]. Nisin (MIC: 0.8–51.2 μg/mL) also inhibited *C. difficile* vegetative cell growth and blocked spore outgrowth (log reduction > 4) at a concentration of 3.2 μg/mL after the germination started [111,112] via binding to the lipid II, thus interfering with cell wall biosynthesis and disrupting the spore membrane [110]. However, Le Lay's group showed that only a higher concentration of nisin (25.6 μg/mL) directly decreased viability of *C. difficile* spores to 40–50% [111].

Degradation of bacterial cell wall as an anti-CDI strategy has also been extensively explored. Cell wall hydrolase (CWH) encoded by bacteriophages provokes degradation of bacterial cell wall peptidoglycan [113]. Mondal et al. found that a catalytic domain (glucosaminidase and Nlp60 domain) CWH351-656of the hydrolase encoded by *C. difficile* phage phiMMP01 presented lytic activity higher than the full-length CWH. The fragment killed 100% of *C. difficile* vegetative cells and completely inhibited their spores' outgrowth at a concentration of 200 μg/mL [113]. Although CWH351-656may have therapeutic potential against CDI, further biocompatibility, immunological, and clinical studies are required.

5. Emergent Roles for Nanotechnology in Infectious Diseases

Infectious diseases have emerged as a serious global public health concern, underscored by the rapidly increasing number of drug-resistant strains of existing pathogens and the emergence of new pathogens [114]. Multiple challenges must be overcome in the effective management of infectious diseases. These include the lack of safe and effective medications central for disease treatment. The recent development of nanotechnology attracted significant attention due to its potential for transforming both disease diagnostics and therapeutics. Over the past few decades, intensive research in the field enabled the birth of more and more FDA-approved items in chemotherapeutics, anesthetics, imaging contrast agents, nutritional supplements and others [115]. Infectious diseases are also a major focus in nanomedicine.

The use of nanotechnology to defeat multidrug resistance gained significant global attention as new effective antibiotic development is extremely challenging and costly. Modifications in nanoparticles (NPs) could enable multifunctional purposes and bring about advanced applications in medicine. Nanomaterials could be modified with specific targeting moieties such as antibodies or aptamers, to enhance the therapeutic specificity and minimize collateral damage to healthy tissues [116]. Various types of nanomaterials have been shown to deliver drugs with good releasing profile and improve efficacy. These nanomedicines have been extensively explored for applications in the infectious disease area as well [117,118].

Organic nanoparticles (e.g., liposomes, polymeric, micelles and ferritin) have been used to enhance the bioavailability of therapeutic compounds and to increase their delivery and efficacy [119]. They were developed as drug delivery systems, offering a controlled-release profile and targeting the desired tissues or cells. These nanocarrier systems may control drug release by an excipient that enabled slow dissolution of poorly soluble drug crystals, from the core compartment to the interstitial space. Sustained release can also be obtained by encapsulating drugs in nanocarriers capable of loading both hydrophobic and hydrophilic drugs. Organic nanocarrier systems have been evaluated for the treatment of local infections of the female reproductive tract, lungs and skin. Injectable nanocarriers have also been explored for the systemic delivery of drugs [120]. Regarding the types of pathogens targeted, nanoparticles have also been extensively explored for treating fungal [121], bacterial [120] and viral infections, including by *Candida albicans* and severe acute respiratory syndrome 2 (SARS-CoV-2) [122].

Considerable research has focused on polyester-based organic nanosystems that degrade in the presence of physiological esterases (for example, poly (lactide-co-glycolide) (PLGA) and poly (caprolactone)). Modulated by the alteration of the hydrophobicity of the monomer, polymer chain length and particle size, active pharmaceutical ingredients could be released in a predesigned control manner, via bulk degradation of the polymers to enable drug diffusion [123]. Polymers such as poly (anhydrides), poly (orthoesters), poly (cyanoacrylates) and poly (amides) have also been used in the sustained release design [124]. The combination of polymer-based nanoparticles and antibiotics achieved better antibacterial activity than antibiotics alone [125]. Liposomes such as MiKasomes (NeXstar Pharmaceuticals) have also been developed to encapsulate drugs for sustained release in the treatment of bacterial infections including *C. difficile* [126]. These vesicles could also load both hydrophobic and hydrophilic drugs to reduce dosing frequency and ease the dosing regimen.

Inorganic nanoparticles (e.g., metals or metal oxides) have also been investigated for the prevention and treatment of infectious pathogens. Some inorganic nanomaterials were discovered to exhibit diverse activities against multi-drug-resistant pathogens [127]. These include silver (Ag), zinc oxide (ZnO), iron-containing nanoparticles and more. The antibacterial properties of the metallic nanoparticles may be attributed to the generation of reactive oxygen species (ROS), disruption of cell membranes, ability to bind thiol groups (SH-)/disulfide bonds (R-S-S-R) in biomolecules and the release of soluble metal ions [128,129]. The most widely studied metallic materials in infection control are silver (Ag) nanoparticles. The antimicrobial mechanisms of Ag nanoparticles are associated with ROS generation and silver ion release from the nanoparticles. Ag nanoparticles and ions interact with the thiol group, sulfur and phosphorus in the microbial cells subsequently bringing about DNA damage and protein dysfunction [130]. In addition, Ag nanoparticles could also anchor to the bacterial cell wall and cause structural changes in the cell membrane, thus radically affecting cell membrane permeability and inducing cell death. Free radicals generated by Ag nanoparticles upon contact with the bacterial cell membrane are another important mechanism for their anti-microbial activity, as confirmed by electron spin resonance analysis [130]. Compared to their bulk state, Ag nanoparticles also display efficient antimicrobial properties due to their large surface-to-volume ratio, providing better contact interface with the microorganisms [131].

Moreover, nanomaterials responsive to photoactivation have especially been applied for photodynamic, photothermal and photoactivation of chemotherapeutics or their combination. Photoactivation mechanisms could be placed in the payload of the nanocarriers or inside the nanomaterials, as an endogenous property [132]. Photodynamic therapy (PDT) combines special drugs, so-called photosensitizing agents, with light to destroy microorganisms for the management of infectious diseases [133]. The irradiated light activates photosensitizers (PS) to induce the generation of ROS (e.g., peroxides, superoxide, hydroxyl radical, singlet oxygen ($^1O_2$)) that in turn induce cell death [134]. Despite only relatively low laser power being required, successful treatment is dependent upon sufficient oxygen supply to the target tissues. As most PSs are hydrophobic compounds with limited accumulation in the target regions, nanoformulation may provide a solution [135]. On the other hand, photothermal modulation utilizes photo-absorbers to convert photon energy into heat [136]. In this application, high laser power is required and prevention of other side effects such as overheating, which could induce excessive inflammation, should be considered. For photoactivation, photon irradiation was applied to induce a change in the chemical structure, leading to the cleavage of certain functional groups and release of the active pharmaceutical ingredients from the carriers [137]. Over the years, the use of nanomaterials in photothermal therapy has received considerable attention. Inorganic nanoparticles such as zinc oxide (ZnO) and copper oxide nanomaterials have also been reported to harbor strong anti-microbial activities and have been incorporated into a variety of medical applications including skin dressing materials. ZnO has excellent photocatalytic activity [138] and could be accumulated in the microorganisms to cause efficient inhibition of their growth at concentrations between 3 and 10 mM [139]. The lipid bilayer of bacteria is extremely sensitive to ROS. Therefore, photon-induced hydrogen peroxide generation by ZnO plays a primary role in killing bacteria, together with penetration of the cell envelope and disorganization of the cell membrane upon contact with nanoparticles [140].

Nanotechnology has also been applied to disease prevention in vaccine formulation, the so called nanovaccinology. Over the past decade, nanoscale size materials such as virus-like particles (VLPs), liposomes, polymeric, inorganic nanoparticles and emulsions have gained attention as potential delivery vehicles for vaccine antigens, which can both stabilize vaccine antigens and act as adjuvants [141]. These advantages are attributable to the nanoscale particle size, which facilitates uptake by antigen-presenting cells (APCs), leading to efficient antigen recognition and presentation. Modifying the surfaces of nanoparticles with different targeting moieties permits the delivery of antigens to specific receptors on the cell surface, thereby stimulating selective and specific immune responses [142]. The most well-known example is the liposome applied for encapsulating modified mRNAs and stimulating host immune response in SARS-CoV-2 vaccines developed by Moderna and Pfizer-BioNTech [143]. Nanoparticles in the vaccine formulations allow for enhanced immunogenicity and stability of the payload (antigen or nucleic acids encoding the expression of antigen), but also targeted delivery and slow release for longer immunostimulation [144].

Three parenterally delivered vaccines for the prevention of *C. difficile* infection have been developed. These vaccines were based on detoxified or recombinant forms of TcdA and TcdB and are expected to generate high titers of toxin neutralizing antibodies in clinical trials [145]. However, improvements of existing vaccine formulations are necessary. Strategies may include addition of more antigens to limit colonization or sporulation, or integration with treatment regimens. The use of nanotechnology in vaccine development against CDI was first reported in 2017 by Liu's group using poly-γ-glutamic acid (γ-PGA) and chitosan to form biodegradable nanoparticles [146]. The particle was used to encapsulate recombinant receptor binding domains of TcdB. This strategy successfully induced the production of TcdB neutralizing antibodies in vaccinated mice. The vaccinated mice had low-level inflammation, and all survived the lethal dose of *C. difficile* spore challenge [146]. A nanovaccine for CDI is currently under phase I clinical trial in the USA.

6. Nanomaterials for CDI Therapeutics

Organic nanoparticles for the delivery of anti-sense anti-microbial oligonucleotides have been reported recently for anti-CDI therapy [147]. The modified anti-sense oligonucleotides can specifically target five essential *C. difficile* genes simultaneously. They used three (APDE-8, CODE-9, CYDE-21) novel cationic amphiphilic bolaamphiphiles (CABs) to form nano-sized vesicles or vesicle-like aggregates (CABVs) and encapulate 25-mer antisense oligonucleotides (ASO). The empty CABVs had little effect on *C. difficile* growth and could deliver an effective amount of ASO against *C. difficile.* Through encapsulation by bolaamphiphile-based nanocomplex, the oligonucleotides could be effectively transported into *C. difficile* to modulate the translation of specific mRNA which achieved inhibitory concentrations in *C. difficile* without affecting normal microbiota [148,149].

There are reports showing most antibacterial metallic nanomaterials are non-selective generic biocidal agents, mainly against vegetative cells. Their sporicidal activity was explored in only a few studies under high concentrations [150,151]. Ag nanoparticles synthesized by *Streptomyces* sp. have also been reported to exhibit anti-spore potency against *C. difficile* at 75 μg/mL [152]. According to Gopinath's report, these Ag nanoparticles adhered to the entire spore coat followed by surface protein denaturation and pit formation [152]. Surface modification of Ag nanoparticles with chitosan also showed antibacterial activity against *B. subtilis* vegetative cells and spores [153]. Their activity against *C. difficile* spores remains to be validated. However, the safety for the use of Ag nanoparticles in the human body is still an important concern, as it has been reported that Ag nanoparticles could compromise cell viability and induce pathological damages in animal models [154]. In a clinical study reported by Munger, orally administered Ag nanoparticles (32 ppm) followed by a 2-week observation period presented no clinically important changes in metabolic, hematologic, or urinalysis measures [155]. There were also no detectable morphological changes in the lungs, heart or abdominal organs. ROS formation and subsequent pro-inflammatory cytokine generation commonly associated with Ag nanoparticles were not noted [155]. However, the chronic toxicity of Ag nanoparticles still remains to be further studied [156].

Polyurethane containing crystal violet (CV) and 3–4 nm ZnO nanoparticles have been reported to present bactericidal activity against hospital-acquired pathogens including multidrug-resistant *E. coli*, *Pseudomonas aeruginosa*, methicillin-resistant *S. aureus* (MRSA) and even highly resistant endospores of *C. difficile* [157]. However, recent studies showed that ZnO nanoparticles may affect other microorganisms and impact normal intestinal microflora despite their widespread use in biomedicine [158]. DNA damage induced by ZnO also limits its biomedical application in clinical settings [159]. Other types of nanomaterials responsive to photonic energy (e.g., photodynamic or photothermal therapy) have also been developed for anti-microbial therapy, to enhance drug delivery and local activation. However, the gastrointestinal tract is not the ideal organ for light illumination.

Iron is the most abundant transition metal in the human body and participates in important physiological functions such as oxygen transport and electron transfer. The human body has developed sophisticated systems for the uptake, transport, storage and metabolism of iron. Iron-containing nanoparticles usually exhibited magnetic properties and are among the pioneer nanomaterials used in a wide variety of biomedical and bioengineering applications. Many iron-containing nanoparticles have been evaluated in preclinical and clinical trials, and some of those have reached the market. Zero-valent-iron (ZVI) nanoparticles exhibited excellent biocompatibility while harboring prominently bactericidal efficacy against *E. coli*. Iron oxide nanoparticles also have been widely used for biomedical applications, including hyperthermia therapy and magnetic resonance imagining [160]. There are reports describing that iron oxide nanoparticles have reduced bacterial biofilm formation and viability via an increase in oxidative stress [161,162]. The anti-bacterial mechanisms of these metallic nanoparticles are attributed to their ability to generate reactive oxygen species, disrupt cell membranes, bind thiol groups and release toxic ions. Iron oxide nanoparticles, widely used as T2 weighed MRI imaging contrast agents, were recently used in CDI treatment. The $Fe_{3-\delta}O_4$ magnetite nanoparticles (500 μg/mL) were reported to display sporicidal activity against *C. difficile* spores without adversely affecting the gut microbiota of experimental mice [163]. $Fe_{3-\delta}O_4$ magnetite nanoparticles bind to the surface of *C. difficile* spores, decreasing Ca-DPA release from the spores. The nanoparticles eventually inhibited spore viability in vitro and attenuated *C. difficile*-induced colitis in this mouse model. However, $Fe_{3-\delta}O_4$ nanoparticles did not kill the vegetative cells. A ZVI signal, detected in the $Fe_{3-\delta}O_4$ nanoparticles by X-ray diffraction, has been reported to involve the induction of intracellular oxidative stress and depleting mitochondrial membrane potential in malignant cells [164,165]. Generation of ROS may contribute to the inhibition of *C. difficile* spore germination. As the $Fe_{3-\delta}O_4$ nanoparticles only showed efficacy in anti-spore germination without killing the vegetative form of *C. difficile*, vancomycin-loaded $Fe_{3-\delta}O_4$ nanoparticles (van-IONPs) were synthesized to further enhance CDI control. These nanoparticles demonstrated the ability to inhibit both vegetative cell growth and spore germination [163,166] through direct binding to *C. difficile* spores and blocking their germination, while inhibiting vegetative cells by releasing antibiotics in a synchronized manner (Figure 2). Moreover, van-IONPs protected the intestinal mucosa from *C. difficile* spore adhesion and significantly decreased the level of *C. difficile*-induced inflammation in mice. These nanoparticles outperform both $Fe_{3-\delta}O_4$ nanoparticles and free vancomycin in overall anti-CDI efficacy, due to the dual-function activities of targeting both spores and vegetative cells [166]. ROS production has also been reported as the cause for the anti-bacterial properties of another type of $Fe_{3-\delta}O_4$ nanoparticles [167]. One important advantage of these iron-based nanoparticles in CDI control is their selectivity for *C. difficile* spores and biocompatibility to intestinal mucosa cells. Such properties preserved the normal intestinal flora critical for preventing invasion by other pathogens and protecting the host from recurrence [168].

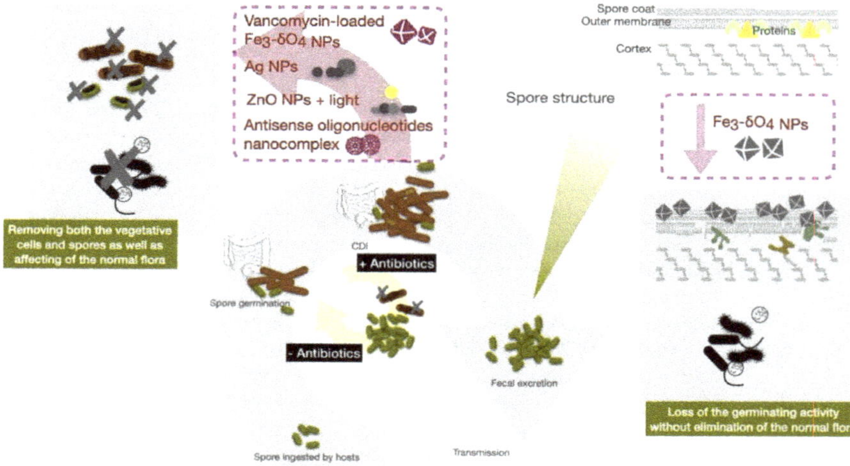

Figure 2. Schematic illustration of nanoparticles (NPs) targeting essential pathways of *C. difficile* infection, including the life cycle of vegetative cells and spores.

7. Conclusions

Clostridioides difficile accounts for about 20% of antibiotic-associated diarrhea, with global incidence increasing significantly between 2001 and 2016. CDI is a common healthcare-associated infection and about 30% of these infections are transmitted within hospitals. Antibiotic therapy is still the major treatment of choice for CDI, despite severe side effects and resistance remaining unsolved. Alternative therapeutic approaches, including FMT, probiotics and other microbiome-based therapeutics delivered through various routes, have been extensively investigated. While novel antimicrobials are being developed against the vegetative cells of the pathogen, non-selective inhibition of bacterial growth may lead to the imbalance of normal intestinal microbiota, leading to recurrent disease and therapeutic resistance. Targeting the spores is a new strategy emerging against CDI, as the *C. difficile* spores are notorious for their resistance to various antibiotic treatments, chemical and physical disinfections, and can survive extremely harsh environment for disease transmission. In this article, we reviewed the efficacy of regimens targeting spore germination, including compounds mimicking bile acids to serve as a decoy to block their germination process, anti-microbial peptides and their bio-mimetic compounds, as well as enzyme fragments to degrade the bacterial cell wall. Nanomaterials provide opportunities to integrate anti-vegetative cell strategies with those targeting spores, while managing toxins produced by these pathogens. While nanomaterials have demonstrated excellent antibacterial capability, they also showed potential adverse effects for gut microbiota, which is important in preventing CDI. Interestingly, iron-containing nanoparticles were recently described by several groups to harbor both antibacterial properties and excellent biocompatibility to intestinal mucosa cells and normal flora. $Fe_{3-\delta}O_4$ nanoparticles have especially showed specific pathogen targeting capability and effective inhibition of spore outgrowth. The next generation of $Fe_{3-\delta}O_4$ nanoparticles carrying vancomycin (van-IONPs) have demonstrated simultaneous targeted inhibition of vegetative cell growth, spore germination and toxin production in a superior fashion to the antibiotics or nanoparticles alone. These advancements prove the great potential of nanomedicine as a novel strategy in the future clinical management of CDI. Tailor-designed nanomedicine will provide new insights and opportunities for precision medicine in the prevention and treatment of emerging infectious diseases.

Author Contributions: Writing—original draft preparation, P.-W.W. and W.-T.L.; writing—review and editing, P.-W.W., W.-T.L., Y.-N.W. and D.-B.S.; visualization, Y.-N.W.; supervision, D.-B.S.; project administration, D.-B.S.; funding acquisition, D.-B.S. All authors have read and agreed to the published version of the manuscript.

Funding: This work was supported by the Center of Applied Nanomedicine, National Cheng Kung University, Featured Areas Research Center Program, Higher Education Sprout Project of the Taiwan Ministry of Education (MOE), and by grants from the Taiwan Ministry of Science and Technology (MOST 108-2314-B-006 -009 -MY3).

Conflicts of Interest: The authors declare no conflict of interest.

References

1. Hall, I.C.; O'toole, E. Intestinal flora in new-born infants: With a description of a new pathogenic anaerobe, *Bacillus difficilis*. *Am. J. Dis. Child.* **1935**, *49*, 390–402. [CrossRef]
2. Bloomfield, L.E.; Riley, T.V. Epidemiology and risk factors for community-associated *Clostridium difficile* infection: A narrative review. *Infect. Dis. Ther.* **2016**, *5*, 231–251. [CrossRef]
3. Kochan, T.J.; Foley, M.H.; Shoshiev, M.S.; Somers, M.J.; Carlson, P.E.; Hanna, P.C. Updates to *Clostridium difficile* spore germination. *J. Bacteriol.* **2018**, *200*, e00218-18. [CrossRef] [PubMed]
4. Brown, K.A.; Khanafer, N.; Daneman, N.; Fisman, D.N. Meta-analysis of antibiotics and the risk of community-associated *Clostridium difficile* infection. *Antimicrob. Agents Chemother.* **2013**, *57*, 7. [CrossRef]
5. Jump, R.L. *Clostridium difficile* infection in older adults. *Aging Health* **2013**, *9*, 403–414. [CrossRef]
6. Poutanen, S.M.; Simor, A.E. *Clostridium difficile*—Associated diarrhea in adults. *CMAJ* **2004**, *171*, 51–58. [CrossRef]
7. Public Health England. *Annual Epidemiological Commentary: Gram-Negative Bacteraemia, MRSA Bacteraemia, MSSA Bacteraemia and C. difficile Infections, up to and Including Financial Year April 2019 to March 2020*; Public Health England: London, UK, 2020.
8. Guh, A.Y.; Mu, Y.; Winston, L.G.; Johnston, H.; Olson, D.; Farley, M.M.; Wilson, L.E.; Holzbauer, S.M.; Phipps, E.C.; Dumyati, G.K. Trends in US burden of *Clostridioides difficile* infection and outcomes. *N. Engl. J. Med.* **2020**, *382*, 1320–1330. [CrossRef]
9. Collins, J.; Robinson, C.; Danhof, H.; Knetsch, C.; Van Leeuwen, H.; Lawley, T.; Auchtung, J.; Britton, R. Dietary trehalose enhances virulence of epidemic *Clostridium difficile*. *Nature* **2018**, *553*, 291–294. [CrossRef]
10. Akerlund, T.; Persson, I.; Unemo, M.; Norén, T.R.; Svenungsson, B.; Wullt, M.; Burman, L.G. Increased sporulation rate of epidemic *Clostridium difficile* type 027/NAP1. *J. Clin. Microbiol.* **2008**, *46*, 1530–1533. [CrossRef]
11. Vitucci, J.C.; Pulse, M.; Tabor-Simecka, L.; Simecka, J. Epidemic ribotypes of *Clostridium* (now *Clostridioides*) *difficile* are likely to be more virulent than non-epidemic ribotypes in animal models. *BMC Microbiol.* **2020**, *20*, 27. [CrossRef] [PubMed]
12. Weaver, L.; Michels, H.; Keevil, C. Survival of *Clostridium difficile* on copper and steel: Futuristic options for hospital hygiene. *J. Hosp. Infect.* **2008**, *68*, 145–151. [CrossRef]
13. Ragusa, R.; Giorgianni, G.; Lupo, L.; Sciacca, A.; Rametta, S.; La Verde, M.; Mulè, S.; Marranzano, M. Healthcare-associated *Clostridium difficile* infection: Role of correct hand hygiene in cross-infection control. *J. Prev. Med. Hyg.* **2018**, *59*, E145. [PubMed]

14. Scaria, E.; Barker, A.K.; Alagoz, O.; Safdar, N. Association of Visitor Contact Precautions with Estimated Hospital-Onset *Clostridioides difficile* Infection Rates in Acute Care Hospitals. *JAMA Netw. Open* **2021**, *4*, e210361. [CrossRef]
15. Jabbar, U.; Leischner, J.; Kasper, D.; Gerber, R.; Sambol, S.P.; Parada, J.P.; Johnson, S.; Gerding, D.N. Effectiveness of alcohol-based hand rubs for removal of *Clostridium difficile* spores from hands. *Infect. Control Hosp. Epidemiol.* **2010**, *31*, 565. [CrossRef] [PubMed]
16. Boyce, J.M.; Pittet, D. Guideline for hand hygiene in health-care settings: Recommendations of the Healthcare Infection Control Practices Advisory Committee and the HICPAC/SHEA/APIC/IDSA Hand Hygiene Task Force. *Am. J. Infect. Control.* **2002**, *30*, S1–S46. [CrossRef] [PubMed]
17. Barbut, F. Comparison of the efficacy of a hydrogen peroxide dry-mist disinfection system and sodium hypochlorite solution for eradication of *Clostridium difficile* spores. *Infect. Control Hosp. Epidemiol.* **2009**, *30*, 507–514. [CrossRef] [PubMed]
18. Leggett, M.J.; McDonnell, G.; Denyer, S.P.; Setlow, P.; Maillard, J.Y. Bacterial spore structures and their protective role in biocide resistance. *J. Appl. Microbiol.* **2012**, *113*, 485–498. [CrossRef] [PubMed]
19. Barra-Carrasco, J.; Olguín-Araneda, V.; Plaza-Garrido, Á.; Miranda-Cárdenas, C.; Cofré-Araneda, G.; Pizarro-Guajardo, M.; Sarker, M.R.; Paredes-Sabja, D. The *Clostridium difficile* exosporium cysteine (CdeC)-rich protein is required for exosporium morphogenesis and coat assembly. *J. Bacteriol.* **2013**, *195*, 3863. [CrossRef]
20. Mora-Uribe, P.; Miranda-Cárdenas, C.; Castro-Córdova, P.; Gil, F.; Calderón, I.; Fuentes, J.A.; Rodas, P.I.; Banawas, S.; Sarker, M.R.; Paredes-Sabja, D. Characterization of the adherence of *Clostridium difficile* spores: The integrity of the outermost layer affects adherence properties of spores of the epidemic strain R20291 to components of the intestinal mucosa. *Front. Cell. Infect. Microbiol.* **2016**, *6*, 99. [CrossRef]
21. Calderón-Romero, P.; Castro-Córdova, P.; Reyes-Ramírez, R.; Milano-Céspedes, M.; Guerrero-Araya, E.; Pizarro-Guajardo, M.; Olguín-Araneda, V.; Gil, F.; Paredes-Sabja, D. *Clostridium difficile* exosporium cysteine-rich proteins are essential for the morphogenesis of the exosporium layer, spore resistance, and affect *C. difficile* pathogenesis. *PLoS Pathog.* **2018**, *14*, e1007199. [CrossRef]
22. Permpoonpattana, P.; Phetcharaburanin, J.; Mikelsone, A.; Dembek, M.; Tan, S.; Brisson, M.-C.; La Ragione, R.; Brisson, A.R.; Fairweather, N.; Hong, H.A. Functional characterization of *Clostridium difficile* spore coat proteins. *J. Bacteriol.* **2013**, *195*, 1492. [CrossRef]
23. Sunde, E.P.; Setlow, P.; Hederstedt, L.; Halle, B. The physical state of water in bacterial spores. *Proc. Natl. Acad. Sci. USA* **2009**, *106*, 19334–19339. [CrossRef]
24. Bressuire-Isoard, C.; Broussolle, V.; Carlin, F. Sporulation environment influences spore properties in *Bacillus*: Evidence and insights on underlying molecular and physiological mechanisms. *FEMS Microbiol. Rev.* **2018**, *42*, 614–626. [CrossRef]
25. Paredes-Sabja, D.; Shen, A.; Sorg, J.A. *Clostridium difficile* spore biology: Sporulation, germination, and spore structural proteins. *Trends Microbiol.* **2014**, *22*, 406–416. [CrossRef] [PubMed]
26. Jamroskovic, J.; Chromikova, Z.; List, C.; Bartova, B.; Barak, I.; Bernier-Latmani, R. Variability in DPA and calcium content in the spores of *Clostridium* species. *Front. Microbiol.* **2016**, *7*, 1791. [CrossRef] [PubMed]
27. Rutala, W.A.; Gergen, M.F.; Tande, B.M.; Weber, D.J. Rapid hospital room decontamination using ultraviolet (UV) light with a nanostructured UV-reflective wall coating. *Infect. Control Hosp. Epidemiol.* **2013**, *34*, 527–529. [CrossRef] [PubMed]
28. Rodriguez-Palacios, A.; LeJeune, J.T. Moist heat resistance, spore aging, and superdormancy in *Clostridium difficile*. *Appl. Environ. Microbiol.* **2011**, *77*, 3085–3091. [CrossRef] [PubMed]
29. Gerding, D.N.; Muto, C.A.; Owens, R.C. Measures to control and prevent *Clostridium difficile* infection. *Clin. Infect. Dis.* **2008**, *46*, S43–S49. [CrossRef] [PubMed]
30. Shapey, S.; Machin, K.; Levi, K.; Boswell, T. Activity of a dry mist hydrogen peroxide system against environmental *Clostridium difficile* contamination in elderly care wards. *J. Hosp. Infect.* **2008**, *70*, 136–141. [CrossRef]
31. Lawley, T.D.; Clare, S.; Deakin, L.J.; Goulding, D.; Yen, J.L.; Raisen, C.; Brandt, C.; Lovell, J.; Cooke, F.; Clark, T.G. Use of purified *Clostridium difficile* spores to facilitate evaluation of health care disinfection regimens. *Appl. Environ. Microbiol.* **2010**, *76*, 6895. [CrossRef]
32. Rupnik, M.; Wilcox, M.H.; Gerding, D.N. *Clostridium difficile* infection: New developments in epidemiology and pathogenesis. *Nat. Rev. Microbiol.* **2009**, *7*, 526–536. [CrossRef] [PubMed]
33. Sorg, J.A.; Sonenshein, A.L. Bile salts and glycine as cogerminants for *Clostridium difficile* spores. *J. Bacteriol.* **2008**, *190*, 2505. [CrossRef] [PubMed]
34. Kochan, T.J.; Shoshiev, M.S.; Hastie, J.L.; Somers, M.J.; Plotnick, Y.M.; Gutierrez-Munoz, D.F.; Foss, E.D.; Schubert, A.M.; Smith, A.D.; Zimmerman, S.K. Germinant synergy facilitates *Clostridium difficile* spore germination under physiological conditions. *mSphere* **2018**, *3*. [CrossRef]
35. Francis, M.B.; Allen, C.A.; Shrestha, R.; Sorg, J.A. Bile acid recognition by the *Clostridium difficile* germinant receptor, CspC, is important for establishing infection. *PLoS Pathog.* **2013**, *9*, e1003356. [CrossRef]
36. Lawler, A.J.; Lambert, P.A.; Worthington, T. A Revised Understanding of *Clostridioides difficile* Spore Germination. *Trends Microbiol.* **2020**, *28*, 744–752. [CrossRef] [PubMed]
37. Bhattacharjee, D.; Francis, M.B.; Ding, X.; McAllister, K.N.; Shrestha, R.; Sorg, J.A. Reexamining the germination phenotypes of several *Clostridium difficile* strains suggests another role for the CspC germinant receptor. *J. Bacteriol.* **2015**, *198*, 777–786. [CrossRef] [PubMed]

38. Fimlaid, K.A.; Jensen, O.; Donnelly, M.L.; Francis, M.B.; Sorg, J.A.; Shen, A. Identification of a novel lipoprotein regulator of *Clostridium difficile* spore germination. *PLoS Pathog.* **2015**, *11*, e1005239. [CrossRef] [PubMed]
39. Francis, M.B.; Allen, C.A.; Sorg, J.A. Spore cortex hydrolysis precedes dipicolinic acid release during *Clostridium difficile* spore germination. *J. Bacteriol.* **2015**, *197*, 2276–2283. [CrossRef]
40. Paredes-Sabja, D.; Bond, C.; Carman, R.J.; Setlow, P.; Sarker, M.R. Germination of spores of *Clostridium difficile* strains, including isolates from a hospital outbreak of *Clostridium difficile*-associated disease (CDAD). *Microbiology* **2008**, *154*, 2241–2250. [CrossRef] [PubMed]
41. Wang, S.; Shen, A.; Setlow, P.; Li, Y.-Q. Characterization of the dynamic germination of individual *Clostridium difficile* spores using Raman spectroscopy and differential interference contrast microscopy. *J. Bacteriol.* **2015**, *197*, 2361. [CrossRef]
42. Govind, R.; Dupuy, B. Secretion of *Clostridium difficile* toxins A and B requires the holin-like protein TcdE. *PLoS Pathog.* **2012**, *8*, e1002727. [CrossRef] [PubMed]
43. Abt, M.C.; McKenney, P.T.; Pamer, E.G. *Clostridium difficile* colitis: Pathogenesis and host defence. *Nat. Rev. Microbiol.* **2016**, *14*, 609–620. [CrossRef]
44. Fletcher, J.R.; Pike, C.M.; Parsons, R.J.; Rivera, A.J.; Foley, M.H.; McLaren, M.R.; Montgomery, S.A.; Theriot, C.M. *Clostridioides difficile* exploits toxin-mediated inflammation to alter the host nutritional landscape and exclude competitors from the gut microbiota. *Nat. Commun.* **2021**, *12*, 462. [CrossRef]
45. Tao, L.; Zhang, J.; Meraner, P.; Tovaglieri, A.; Wu, X.; Gerhard, R.; Zhang, X.; Stallcup, W.B.; Miao, J.; He, X. Frizzled proteins are colonic epithelial receptors for *C. difficile* toxin B. *Nature* **2016**, *538*, 350–355. [CrossRef] [PubMed]
46. Papatheodorou, P.; Zamboglou, C.; Genisyuerek, S.; Guttenberg, G.; Aktories, K. Clostridial glucosylating toxins enter cells via clathrin-mediated endocytosis. *PLoS ONE* **2010**, *5*, e10673. [CrossRef]
47. Hirota, S.A.; Iablokov, V.; Tulk, S.E.; Schenck, L.P.; Becker, H.; Nguyen, J.; Al Bashir, S.; Dingle, T.C.; Laing, A.; Liu, J. Intrarectal instillation of *Clostridium difficile* toxin A triggers colonic inflammation and tissue damage: Development of a novel and efficient mouse model of *Clostridium difficile* toxin exposure. *Infect. Immun.* **2012**, *80*, 4474–4484. [CrossRef]
48. Chen, P.; Lam, K.-h.; Liu, Z.; Mindlin, F.A.; Chen, B.; Gutierrez, C.B.; Huang, L.; Zhang, Y.; Hamza, T.; Feng, H. Structure of the full-length *Clostridium difficile* toxin B. *Nat. Struct. Mol. Biol.* **2019**, *26*, 712–719. [CrossRef]
49. Orrell, K.E.; Zhang, Z.; Sugiman-Marangos, S.N.; Melnyk, R.A. *Clostridium difficile* toxins A and B: Receptors, pores, and translocation into cells. *Crit. Rev. Biochem. Mol. Biol.* **2017**, *52*, 461–473. [CrossRef]
50. Pfeifer, G.; Schirmer, J.; Leemhuis, J.; Busch, C.; Meyer, D.K.; Aktories, K.; Barth, H. Cellular uptake of *Clostridium difficile* toxin B translocation of the N-terminal catalytic domain into the cytosol of eukaryotic cells. *J. Biol. Chem.* **2003**, *278*, 44535–44541. [CrossRef]
51. Pettit, L.J.; Browne, H.P.; Yu, L.; Smits, W.K.; Fagan, R.P.; Barquist, L.; Martin, M.J.; Goulding, D.; Duncan, S.H.; Flint, H.J. Functional genomics reveals that *Clostridium difficile* Spo0A coordinates sporulation, virulence and metabolism. *BMC Genomics* **2014**, *15*, 160. [CrossRef] [PubMed]
52. Pereira, F.C.; Saujet, L.; Tomé, A.R.; Serrano, M.; Monot, M.; Couture-Tosi, E.; Martin-Verstraete, I.; Dupuy, B.; Henriques, A.O. The spore differentiation pathway in the enteric pathogen *Clostridium difficile*. *PLoS Genet.* **2013**, *9*, e1003782. [CrossRef]
53. Fimlaid, K.A.; Bond, J.P.; Schutz, K.C.; Putnam, E.E.; Leung, J.M.; Lawley, T.D.; Shen, A. Global analysis of the sporulation pathway of *Clostridium difficile*. *PLoS Genet.* **2013**, *9*, e1003660. [CrossRef]
54. Aithinne, K.A.; Cooper, C.W.; Lynch, R.A.; Johnson, D.L. Toilet plume aerosol generation rate and environmental contamination following bowl water inoculation with *Clostridium difficile* spores. *Am. J. Infect. Control.* **2019**, *47*, 515–520. [CrossRef] [PubMed]
55. Fekety, R.; Kim, K.-H.; Brown, D.; Batts, D.H.; Cudmore, M.; Silva, J., Jr. Epidemiology of antibiotic-associated colitis: Isolation of *Clostridium difficile* from the hospital environment. *Am. J. Med.* **1981**, *70*, 906–908. [CrossRef]
56. Jump, R.L.; Pultz, M.J.; Donskey, C.J. Vegetative *Clostridium difficile* survives in room air on moist surfaces and in gastric contents with reduced acidity: A potential mechanism to explain the association between proton pump inhibitors and *C. difficile*-associated diarrhea? *Antimicrob. Agents Chemother.* **2007**, *51*, 2883–2887. [CrossRef]
57. Pokrywka, M.; Feigel, J.; Douglas, B.; Grossberger, S.; Hensler, A.; Weber, D. A bundle strategy including patient hand hygiene to decrease *Clostridium difficile* infections. *Medsurg Nurs.* **2014**, *23*, 145. [PubMed]
58. Furuya-Kanamori, L.; Marquess, J.; Yakob, L.; Riley, T.V.; Paterson, D.L.; Foster, N.F.; Huber, C.A.; Clements, A.C. Asymptomatic *Clostridium difficile* colonization: Epidemiology and clinical implications. *BMC Infect. Dis.* **2015**, *15*, 516. [CrossRef] [PubMed]
59. Garneau, J.R.; Valiquette, L.; Fortier, L.-C. Prevention of *Clostridium difficile* spore formation by sub-inhibitory concentrations of tigecycline and piperacillin/tazobactam. *BMC Infect. Dis.* **2014**, *14*, 29. [CrossRef] [PubMed]
60. Dapa, T.; Unnikrishnan, M. Biofilm formation by *Clostridium difficile*. *Gut Microbes* **2013**, *4*, 397–402. [CrossRef]
61. Normington, C.; Moura, I.B.; Bryant, J.A.; Ewin, D.J.; Clark, E.V.; Kettle, M.J.; Harris, H.C.; Spittal, W.; Davis, G.; Henn, M.R. Biofilms harbour *Clostridioides difficile*, serving as a reservoir for recurrent infection. *NPJ Biofilms Microbiomes* **2021**, *7*, 16. [CrossRef]
62. Frost, L.R.; Cheng, J.K.; Unnikrishnan, M. *Clostridioides difficile* biofilms: A mechanism of persistence in the gut? *PLoS Pathog.* **2021**, *17*, e1009348. [CrossRef] [PubMed]
63. Uruén, C.; Chopo-Escuin, G.; Tommassen, J.; Mainar-Jaime, R.C.; Arenas, J. Biofilms as Promoters of Bacterial Antibiotic Resistance and Tolerance. *Antibiotics* **2021**, *10*, 3. [CrossRef]
64. Ananthakrishnan, A.N. *Clostridium difficile* infection: Epidemiology, risk factors and management. *Nat. Rev. Gastroenterol. Hepatol.* **2011**, *8*, 17. [CrossRef] [PubMed]

65. Stevens, V.W.; Nelson, R.E.; Schwab-Daugherty, E.M.; Khader, K.; Jones, M.M.; Brown, K.A.; Greene, T.; Croft, L.D.; Neuhauser, M.; Glassman, P. Comparative effectiveness of vancomycin and metronidazole for the prevention of recurrence and death in patients with *Clostridium difficile* infection. *JAMA Intern. Med.* **2017**, *177*, 546–553. [CrossRef] [PubMed]
66. Lübbert, C.; Zimmermann, L.; Borchert, J.; Hörner, B.; Mutters, R.; Rodloff, A.C. Epidemiology and recurrence rates of *Clostridium difficile* infections in Germany: A secondary data analysis. *Infect. Dis. Ther.* **2016**, *5*, 545–554. [CrossRef] [PubMed]
67. Vitucci, J.C.; Pulse, M.; Simecka, J. *Clostridium* (Now *Closteroides*) *difficile* Spore Formation Is Higher in Epidemic Isolates When Treated With Vancomycin in Vivo and in Vitro. *Arch. Microbiol. Immunol.* **2019**, *3*, 161–172. [CrossRef]
68. Thorpe, C.; McDermott, L.; Tran, M.; Chang, J.; Jenkins, S.; Goldstein, E.; Patel, R.; Forbes, B.; Johnson, S.; Gerding, D. US-based national surveillance for fidaxomicin susceptibility of *Clostridioides difficile*-associated diarrheal isolates from 2013 to 2016. *Antimicrob. Agents Chemother.* **2019**, *63*, e00391-19. [CrossRef]
69. Peng, Z.; Addisu, A.; Alrabaa, S.; Sun, X. Antibiotic resistance and toxin production of *Clostridium difficile* isolates from the hospitalized patients in a large hospital in Florida. *Front. Microbiol.* **2017**, *8*, 2584. [CrossRef]
70. Louie, T.J.; Miller, M.A.; Mullane, K.M.; Weiss, K.; Lentnek, A.; Golan, Y.; Gorbach, S.; Sears, P.; Shue, Y.-K. Fidaxomicin versus vancomycin for *Clostridium difficile* infection. *N. Engl. J. Med.* **2011**, *364*, 422–431. [CrossRef]
71. Babakhani, F.; Bouillaut, L.; Gomez, A.; Sears, P.; Nguyen, L.; Sonenshein, A.L. Fidaxomicin inhibits spore production in *Clostridium difficile. Clin. Infect. Dis.* **2012**, *55*, S162–S169. [CrossRef]
72. Davies, K.; Mawer, D.; Walker, A.S.; Berry, C.; Planche, T.; Stanley, P.; Goldenberg, S.; Sandoe, J.; Wilcox, M.H. An Analysis of *Clostridium difficile* Environmental Contamination During and After Treatment for *C. difficile* Infection. *Open Forum Infect. Dis.* **2020**, *7*, ofaa362. [CrossRef]
73. Sholeh, M.; Krutova, M.; Forouzesh, M.; Mironov, S.; Sadeghifard, N.; Molaeipour, L.; Maleki, A.; Kouhsari, E. Antimicrobial resistance in *Clostridioides* (*Clostridium*) *difficile* derived from humans: A systematic review and meta-analysis. *Antimicrob. Resist. Infect. Control.* **2020**, *9*, 158. [CrossRef] [PubMed]
74. Kwak, S.; Choi, J.; Hink, T.; Reske, K.A.; Blount, K.; Jones, C.; Bost, M.H.; Sun, X.; Burnham, C.-A.D.; Dubberke, E.R. Impact of investigational microbiota therapeutic RBX2660 on the gut microbiome and resistome revealed by a placebo-controlled clinical trial. *Microbiome* **2020**, *8*, 125. [CrossRef] [PubMed]
75. Eiseman, B.; Silen, W.; Bascom, G.S.; Kauvar, A.J. Fecal enema as an adjunct in the treatment of pseudomembranous enterocolitis. *Surgery* **1958**, *44*, 854–859. [PubMed]
76. Aas, J.; Gessert, C.E.; Bakken, J.S. Recurrent *Clostridium difficile* colitis: Case series involving 18 patients treated with donor stool administered via a nasogastric tube. *Clin. Infect. Dis.* **2003**, *36*, 580–585. [CrossRef] [PubMed]
77. Youngster, I.; Sauk, J.; Pindar, C.; Wilson, R.G.; Kaplan, J.L.; Smith, M.B.; Alm, E.J.; Gevers, D.; Russell, G.H.; Hohmann, E.L. Fecal microbiota transplant for relapsing *Clostridium difficile* infection using a frozen inoculum from unrelated donors: A randomized, open-label, controlled pilot study. *Clin. Infect. Dis.* **2014**, *58*, 1515–1522. [CrossRef] [PubMed]
78. Seekatz, A.M.; Theriot, C.M.; Molloy, C.T.; Wozniak, K.L.; Bergin, I.L.; Young, V.B. Fecal microbiota transplantation eliminates *Clostridium difficile* in a murine model of relapsing disease. *Infect. Immun.* **2015**, *83*, 3838–3846. [CrossRef]
79. Wu, K.-S.; Syue, L.-S.; Cheng, A.; Yen, T.-Y.; Chen, H.-M.; Chiu, Y.-H.; Hsu, Y.-L.; Chiu, C.-H.; Su, T.-Y.; Tsai, W.-L. Recommendations and guidelines for the treatment of *Clostridioides difficile* infection in Taiwan. *J. Microbiol. Immunol. Infect.* **2020**, *53*, 191–208. [CrossRef]
80. Khoruts, A.; Sadowsky, M.J. Understanding the mechanisms of faecal microbiota transplantation. *Nat. Rev. Gastroenterol. Hepatol.* **2016**, *13*, 508–516. [CrossRef] [PubMed]
81. Weingarden, A.R.; Chen, C.; Bobr, A.; Yao, D.; Lu, Y.; Nelson, V.M.; Sadowsky, M.J.; Khoruts, A. Microbiota transplantation restores normal fecal bile acid composition in recurrent *Clostridium difficile* infection. *Am. J. Physiol. Gastrointest. Liver Physiol.* **2014**, *306*, G310–G319. [CrossRef]
82. Dailey, F.E.; Turse, E.P.; Daglilar, E.; Tahan, V. The dirty aspects of fecal microbiota transplantation: A review of its adverse effects and complications. *Curr. Opin. Pharmacol.* **2019**, *49*, 29–33. [CrossRef]
83. Kim, K.O.; Gluck, M. Fecal microbiota transplantation: An update on clinical practice. *Clin. Endosc.* **2019**, *52*, 137. [CrossRef]
84. Lin, T.-C.; Hung, Y.-P.; Ko, W.-C.; Ruan, J.-W. Fecal microbiota transplantation for *Clostridium difficile* infection in Taiwan: Establishment and implementation. *J. Microbiol. Immunol. Infect.* **2019**, *52*, 841–850. [CrossRef]
85. Mills, J.P.; Rao, K.; Young, V.B. Probiotics for prevention of *Clostridium difficile* infection. *Curr. Opin. Gastroenterol.* **2018**, *34*, 3–10. [CrossRef]
86. Kwoji, I.D.; Aiyegoro, O.A.; Okpeku, M.; Adeleke, M.A. Multi-Strain Probiotics: Synergy among Isolates Enhances Biological Activities. *Biology* **2021**, *10*, 322. [CrossRef]
87. Gould, L.H.; Limbago, B. *Clostridium difficile* in food and domestic animals: A new foodborne pathogen? *Clin. Infect. Dis.* **2010**, *51*, 577–582. [CrossRef] [PubMed]
88. Egan, K.; Field, D.; Rea, M.C.; Ross, R.P.; Hill, C.; Cotter, P.D. Bacteriocins: Novel solutions to age old spore-related problems? *Front. Microbiol.* **2016**, *7*, 461. [CrossRef] [PubMed]
89. Durnaś, B.; Wnorowska, U.; Pogoda, K.; Deptuła, P.; Wątek, M.; Piktel, E.; Głuszek, S.; Gu, X.; Savage, P.B.; Niemirowicz, K. Candidacidal activity of selected ceragenins and human cathelicidin LL-37 in experimental settings mimicking infection sites. *PLoS ONE* **2016**, *11*, e0157242. [CrossRef] [PubMed]

90. Güzel, Ç.B.; Nevin Meltem, A.; Savage, P. In Vitro Activities of the Cationic Steroid Antibiotics CSA-13, CSA-131, CSA-138, CSA-142, and CSA-192 Against Carbapenem-resistant *Pseudomonas aeruginosa*. *Turk. J. Pharm. Sci.* **2020**, *17*, 63. [CrossRef]
91. Wnorowska, U.; Piktel, E.; Durnaś, B.; Fiedoruk, K.; Savage, P.B.; Bucki, R. Use of ceragenins as a potential treatment for urinary tract infections. *BMC Infect. Dis.* **2019**, *19*, 369. [CrossRef]
92. Piktel, E.; Pogoda, K.; Roman, M.; Niemirowicz, K.; Tokajuk, G.; Wróblewska, M.; Szynaka, B.; Kwiatek, W.M.; Savage, P.B.; Bucki, R. Sporicidal activity of ceragenin CSA-13 against *Bacillus subtilis*. *Sci. Rep.* **2017**, *7*, 44452. [CrossRef]
93. Wang, J.; Ghali, S.; Xu, C.; Mussatto, C.C.; Ortiz, C.; Lee, E.C.; Tran, D.H.; Jacobs, J.P.; Lagishetty, V.; Faull, K.F. Ceragenin CSA13 reduces *Clostridium difficile* infection in mice by modulating the intestinal microbiome and metabolites. *Gastroenterology* **2018**, *154*, 1737–1750. [CrossRef]
94. Saha, S.; Savage, P.; Bal, M. Enhancement of the efficacy of erythromycin in multiple antibiotic-resistant gram-negative bacterial pathogens. *J. Appl. Microbiol.* **2008**, *105*, 822–828. [CrossRef]
95. Weingarden, A.R.; Chen, C.; Zhang, N.; Graiziger, C.T.; Dosa, P.I.; Steer, C.J.; Shaughnessy, M.K.; Johnson, J.R.; Sadowsky, M.J.; Khoruts, A. Ursodeoxycholic acid inhibits *Clostridium difficile* spore germination and vegetative growth, and prevents recurrence of ileal pouchitis associated with the infection. *J. Clin. Gastroenterol.* **2016**, *50*, 624–630. [CrossRef] [PubMed]
96. Sorg, J.A.; Sonenshein, A.L. Inhibiting the initiation of *Clostridium difficile* spore germination using analogs of chenodeoxycholic acid, a bile acid. *J. Bacteriol.* **2010**, *192*, 4983–4990. [CrossRef]
97. Stoltz, K.L.; Erickson, R.; Staley, C.; Weingarden, A.R.; Romens, E.; Steer, C.J.; Khoruts, A.; Sadowsky, M.J.; Dosa, P.I. Synthesis and biological evaluation of bile acid analogues inhibitory to *Clostridium difficile* spore germination. *J. Med. Chem.* **2017**, *60*, 3451–3471. [CrossRef]
98. Tam, J.; Icho, S.; Utama, E.; Orrell, K.E.; Gómez-Biagi, R.F.; Theriot, C.M.; Kroh, H.K.; Rutherford, S.A.; Lacy, D.B.; Melnyk, R.A. Intestinal bile acids directly modulate the structure and function of *C. difficile* TcdB toxin. *Proc. Natl. Acad. Sci. USA* **2020**, *117*, 6792–6800. [CrossRef] [PubMed]
99. Farver, D.K.; Hedge, D.D.; Lee, S.C. Ramoplanin: A lipoglycodepsipeptide antibiotic. *Ann. Pharmacother.* **2005**, *39*, 863–868. [CrossRef]
100. Freeman, J.; Baines, S.D.; Jabes, D.; Wilcox, M.H. Comparison of the efficacy of ramoplanin and vancomycin in both in vitro and in vivo models of clindamycin-induced *Clostridium difficile* infection. *J. Antimicrob. Chemother.* **2005**, *56*, 717–725. [CrossRef] [PubMed]
101. Kraus, C.N.; Lyerly, M.W.; Carman, R.J. Ambush of *Clostridium difficile* spores by ramoplanin: Activity in an in vitro model. *Antimicrob. Agents Chemother.* **2015**, *59*, 2525–2530. [CrossRef]
102. Mowery, B.P.; Lindner, A.H.; Weisblum, B.; Stahl, S.S.; Gellman, S.H. Structure—Activity relationships among random nylon-3 copolymers that mimic antibacterial host-defense peptides. *J. Am. Chem. Soc.* **2009**, *131*, 9735–9745. [CrossRef]
103. Hovakeemian, S.G.; Liu, R.; Gellman, S.H.; Heerklotz, H. Correlating antimicrobial activity and model membrane leakage induced by nylon-3 polymers and detergents. *Soft Matter.* **2015**, *11*, 6840–6851. [CrossRef]
104. Liu, R.; Suárez, J.M.; Weisblum, B.; Gellman, S.H.; McBride, S.M. Synthetic polymers active against *Clostridium difficile* vegetative cell growth and spore outgrowth. *J. Am. Chem. Soc.* **2014**, *136*, 14498–14504. [CrossRef]
105. Taylor, L.Y.; Cann, D.D.; Welch, B.J. Antibotulinal properties of nisin in fresh fish packaged in an atmosphere of carbon dioxide. *J. Food Prot.* **1990**, *53*, 953–957. [CrossRef] [PubMed]
106. Shin, J.M.; Gwak, J.W.; Kamarajan, P.; Fenno, J.C.; Rickard, A.H.; Kapila, Y.L. Biomedical applications of nisin. *J. Appl. Microbiol.* **2016**, *120*, 1449–1465. [CrossRef]
107. Twomey, E.; Hill, C.; Field, D.; Begley, M. Bioengineered Nisin Derivative M17Q Has Enhanced Activity against *Staphylococcus epidermidis*. *Antibiotics* **2020**, *9*, 305. [CrossRef]
108. Lewies, A.; Wentzel, J.F.; Jordaan, A.; Bezuidenhout, C.; Du Plessis, L.H. Interactions of the antimicrobial peptide nisin Z with conventional antibiotics and the use of nanostructured lipid carriers to enhance antimicrobial activity. *Int. J. Pharm.* **2017**, *526*, 244–253. [CrossRef]
109. Scott, V.N.; Taylor, S.L. Temperature, pH, and spore load effects on the ability of nisin to prevent the outgrowth of *Clostridium botulinum* spores. *J. Food Sci.* **1981**, *46*, 121–126. [CrossRef]
110. Gut, I.M.; Blanke, S.R.; Van Der Donk, W.A. Mechanism of inhibition of *Bacillus anthracis* spore outgrowth by the lantibiotic nisin. *ACS Chem. Biol.* **2011**, *6*, 744–752. [CrossRef] [PubMed]
111. Le Lay, C.; Dridi, L.; Bergeron, M.G.; Ouellette, M. Nisin is an effective inhibitor of *Clostridium difficile* vegetative cells and spore germination. *J. Med. Microbiol.* **2016**, *65*, 169–175. [CrossRef]
112. Nerandzic, M.M.; Donskey, C.J. Activate to eradicate: Inhibition of *Clostridium difficile* spore outgrowth by the synergistic effects of osmotic activation and nisin. *PLoS ONE* **2013**, *8*, e54740. [CrossRef]
113. Vermassen, A.; Leroy, S.; Talon, R.; Provot, C.; Popowska, M.; Desvaux, M. Cell wall hydrolases in bacteria: Insight on the diversity of cell wall amidases, glycosidases and peptidases toward peptidoglycan. *Front. Microbiol.* **2019**, *10*, 331. [CrossRef] [PubMed]
114. Rao, L.; Tian, R.; Chen, X. Cell-membrane-mimicking nanodecoys against infectious diseases. *ACS Nano* **2020**, *14*, 2569–2574. [CrossRef]
115. Anselmo, A.C.; Mitragotri, S. Nanoparticles in the clinic. *Bioeng. Translat.* **2016**, *1*, 10–29. [CrossRef] [PubMed]

116. Amin, M.L.; Joo, J.Y.; Yi, D.K.; An, S.S.A. Surface modification and local orientations of surface molecules in nanotherapeutics. *J. Control Release* **2015**, *207*, 131–142. [CrossRef]
117. De Jong, W.H.; Borm, P.J. Drug delivery and nanoparticles: Applications and hazards. *Int. J. Nanomed.* **2008**, *3*, 133–149. [CrossRef] [PubMed]
118. Gao, W.; Chan, J.M.; Farokhzad, O.C. pH-responsive nanoparticles for drug delivery. *Mol. Pharm.* **2010**, *7*, 1913–1920. [CrossRef]
119. Yetisgin, A.A.; Cetinel, S.; Zuvin, M.; Kosar, A.; Kutlu, O. Therapeutic nanoparticles and their targeted delivery applications. *Molecules* **2020**, *25*, 2193. [CrossRef] [PubMed]
120. Kirtane, A.R.; Verma, M.; Karandikar, P.; Furin, J.; Langer, R.; Traverso, G. Nanotechnology approaches for global infectious diseases. *Nat. Nanotechnol.* **2021**, *16*, 369–384. [CrossRef]
121. Mba, I.E.; Nweze, E.I. The use of nanoparticles as alternative therapeutic agents against *Candida* infections: An up-to-date overview and future perspectives. *World J. Microbiol. Biotechnol.* **2020**, *36*, 163. [CrossRef]
122. Mba, I.E.; Sharndama, H.C.; Osondu-Chuka, G.O.; Okeke, O.P. Immunobiology and nanotherapeutics of severe acute respiratory syndrome 2 (SARS-CoV-2): A current update. *Infect. Dis.* **2021**, *53*, 559–580. [CrossRef]
123. Makadia, H.K.; Siegel, S.J. Poly lactic-co-glycolic acid (PLGA) as biodegradable controlled drug delivery carrier. *Polymers* **2011**, *3*, 1377–1397. [CrossRef]
124. Sung, Y.K.; Kim, S.W. Recent advances in polymeric drug delivery systems. *Biomater. Res.* **2020**, *24*, 12. [CrossRef]
125. Spirescu, V.A.; Chircov, C.; Grumezescu, A.M.; Andronescu, E. Polymeric Nanoparticles for Antimicrobial Therapies: An up-to-date Overview. *Polymers* **2021**, *13*, 724. [CrossRef] [PubMed]
126. Azzopardi, E.A.; Ferguson, E.L.; Thomas, D.W. The enhanced permeability retention effect: A new paradigm for drug targeting in infection. *J. Antimicrob. Chemother.* **2013**, *68*, 257–274. [CrossRef] [PubMed]
127. Turner, R.J. Metal-based antimicrobial strategies. *Microb. Biotechnol.* **2017**, *10*, 1062–1065. [CrossRef] [PubMed]
128. Slavin, Y.N.; Asnis, J.; Häfeli, U.O.; Bach, H. Metal nanoparticles: Understanding the mechanisms behind antibacterial activity. *J. Nanobiotechnol.* **2017**, *15*, 65. [CrossRef] [PubMed]
129. Shaikh, S.; Nazam, N.; Rizvi, S.M.D.; Ahmad, K.; Baig, M.H.; Lee, E.J.; Choi, I. Mechanistic insights into the antimicrobial actions of metallic nanoparticles and their implications for multidrug resistance. *Int. J. Mol. Sci.* **2019**, *20*, 2468. [CrossRef]
130. Prabhu, S.; Poulose, E.K. Silver nanoparticles: Mechanism of antimicrobial action, synthesis, medical applications, and tox-icity effects. *Int. Nano Lett.* **2012**, *2*, 32. [CrossRef]
131. Lin, Z.; Monteiro-Riviere, N.A.; Riviere, J.E. Pharmacokinetics of metallic nanoparticles. *Wiley Interdiscip. Rev. Nanomed. Nanobiotechnol.* **2015**, *7*, 189–217. [CrossRef]
132. Thang, D.T.; Wang, Z.; Lu, X.; Xing, B. Precise cell behaviors manipulation through light-responsive nano-regulators: Recent advance and perspective. *Theranostics* **2019**, *9*, 3308. [CrossRef]
133. Shi, X.; Zhang, C.Y.; Gao, J.; Wang, Z. Recent advances in photodynamic therapy for cancer and infectious diseases. *Wiley Interdiscip. Rev. Nanomed. Nanobiotechnol.* **2019**, *11*, e1560. [CrossRef]
134. Issa, M.C.A.; Manela-Azulay, M. Photodynamic therapy: A review of the literature and image documentation. *An. Bras. Dermatol.* **2010**, *85*, 501–511. [CrossRef]
135. Huang, Z.; Xu, H.; Meyers, A.D.; Musani, A.I.; Wang, L.; Tagg, R.; Barqawi, A.B.; Chen, Y.K. Photodynamic therapy for treatment of solid tumors—potential and technical challenges. *Technol. Cancer Res. Treat.* **2008**, *7*, 309–320. [CrossRef]
136. Jaque, D.; Maestro, L.M.; Del Rosal, B.; Haro-Gonzalez, P.; Benayas, A.; Plaza, J.L.; Rodríguez, E.M.; Solé, J.G. Nanoparticles for photothermal therapies. *Nanoscale* **2014**, *6*, 9494–9530. [CrossRef]
137. Linsley, C.S.; Wu, B.M. Recent advances in light-responsive on-demand drug-delivery systems. *Ther. Deliv.* **2019**, *8*, 89–107. [CrossRef] [PubMed]
138. Tong, D.; Wu, P.; Su, P.; Wang, D.; Tian, H. Preparation of zinc oxide nanospheres by solution plasma process and their optical property, photocatalytic and antibacterial activities. *Mater. Lett.* **2012**, *70*, 94–97. [CrossRef]
139. Swaminathan, M.; Sharma, N.K. *Handbook of Ecomaterials, eBook*; Springer: Cham, Switzerland, 2019; pp. 549–563.
140. Pasquet, J.; Chevalier, Y.; Couval, E.; Bouvier, D.; Noizet, G.; Morlière, C.; Bolzinger, M.-A. Antimicrobial activity of zinc oxide particles on five micro-organisms of the Challenge Tests related to their physicochemical properties. *Int. J. Pharm.* **2014**, *460*, 92–100. [CrossRef] [PubMed]
141. Kreuter, J. Nanoparticles as adjuvants for vaccines. *Vaccine Design.* **1995**, 463–472.
142. Mehrabi, M.; Dounighi, N.M.; Mohammadi, M.; Masoudi, A. Nanoparticles and vaccine development. *Pharm. Nanotechnol.* **2020**, *8*, 6–21.
143. Shin, M.D.; Shukla, S.; Chung, Y.H.; Beiss, V.; Chan, S.K.; Ortega-Rivera, O.A.; Wirth, D.M.; Chen, A.; Sack, M.; Pokorski, J.K.; et al. COVID-19 vaccine development and a potential nanomaterial path forward. *Nat. Nanotechnol.* **2020**, *15*, 646–655. [CrossRef]
144. Demento, S.L.; Cui, W.; Criscione, J.M.; Stern, E.; Tulipan, J.; Kaech, S.M.; Fahmy, T.M. Role of sustained antigen release from nanoparticle vaccines in shaping the T cell memory phenotype. *Biomaterials* **2012**, *33*, 4957–4964. [CrossRef]
145. Riley, T.V.; Lyras, D.; Douce, G.R. Status of vaccine research and development for *Clostridium difficile*. *Vaccine* **2019**, *37*, 7300–7306. [CrossRef]
146. Liu, Y.W.; Chen, Y.H.; Chen, J.W.; Tsai, P.J.; Huang, I. Immunization with recombinant TcdB-encapsulated nanocomplex induces protection against *Clostridium difficile* challenge in a mouse model. *Front. Microbiol.* **2017**, *8*, 1411. [CrossRef] [PubMed]
147. Stewart, D.B. Anti-sense antibiotic agents as treatment for bacterial infections. *Surg. Infect.* **2018**, *19*, 831–835. [CrossRef]

148. Sharma, A.K.; Krzeminski, J.; Weissig, V.; Hegarty, J.P.; Stewart, D.B. Cationic amphiphilic bolaamphiphile-based delivery of antisense oligonucleotides provides a potentially microbiome sparing treatment for *C. difficile*. *J. Antibiot.* **2018**, *71*, 713–721. [CrossRef]
149. Hegarty, J.P.; Krzeminski, J.; Sharma, A.K.; Guzman-Villanueva, D.; Weissig, V.; Stewart Sr, D.B. Bolaamphiphile-based nanocomplex delivery of phosphorothioate gapmer antisense oligonucleotides as a treatment for *Clostridium difficile*. *Int. J. Nanomed.* **2016**, *11*, 3607. [CrossRef]
150. Hamal, D.B.; Haggstrom, J.A.; Marchin, G.L.; Ikenberry, M.A.; Hohn, K.; Klabunde, K.J. A multifunctional biocide/sporocide and photocatalyst based on titanium dioxide (TiO_2) codoped with silver, carbon, and sulfur. *Langmuir* **2009**, *26*, 2805–2810. [CrossRef] [PubMed]
151. Imani, S.; Saadati, M.; Honari, H.; Rezaei-Zarchi, S.; Javid, A.; Zareh, M.; Doroudian, M. Comprehensive study of sporicidal and sporstatic effect of CuO and AgO metal nanoparticles upon spore of *Clostridium botulinum* type E. *Afr. J. Microbiol. Res.* **2012**, *6*, 1417–1422.
152. Gopinath, P.M.; Ranjani, A.; Dhanasekaran, D.; Thajuddin, N.; Archunan, G.; Akbarsha, M.A.; Gulyás, B.; Padmanabhan, P. Multi-functional nano silver: A novel disruptive and theranostic agent for pathogenic organisms in real-time. *Sci. Rep.* **2016**, *6*, 34058. [CrossRef]
153. Alfaro-González, B.; Ulate, D.; Alvarado, R.; Argüello-Miranda, O. Chitosan-silver nanoparticles as an approach to control bacterial proliferation, spores and antibiotic-resistant bacteria. *Biomed. Phys. Eng. Express.* **2018**, *4*, 035011. [CrossRef]
154. Ferdous, Z.; Nemmar, A. Health impact of silver nanoparticles: A review of the biodistribution and toxicity following various routes of exposure. *Int. J. Mol. Sci.* **2020**, *21*, 2375. [CrossRef]
155. Munger, M.A.; Radwanski, P.; Hadlock, G.C.; Stoddard, G.; Shaaban, A.; Falconer, J.; Grainger, D.W.; Deering-Rice, C.E. *In vivo* human time-exposure study of orally dosed commercial silver nanoparticles. *Nanomedicine* **2014**, *10*, 1–9. [CrossRef] [PubMed]
156. Mathur, P.; Jha, S.; Ramteke, S.; Jain, N. Pharmaceutical aspects of silver nanoparticles. *Artif. Cells Nanomed. Biotechnol.* **2018**, *46*, 115–126. [CrossRef]
157. Sehmi, S.K.; Lourenco, C.; Alkhuder, K.; Pike, S.D.; Noimark, S.; Williams, C.K.; Shaffer, M.S.; Parkin, I.P.; MacRobert, A.J.; Allan, E. Antibacterial surfaces with activity against antimicrobial resistant bacterial pathogens and endospores. *ACS Infect. Dis.* **2020**, *6*, 939–946. [CrossRef] [PubMed]
158. Elshama, S.S.; Abdallah, M.E.; Abdel-Karim, R.I. Zinc oxide nanoparticles: Therapeutic benefits and toxicological hazards. *Open Nanomed. J.* **2018**, *5*, 16–22. [CrossRef]
159. Hemeg, H.A. Nanomaterials for alternative antibacterial therapy. *Int. J. Nanomed.* **2017**, *12*, 8211. [CrossRef]
160. Arias, L.S.; Pessan, J.P.; Vieira, A.P.M.; Lima, T.M.T.d.; Delbem, A.C.B.; Monteiro, D.R. Iron oxide nanoparticles for biomedical applications: A perspective on synthesis, drugs, antimicrobial activity, and toxicity. *Antibiotics* **2018**, *7*, 46. [CrossRef]
161. Jamzad, M.; Bidkorpeh, M.K. Green synthesis of iron oxide nanoparticles by the aqueous extract of *Laurus nobilis* L. leaves and evaluation of the antimicrobial activity. *J. Nanostruct. Chem.* **2020**, *10*, 193–201. [CrossRef]
162. Thukkaram, M.; Sitaram, S.; Subbiahdoss, G. Antibacterial efficacy of iron-oxide nanoparticles against biofilms on different biomaterial surfaces. *Int. J. Biomater.* **2014**, *2014*, 716080. [CrossRef] [PubMed]
163. Lee, W.-T.; Wu, Y.-N.; Chen, Y.-H.; Wu, S.-R.; Shih, T.-M.; Li, T.-J.; Yang, L.-X.; Yeh, C.-S.; Tsai, P.-J.; Shieh, D.-B. Octahedron iron oxide nanocrystals prohibited *Clostridium difficile* spore germination and attenuated local and systemic inflammation. *Sci. Rep.* **2017**, *7*, 8124. [CrossRef]
164. Huang, C.-C.; Chuang, K.-Y.; Chou, C.-P.; Wu, M.-T.; Sheu, H.-S.; Shieh, D.-B.; Tsai, C.-Y.; Su, C.-H.; Lei, H.-Y.; Yeh, C.-S. Size-control synthesis of structure deficient truncated octahedral $Fe_{3-\delta}O_4$ nanoparticles: High magnetization magnetites as effective hepatic contrast agents. *J. Mater. Chem.* **2011**, *21*, 7472–7479. [CrossRef]
165. Wu, Y.-N.; Chen, D.-H.; Shi, X.-Y.; Lian, C.-C.; Wang, T.-Y.; Yeh, C.-S.; Ratinac, K.R.; Thordarson, P.; Braet, F.; Shieh, D.-B. Cancer-cell-specific cytotoxicity of non-oxidized iron elements in iron core-gold shell NPs. *Nanomedicine* **2011**, *7*, 420–427. [CrossRef] [PubMed]
166. Chen, Y.-H.; Li, T.-J.; Tsai, B.-Y.; Chen, L.-K.; Lai, Y.-H.; Li, M.-J.; Tsai, C.-Y.; Tsai, P.-J.; Shieh, D.-B. Vancomycin-loaded nanoparticles enhance sporicidal and antibacterial efficacy for *Clostridium difficile* infection. *Front. Microbiol.* **2019**, *10*, 1141. [CrossRef]
167. Arakha, M.; Pal, S.; Samantarrai, D.; Panigrahi, T.K.; Mallick, B.C.; Pramanik, K.; Mallick, B.; Jha, S. Antimicrobial activity of iron oxide nanoparticle upon modulation of nanoparticle-bacteria interface. *Sci. Rep.* **2015**, *5*, 14813. [CrossRef] [PubMed]
168. Jandhyala, S.M.; Talukdar, R.; Subramanyam, C.; Vuyyuru, H.; Sasikala, M.; Reddy, D.N. Role of the normal gut microbiota. *World J. Gastroenterol.* **2015**, *21*, 8787–8803. [CrossRef] [PubMed]

MDPI
St. Alban-Anlage 66
4052 Basel
Switzerland
Tel. +41 61 683 77 34
Fax +41 61 302 89 18
www.mdpi.com

Antibiotics Editorial Office
E-mail: antibiotics@mdpi.com
www.mdpi.com/journal/antibiotics

www.ingramcontent.com/pod-product-compliance
Lightning Source LLC
LaVergne TN
LVHW070645100526
838202LV00013B/883
* 9 7 8 3 0 3 6 5 3 8 7 8 5 *